SCARSDALE HOSPITAL

7

Paediatric Neurology

To my mother

Paediatric Neurology

Second Edition

Ingrid Gamstorp, MD
Division of Child Neurology, Department of Paediatrics, University Hospital, Uppsala, Sweden

Butterworths
London Boston Durban Singapore Sydney Toronto Wellington

First edition, 1970
Second edition, 1985

© **Butterworth & Co. (Publishers) Ltd, 1985**

British Library Cataloguing in Publication Data

Gamstorp, Ingrid
   Paediatric neurology.—2nd ed.
   1. Pediatric neurology
   I. Title
   618.9′28   RJ486

   ISBN 0-407-00263-4

Library of Congress Cataloging in Publication Data

Gamstorp, Ingrid, 1924–
   Paediatric neurology.
   Includes bibliographies and index.
   1. Pediatric neurology. I. Title. [DNLM: 1. Nervous
   System Diseases—in infancy & childhood. WS 340 G192p]
   RJ486.G26 1985   618.92′8   84-23157

   ISBN 0-407-00263-4

CDC76

Photoset by Butterworths Litho Preparation Department
Printed in Great Britain at the University Press, Cambridge

Preface

This book was written with the purpose of giving some simple and practical guidelines for the management of neurological disorders in infancy and childhood. The structure of the book is built up from the chief complaints that brings the child to the doctor, thus following the natural way of establishing a diagnosis. The child's symptoms are the starting-point, followed by findings on clinical examination, laboratory studies, and other special examinations leading to a diagnosis, with emphasis on the technique and the normal findings in various ages. Paediatrics is dynamic, never static, and normal findings vary with age. Thus the physician performing a neurological examination on a child must be able to adjust his technique to the age and maturation of the child, and be familiar with the normal child's reactions in various ages. After the establishment of a diagnosis therapy follows (together with its advantages and side-effects) with support to the whole family, and finally the child's prognosis is ascertained. The book tries to follow as closely as possible what is happening in real life in a hospital or a consultation.

The book is written particularly for young physicians who are training to become paediatricians. They may meet these practical problems as neurological and developmental deviations, alleged or proven, which constitute at least one-fifth of paediatric presentations in western countries. My hope is that as well as the paediatrician (who only occasionally sees neurological disorders), the adult neurologist (unused to the problems in childhood, the orthopaedic surgeon), the general practitioner and other physicians who meet a paediatric neurological problem may find some facts which may help them to give the neurologically disabled child and his family better help and understanding.

Ingrid Gamstorp

Acknowledgements

I would like to thank the paediatrician, Dr Gösta Blennow, Hälsingborg, and the neurologist, Dr K.-G. Henriksson, Linköping, both of whom have read the manuscript thoroughly and given me invaluable help through constructive criticism, advice, and suggestions.

Illustrations have kindly been placed at my disposal by Dr Ilmar Sulg, Lund (EEG); Dr Irene Sjögren, Uppsala (echo-encephalography); Dr Mikael Zigmond and Dr Oliver Axen, Jönköping (radiology); and Dr Arne Brun, Lund (neuropathology). For the use of photographs illustrating various diseases discussed in the book, I am indebted to Dr C.-G. Bergstrand, Malmö; Dr Randolph Byers, Boston; Dr Annalise Dupont, Aarhus; Dr Herbert Enell, Hälsingborg; Dr Gösta Holmgren, Umeå; Dr Bengt Kjellman, Lund; Dr Lennart Mannerfelt, Lund; and Dr Bertil Palmgren, Hälsingborg.

My gratitude to all who helped me with the first edition is still valid. The second edition has been made possible through the help of Erik Stålberg, Kjell Bergström, Per Gunnar Lindgren, Paul Enoksson, Sonja Heedh, Kerstin Blom, Inger Bäcklin, and Monica Steen; without their help the manuscript would never have been rewritten and re-illustrated.

Above all my thanks go to the patients and their parents, who have stimulated the writing of this book and cooperated during examinations and photography and who have given me their points of view.

Contents

Introduction

Paediatric neurology includes all those conditions which have their onset before or at adolescence, and which are localized to the nervous system or to the muscular system or which give rise to symptoms predominantly from these systems. This definition also covers what is usually termed *developmental paediatrics,* which deals with children with abnormal or possibly abnormal psychomotor development. In developed countries roughly 20–25 per cent of paediatrics is concerned with neurological disorders. Thus, the general paediatrician needs to have a full knowledge of the techniques of neurological examination and how to use and to interpret the results of many of the special examinations. In many countries there are no paediatric neurologists available; the total care of the neurologically sick child is then the duty of the general paediatrician.

In all age-groups the purpose of the neurological examination is to reveal *abnormalities of one or several neurological functions.* With the anatomical knowledge of where these functions are localized it is possible to tell *where* in the nervous system or the muscular system an injury or a disease is localized, but the neurological findings alone can never give the *cause* of the injury nor the *diagnosis* of the disease. Thus, a diagnosis can never be based on one neurological examination alone. In order to establish a diagnosis it is necessary to obtain, above all, a careful *history,* as well as the results of selected *special examinations* and, when possible, to *follow-up* the child.

In *adulthood* neurological examination can be performed using the same technique in all ages, and the normal findings are basically the same. In *childhood* the nervous system is immature and developing; both technique and evaluation of findings vary with the age of the patient. In childhood the findings on neurological examination can also be used to evaluate the *maturation* of the nervous system. Thus, in infancy and childhood the neurological examination has two purposes: to demonstrate signs of a *localized functional impairment* and to demonstrate *normal or delayed maturation of the child's nervous system.* It is important for the paediatric neurologist to be able to use both of these approaches and to keep them separate.

Paediatric neurology thus requires a knowledge of symptoms and signs from the nervous system and the muscular system at all ages. It also requires a knowledge of the normal child's psychomotor development, and how disturbances within this may be identified. Experience with the normal child's reaction at various ages to the examination situation is also needed. Finally, the paediatric neurologist must have the ability and interest to apply an examination technique in such a way that the best possible cooperation is obtained from every patient at any age. It is (and must be) great fun to play with children.

The neurological disorders of infancy and childhood are usually long-lasting, and occasionally handicapping or even lethal. Such a diagnosis established in a child means a severe blow to the whole family and may impair its functioning. It is absolutely necessary that the diagnosing physician is aware of this emotional reaction and has the knowledge, interest, and empathy to give the family the help and support that it needs.

1

History – general outline

This chapter gives only a general outline of the taking of the history and its evaluation. All special aspects that are relevant to particular diseases described later will be discussed in connection with the disease. A history taken from the parents, as is the general rule in paediatrics, gives better information about family history, pregnancy, neonatal period, and early development than a history taken from the patient. The advantages of a history taken from the parents should be utilized even when the child is old enough to tell about his present symptoms. On the other hand, a history taken from the parents is always second-hand information and should, whenever possible, be supplemented by direct questioning of the child.

FAMILY HISTORY

The simple statement that there are no known diseases in the family is of no value. One must also know the number and sex of healthy family members to judge if there are individuals available who might have shown the abnormal trait. Information about consanguinity is also necessary, as consanguinity between parents increases the probability that the child will have a disease due to an autosomal recessive gene. In some situations tests are now available to diagnose the healthy carriers of an abnormal gene (see Chapter 6).

PREGNANCY

Events that occur during pregnancy may affect the fetus. Various infections, some of which the mother may have unknowingly, may pass to the fetus and cause active disease or permanent damage. Examples of such infections are syphilis, toxoplasmosis, cytomegalic inclusion body disease, rubella, and possibly other viral infections.

The possibility of the toxic influence of drugs became apparent during the 1960s when thalidomide caused malformations in children; this drug is no longer available. Antiepileptic medication, which usually has to be continued throughout pregnancy in a woman with epilepsy, may approximately double the risk of malformation in the child (see page 126), although these malformations do not usually involve the nervous system. Drugs with a cytostatic effect, such as azathioprine and cyclophosphamide, are even more dangerous to the developing fetus. Environmental toxins, particularly ethyl alcohol, may also seriously affect the child (*see* page 126).

Maternal disease, e.g. diabetes, may increase the incidence of malformations in the child, and untreated metabolic conditions, e.g. phenylketonuria (*see* page 127), may impair the development of the fetal brain. Smoking during pregnancy impairs the growth of the child but does not seem to cause malformations. Toxicosis of the mother increases the risk of placental insufficiency and thus the birth of an undernourished small-for-dates child.

Undernourishment of the mother during pregnancy, either general starvation due to lack of food or to lack of appetite and/or vomiting because of serious disease in the mother, or lack of specific substances such as vitamin B_{12} in a diet extremely lacking in all animal protein, may cause irreversible brain damage in the child. The incidence of abnormal children is slightly increased in pregnancies complicated by vaginal bleeding. It is debated whether this bleeding causes abnormalities in the child or whether it should be interpreted as a threatening abortion due to a primary abnormality of the fetus.

An estimation of the duration of the pregnancy, combined with an evaluation of the maturity of the newborn infant, is important. Preterm birth always carries a certain risk of intracranial bleeding and respiratory problems which may lead to asphyxia and brain injury. These risks are small for infants born after 34 or more weeks of pregnancy.

LABOUR AND DELIVERY

All information about labour and delivery is important in the neurological history of a child. Although the incidence of birth injury has diminished with improved obstetric and neonatal care, it still appears to be the most common *single* cause of neurological symptoms and signs during childhood. Although a birth injury may occur when delivery seems entirely normal, its incidence increases when there are complications such as premature birth, abnormal presentation, vacuum extraction, or evidence of fetal stress. It should, however, be emphasized that although the incidence of injuries is statistically increased, only a *small* proportion of infants born under unfavourable conditions will show permanent neurological symptoms and signs.

NEONATAL PERIOD

The neonatal period may be complicated by jaundice, cyanotic spells, respiratory difficulties, apnoeic attacks, or a bleeding tendency, any of which may be an indication of a disorder that may lead to neurological abnormalities. Neurological signs may also have been recorded in the neonatal period, e.g. abnormal cry, apathy, swallowing difficulties, inability to suck, abnormal muscle tone, tremor, or convulsions.

DEVELOPMENT OF THE CHILD

Questions about the psychomotor development of the child are a necessary part of the history. A few 'milestones' of the normal development of the infant born at term are briefly given here (*see also Table 2.1,* page 17). Information about these milestones is a necessary part of the developmental history. The motor development of the prematurely born infant is delayed, particularly during the first weeks and months, when the delay is roughly proportional to the degree of prematurity. The healthy premature baby usually catches up with the baby born at term during the first year of life.

The newborn baby is already able to follow a bright, slowly moving object with his eyes. He also turns his eyes towards the light. The infant starts to fix and give visual contact at the age of 4–6 weeks and to follow an object promptly a few weeks later. The first smile is seen at about the same time. Many newborn infants can lift the head in the prone position; all infants are expected to do so at 6 weeks of age. At 4 months of age the child can lift his head also in the supine position, can balance it when he is held upright, and can lift head and shoulders when lying on his belly. He reaches out for objects but is not yet able to grasp them deliberately; he examines and plays with his hands; he turns his eyes and head towards a sound; he can use his voice to express pleasure. A month or two later he starts to roll over. At the age of 7 months the child sits without support, he can grasp a rather large object in a clumsy way with his whole hand, and can transfer objects from hand to mouth. At 9–10 months of age the child starts to pull himself to standing and to walk holding on to furniture. He can pick up rather small things now, using the pinching grasp, and can transfer from hand to hand.

At 12–14 months of age most children start to walk without support and have a vocabulary of about three to ten words which may be understood by their parents. At 2 years of age the child is expected to be able to put at least two words together in a simple sentence and at 3–4 years to pronounce words distinctly and correctly without having to use baby-talk. The child is usually able to run at 2 years of age and to hop on one leg at 4½ years.

Normal psychomotor development usually seems to occur stepwise rather than smoothly. The normal variation is considerable. Thus, small deviations from the development outlined here should cause no concern. A thorough examination is suggested in the following situations:

1. If the child does not lift his head in the prone position or does not follow an object with his eyes at age 2 months.
2. If the child does not lift his head in the supine position at age 6 months.
3. If the child makes no attempts to sit at age 9 months or to walk at age 18 months.
4. If the child uses no words at all at age 18 months or does not try to form simple sentences at age 3.

The outlined deviations from the usual development do not establish that the child is developing abnormally, only that he is deviating enough to be entitled to a thorough investigation.

In taking the developmental history it is important to note whether a delay is fairly even over all aspects of the psychomotor development, as is seen in the mentally retarded child, or whether the development has proceeded normally in some areas and been severely delayed in others. A deaf child has no speech, but his motor development is normal or, at most, slightly retarded. A child with a disease affecting the peripheral neurones or the muscles may have severely retarded motor development but normal alertness and interest in his surroundings, normal social contact, and normal speech.

ONSET AND COURSE OF THE DISEASE

From the history it is also important to try to form an opinion about the *onset* (acute or insidious) and *course* (stepwise changes, stationary symptoms, steady progression, or steady improvement) of the disease. It is then necessary to keep in mind that the disease is affecting a developing nervous system and that there may be competition between the disease and normal development. A child who loses abilities that he once achieved unequivocally has a progressive disease. If symptoms seem to remain stationary, the disease may still be progressive; in such cases, progression may be slow enough for normal development to balance deterioration.

References

CHUNG, C. S. and MYRIANTHOPOULOUS, N. C. (1975) Factors affecting risks of congenital malformations. I. Epidemiological analysis. Reports from the collaborative perinatal project. Birth Defects: Original Series. The National Foundation March of Dimes. Vol. XI, No 10

HAGBERG, B. (1975) Pre, peri- and postnatal prevention of major neuropediatric handicaps. *Neuropädiatrie*, **6**, 331–338

HAGBERG, B. (1983) Erfolge und Probleme bei der Neugeborenenintensivpflege – eine Analyse der Zerebralparese (CP) in Schweden. *Kinderärzliche Praxis*, **7**, 322–326

HILL, R. M. and STERN, L. (1979) Drugs in pregnancy; effects on the fetus and newborns. *Drugs*, **17**, 182–197

LUNDSTRÖM, R. (1962) Rubella during pregnancy. *Acta Paediatrica* (Uppsala), suppl. 133

NELSON, K. B. and ELLENBERG, J. H. (1981) Apgar scores as predictors of chronic neurologic disability. *Pediatrics*, **68**, 36–44

RUSNAK, S. L. and DRISCOLL, S. G. (1965) Congenital spinal anomalies in infants of diabetic mothers. *Pediatrics*, **35**, 989–995

SEVER, J. L., NELSON, K. B. and GILKESON, M. R. (1965) Rubella epidemic 1964; effects on 6,000 pregnancies. *American Journal of Diseases in Children*, **110**, 395–407

The neurological examination

The neurological examination has the same purpose in all age-groups, i.e. to test various functions of the neuromuscular system. If the tests reveal impaired function, it can be concluded that damage is localized in the part of the neuromuscular system that is normally responsible for this particular function.

Three basic principles are used in the practical performance of a neurological examination in the paediatric age-group. In the newborn period no active cooperation can be expected from the patient. In this age-group one can only *observe the infant's reaction to different tests*. The value of the observation can be increased by the examiner putting the infant in such situations that may bring out abnormal findings. When the infant is some weeks of age he can be enticed to certain actions, the performance of which the examiner wants to study, e.g. the eye movements when the infant follows an object. This technique of *attracting the child's interest and getting him to perform certain actions* begins to take the place of pure observation and forms the main part of the neurological examination of older infants and small children. From 3–4 years of age cooperative children start to obey simple *verbal orders*. This technique then slowly takes the place of tempting the children to do what is wanted until, from 8–10 years of age, the neurological examination can be performed in the same way as in adulthood. However, throughout childhood the best results are obtained if the neurological examination is done as a game and a competition between child and examiner: 'Let us see who can do this best or fastest – you or I'.

Children in the age-group 6 months to 4 years are particularly difficult to examine, because of the following reactions which are normal for this age-group:

1. Fear. The child may be frightened by the new surroundings, by the examiner's unknown face and voice, and by the fact that the examiner touches the child and may even restrain his movements. It is necessary to establish good contact with the parent before starting to examine the child. The examination should begin without undressing the child who is sitting on his parent's lap, and always with movements that can be performed without touching the child and which require the child's attention and active cooperation. The examiner must then sit on a low stool in front of the child, in obedience to the general rule that the examining physician must always be on eye level with his patient (for details, *see* page 18).
2. Boredom. Infants and young children tire easily. Toys must be available and used (preferably with the help of the parent) to keep the child amused during

the part of the examination when no active cooperation is needed. Much information can also be obtained by watching the child undressing himself or being undressed.

Examination of the newborn

Spontaneous posture and activity

The healthy full-term newborn infant has high flexor tone and his normal resting posture is with all joints bent. When lying on his back he keeps his shoulders slightly adducted, elbows flexed, hands loosely clenched with the thumbs half-way across the palm, hips and knees flexed, and ankles in a semiflexed position (*Figure 2.1*). The infant may thus keep his knees and elbows above the bed. He has head

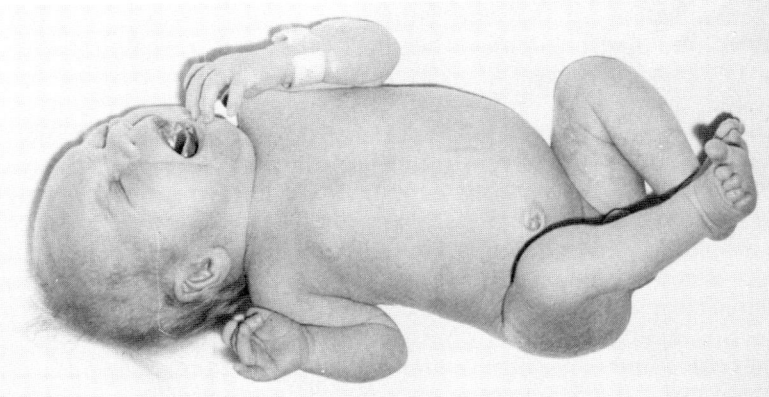

Figure 2.1. A 2-week-old term infant. Note the half-clenched hands with the thumbs half-way across the palms and the flexed position of hips, knees, and elbows. Both knees and one elbow are above the bed.

lag and poor head control, which are demonstrable when an attempt is made to pull him to the sitting position (*Figure 2.2*). The tendency to flexion is also apparent in the prone position (*Figure 2.3*).

The general alertness and spontaneous movements of the infant are noted. A deviation from normal may be either a *depressed* state, when the infant is apathetic, shows a poverty of movements, and has sluggish or no reflexes (*see* page 12), or a *hyperirritable* state, when the infant is aroused by the slightest stimulus and has tremulous, shaky movements and a decreased threshold to the eduction of reflexes, particularly the Moro reflex (*see* page 12); the cry is often high-pitched and intense.

Examination of the head

The tension and size of fontanelles and sutures are evaluated by inspection and palpation. The largest circumference of the head (usually 1–2 cm greater than the measurement recorded by the midwife or obstetrician) is recorded with an unstretchable tape and compared with the value normal for sex and gestational age and possibly also for height. At this age one must rely on one measurement only,

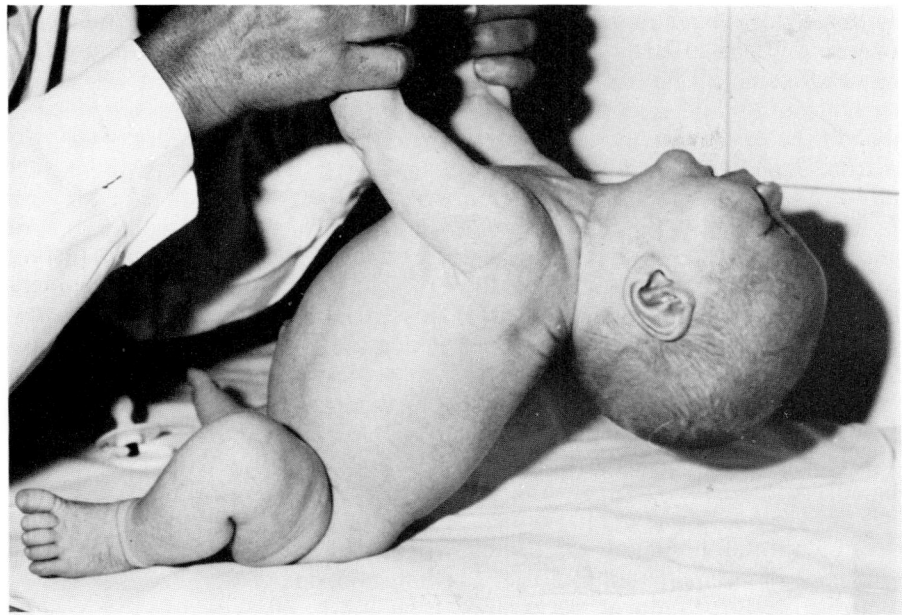

Figure 2.2. A 2-week-old term infant. Note the head lag when an attempt is made to pull the infant to the sitting position

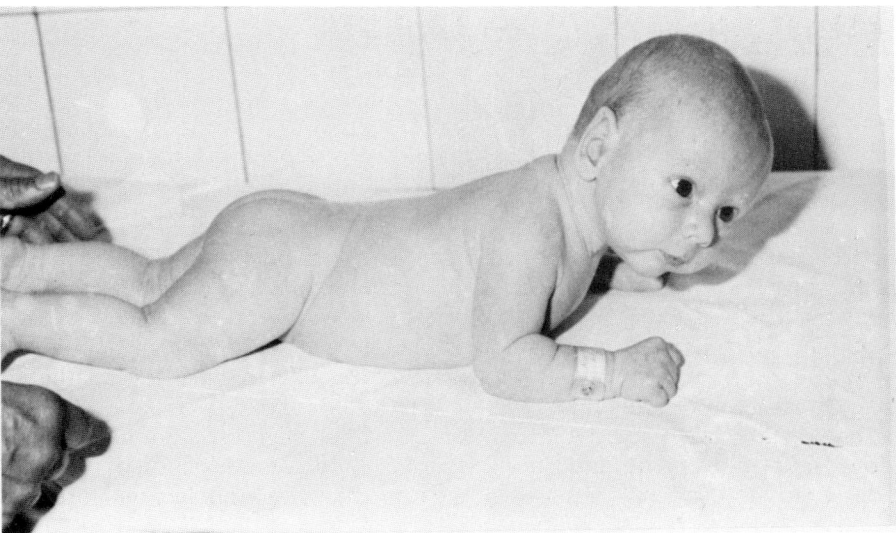

Figure 2.3. A 2-week-old baby in the prone position, lifting his head; elbows, knees, and hips are slightly bent

whereas in the older infant *growth velocity* is more important than an isolated value.

Transillumination of the head is a simple clinical method which can still be used as a screening method but needs confirmation through ultrasound examination or computerized tomography (*see* page 60) before a diagnosis is established. A strong lamp with a thick rubber ring to give a good connection to the skull is used. The examination must be carried out in a dark room by a well-adapted examiner. In a healthy baby a smooth red ring is seen around the rubber attachment where it is pressed against the skull. The ring is usually 1–2 cm broad in the frontal region and roughly half the size in the occipital region. The *ratio* between the width of the ring in the frontal and the occipital region is usually constant, whereas the actual breadth of the ring depends on the brightness of the light and the thickness of the skull bone. Transillumination is equal on left and right sides. Any accumulation of fluid directly under the skull bone will cause a widening of the ring. Thus an abnormal transillumination will raise the suspicion of a subdural hygroma, a porencephalic cyst, or hydranencephaly. This method cannot be used in the immediate neonatal period, as the normal oedema of the scalp will give a false impression of abnormal transillumination; nor is this method helpful when the accumulated fluid is fresh blood, as in an acute subdural haematoma.

The normal nature of oedema and small haemorrhages in the subcutaneous tissue of the scalp, particularly the part leading during delivery, must be recognized. A *cephalhaematoma,* i.e. subperiosteal bleeding, which raises the periosteum over one of the cranial bones, although a benign condition, cannot be considered a normal finding as it indicates a slightly traumatic delivery. It is easily seen (*Figure 2.4*) and palpated as a firm swelling over one cranial bone, usually a parietal bone, with its limits at the sutures. It should be explained to the parents

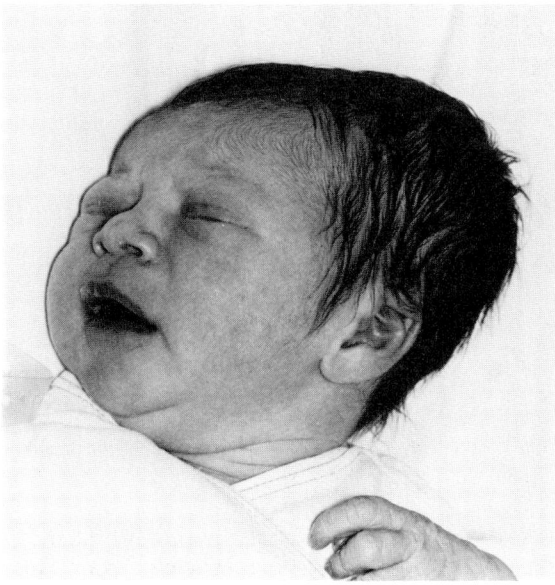

Figure 2.4. A newborn infant with cephalhaematoma in the typical position over one parietal bone

that the bleeding is located *outside* the cranium and cannot therefore endanger the brain. Nothing must be done to a cephalhaematoma, as it disappears spontaneously over several months. An evacuation is at best unnecessary; an attempt at evacuation may under unfortunate circumstances be complicated by infection which can lead to osteitis and meningitis.

Cranial nerves

The newborn infant can already be enticed to follow a slowly moving, fairly big and bright object; thus the child's interest in a visual stimulus and his eye movements can be evaluated. The eye movements may also be evaluated by using the 'doll's head manoeuvre'. In this procedure the infant's head is used as a doll's head and quickly moved from side to side. When the face is turned left the eyes go right, and vice versa, thus allowing the examiner to see a full range of eye movements in the horizontal direction (*Figure 2.5*). The same technique can be used for vertical movements by bending the infant's head up and down, but the response to this stimulus is more difficult to evaluate. On the doll's head manoeuvre the eyes follow each other, unless there is a weakness of one or more of the extraocular muscles, which may thus be revealed; a squint that is present only at rest has no significance in the newborn period.

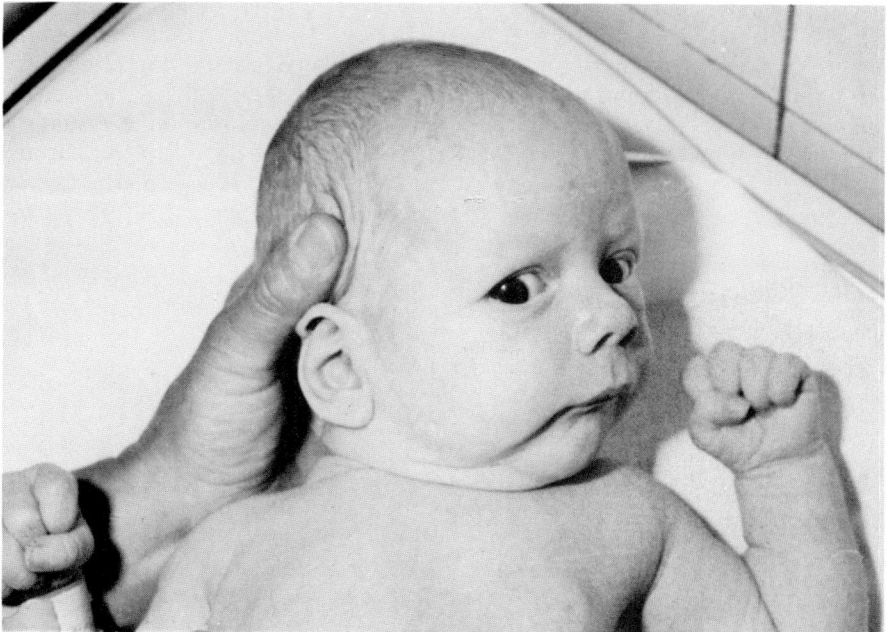

Figure 2.5. Normal horizontal eye movements elicited by the 'doll's head manoeuvre' in a 2-week-old infant

The infant usually opens his eyes when he is lifted up from lying on his back to a sitting position; this is a condition necessary for studying eye movements and also for examination for ptosis (*Figure 2.6*). When the infant is lifted up in this way, the eyes may turn down to reveal a sickle of sclera between the upper eyelid and the upper border of the iris. This is called the *sunset phenomenon* (*Figure 2.7*). It *may* be a normal finding, but is often due to increased intracranial pressure, particularly acute hydrocephalus following neurological damage in the aqueductal region (*see* page 241), which must be excluded. Pupils react more slowly to light at this age than later in life. The healthy seeing neonate reacts to a sudden flash of light by closing his eyes. The absence of this response in a neonate who appears alert and

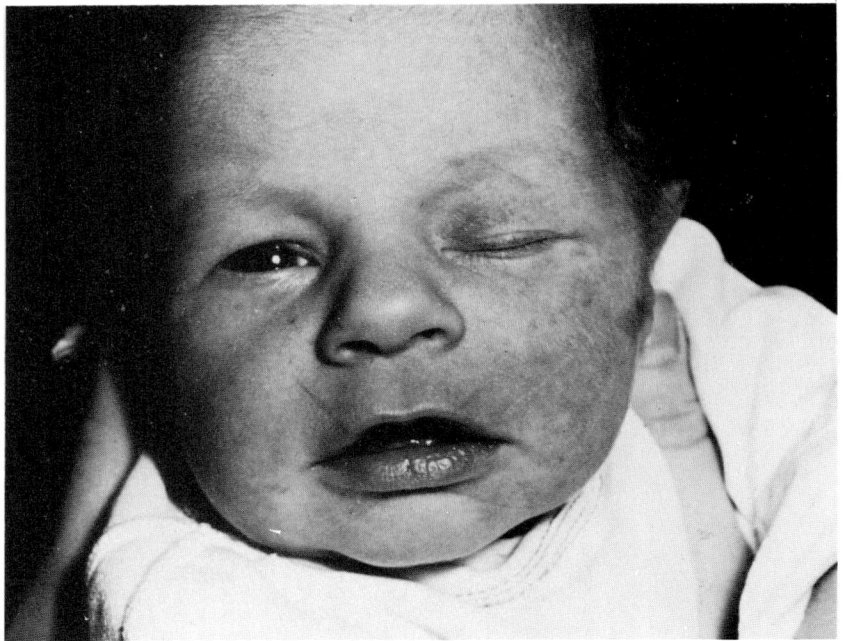

Figure 2.6. Left-sided ptosis in a newborn infant

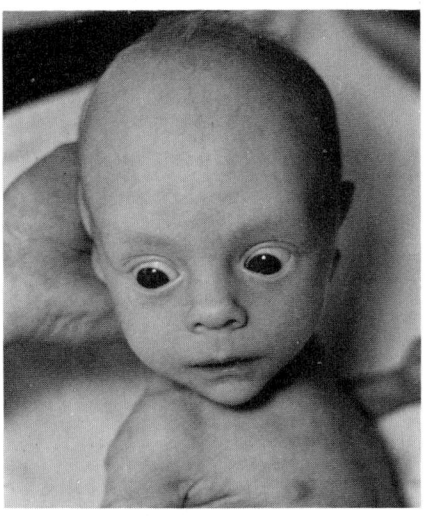

Figure 2.7. 'Sunset phenomenon' in a hydrocephalic infant, aged 1 month. Note the sickle-shaped part of the sclera between the eyelid and the upper margin of the iris

responds to other stimuli should raise the suspicion of impaired vision. The optic discs have a more greyish colour in infants below 6 months of age than later in life. Small retinal haemorrhages are seen in many neonates and have no significance.

Sensation

Sensation can be tested only in a crude way in the newborn. Newborn infants usually respond to a pinprick by withdrawal and crying. However, there is a noticeable delay; a couple of seconds may elapse between the stimulus and the response. It is usually possible to detect complete loss of sensation to pain in a whole limb or below a certain spinal level, but smaller anaesthetic areas cannot be detected and other sensory qualities cannot be examined.

Muscle tone

As described on page 6, the full-term healthy newborn infant has high flexor tone. The joints offer resistance to passive stretching and when this ceases the limb goes rapidly back into the semiflexed position. The head cannot be turned so far to the side that the chin touches the shoulder, and one hand cannot reach beyond the acromion on the other side. The high tone is also felt peripherally and immediately checks the dangling movement of the hand, elicited by shaking the arm.

   This high muscle tone is a typical finding in the healthy full-term baby, and its degree, together with the development of the reflexes (see page 12), constitute the basis for the clinical evaluation of the infant's neurological maturation. The premature infant, even when it is otherwise healthy, has low muscle tone. It lies on

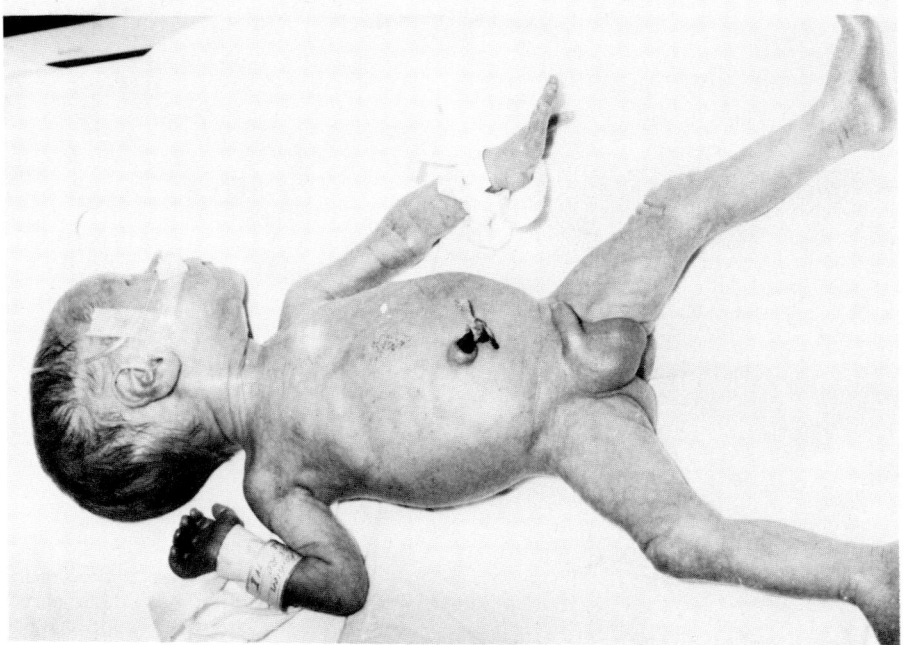

Figure 2.8. A newborn baby, born 8 weeks before term; hips and knees are stretched, elbows and knees are on the bed, and the head can be turned so much that the chin reaches beyond the shoulder

its back, with knees and hips stretched, and elbows and knees on the bed (*Figure 2.8*). Its joints offer no resistance to passive stretching, and the hand dangles unchecked when the arm is shaken. The chin can be turned beyond the shoulder and one hand can reach beyond the acromion on the other side. Diseases causing muscular hypotonia in the newborn period are discussed in Chapter 6.

Reflexes

Muscle reflexes are present in the healthy neonate. Knee jerks, ankle jerks, and biceps reflexes are usually easy to elicit. Ankle clonus may be present and, if so, is not an abnormal sign. Abdominal reflexes are also present, but may be difficult to demonstrate unless the infant is suitably relaxed. The neonatal reflexes – Moro, sucking, and rooting reflexes, and palmar and plantar grasp – are all present in the healthy neonate. Their absence indicates immaturity, temporary depression of the infant due to anaesthesia or analgesics given to the mother, or damage to or disease of the infant.

The Moro reflex can be elicited in many ways. A strong sound or a blow to the bed on both sides of the infant can be used. The best method, however, is a sudden

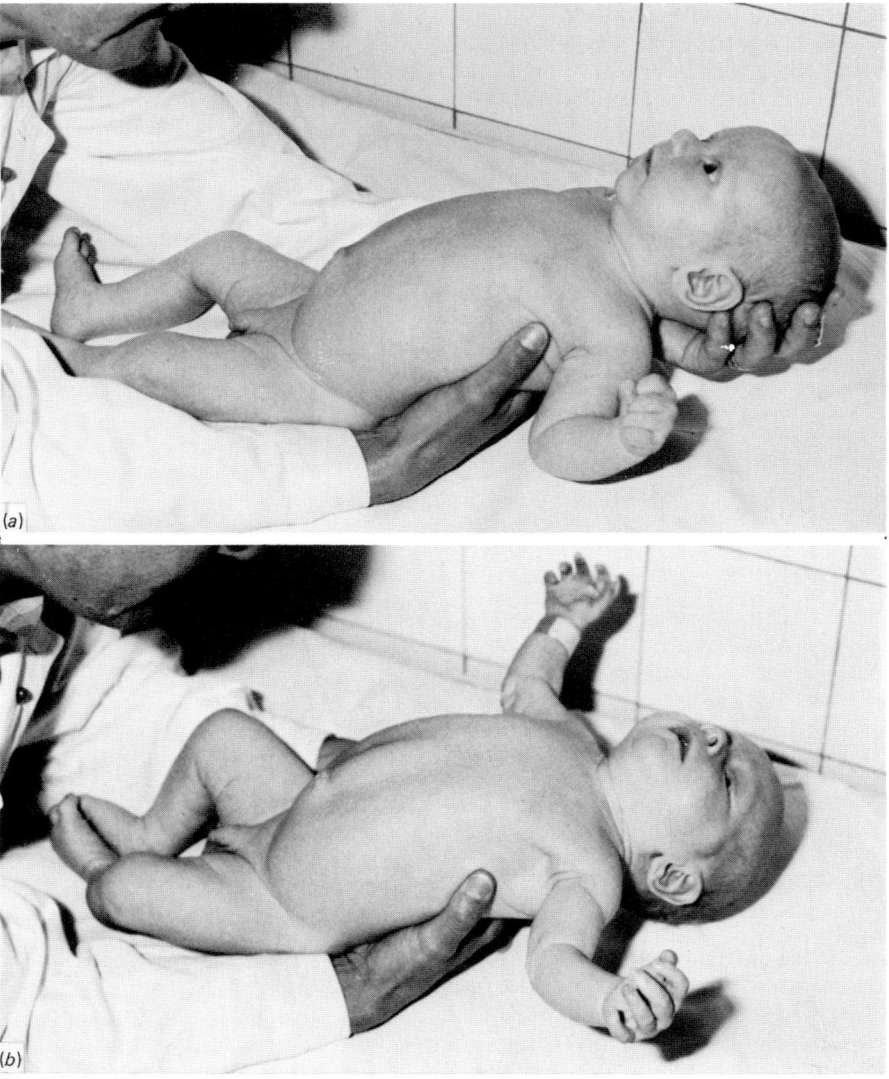

(a)

(b)

Figure 2.9a and *b*. The Moro reflex in a 2-week-old infant controlled drop of the infant's head (*Figure 2.9a*) such that the head is kept in the midline position, because a turn of the head influences the symmetry of the Moro reflex. In response to such a stimulus the infant throws his arms straight out with hands open (*Figure 2.9b*); the arms are then flexed and quickly brought together in a clasping movement. Abnormal findings are lack of or asymmetry of the Moro reflex. A low threshold, i.e. eduction of the reflex by any sound or a light touch, may also be an abnormal finding and is seen in hyperirritable infants (*see* page 6). The reflex must not be elicited in an infant in whom intracranial bleeding is strongly suspected, as this rather rough treatment can worsen the patient's condition.

The sucking reflex is elicited by touching the lip of the child with a soft moist object, e.g. a dummy or the tip of the finger. The infant then shapes his lips and starts to suck (*Figure 2.10*). The rooting reflex, which is closely connected with the sucking reflex, is elicited by touching the cheek of the infant with a soft moist object. The infant then turns his head, grasps the object with his lips, and starts to suck.

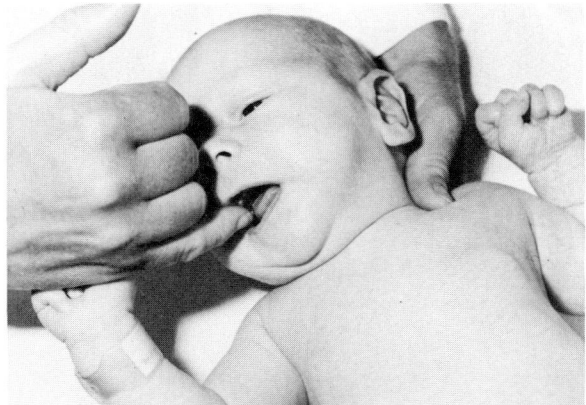

Figure 2.10. The sucking reflex in a 2-week-old infant

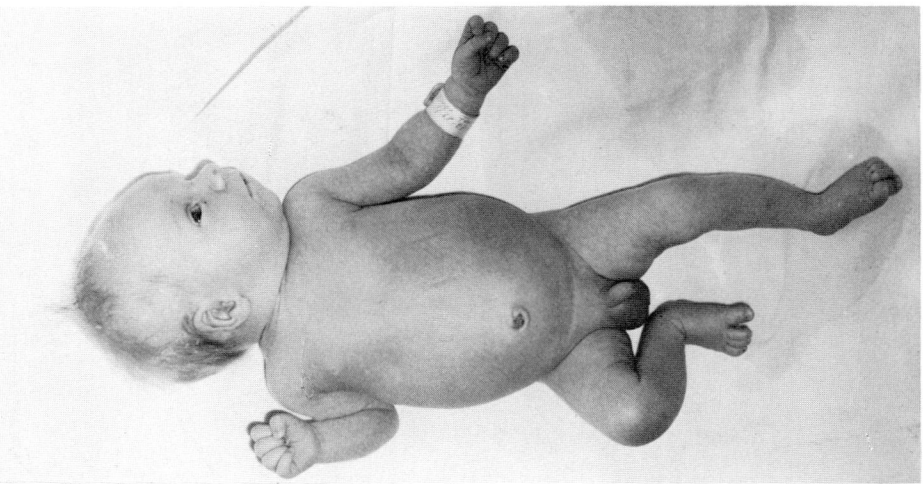

Figure 2.11. The tonic neck reflex in a 2-week-old infant

The tonic neck reflex is elicited by turning the infant's head. In response to this stimulus the arm and the leg extend on the side towards which the face is turned and bend on the opposite side (*Figure 2.11*). The tonic neck reflex is not marked in a normal neonate.

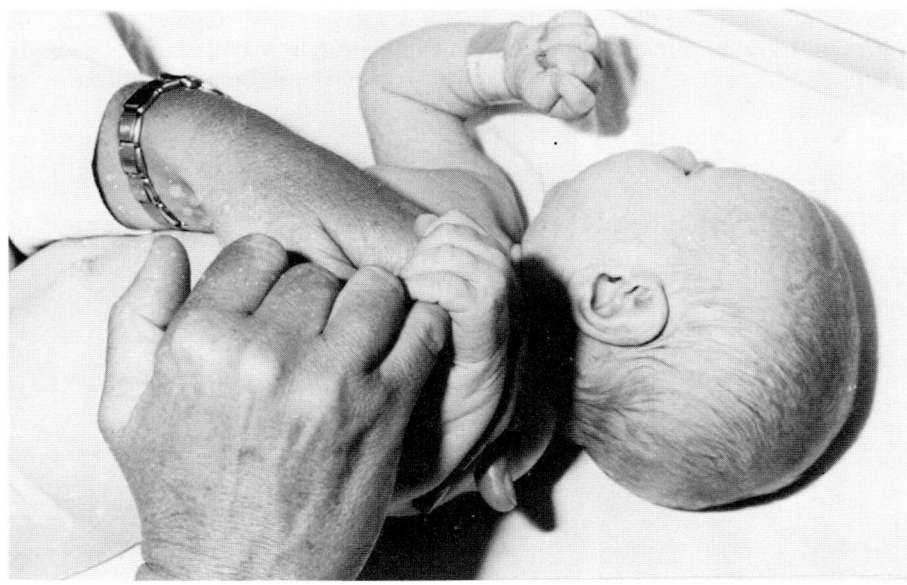

Figure 2.12. The palmar grasp reflex in a 2-week-old infant (*see* page 15)

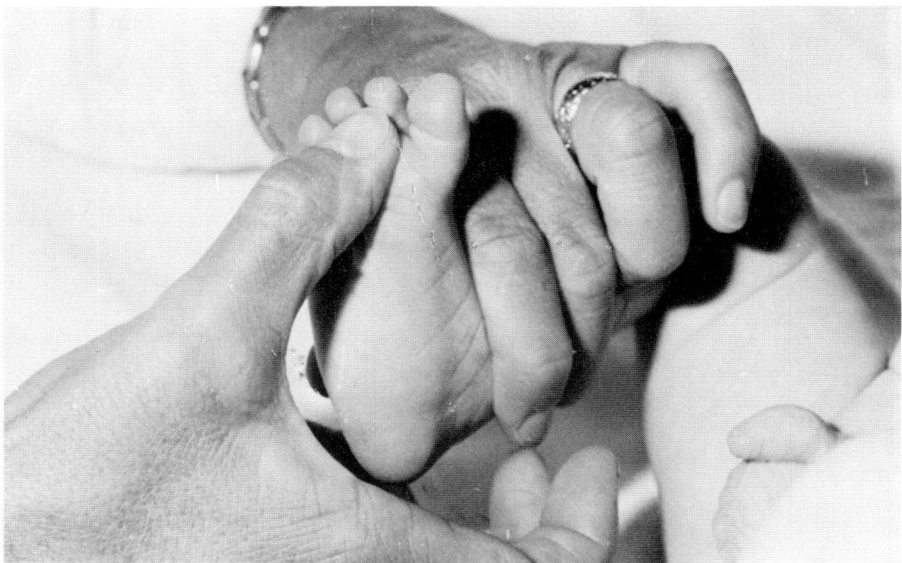

Figure 2.13. The plantar grasp reflex in a 2-week-old infant. The stimulus is the soft tip of the finger, which is gently stroked in the middle of the sole from the heel towards the toes (*see* page 15)

The grasp reflex of the hand is elicited by gently touching the palm of the hand; at this stimulus the hand grasps the touching finger (*Figure 2.12*). The grasp reflex of the foot is elicited by gently stroking the sole of the foot with a broad object (e.g. a finger) from the heel towards the toes; this stimulus elicits a grasping movement of the toes (*Figure 2.13*).

Because of the grasp reflex of the foot, the Babinski sign must always be elicited in a young infant by scratching the sole *from the toes towards the heel.* If the opposite direction is used the response will be made up of a mixture of a grasp reflex and a Babinski sign. The latter reflex is preferably elicited with a fairly sharp

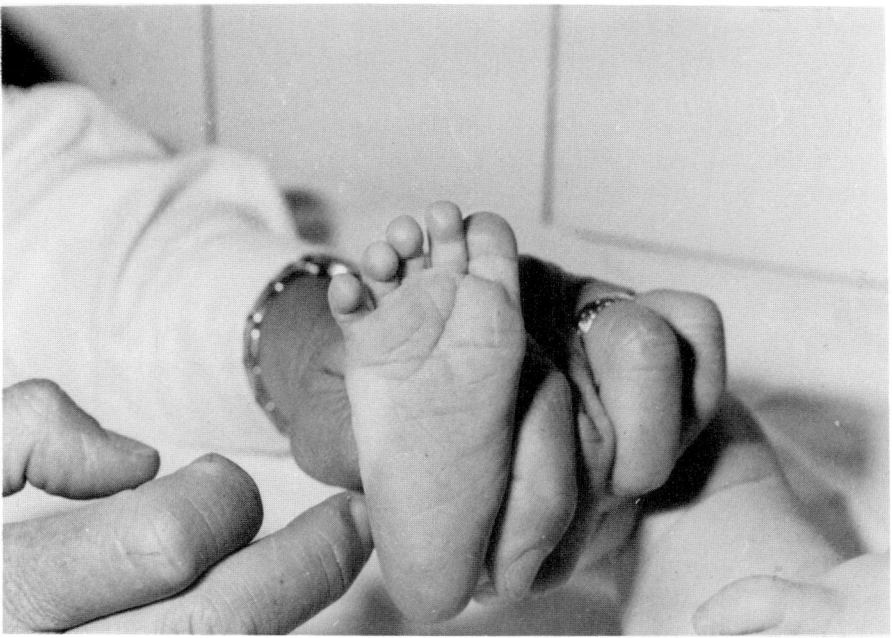

Figure 2.14. The Babinski sign in a 2-week-old infant. The stimulus is the fingernail which scratches the lateral part of the sole from the toes towards the heel

object, such as a fingernail or a knitting needle. In normal neonates the Babinski sign is usually present with an upward movement of the big toe and spreading of the small toes (*Figure 2.14*). It is debated whether this reflex is neurophysiologically identical to the Babinski sign in older children and adults.

Brudzinski's sign

The general neurological examination of a newborn infant also includes a search for evidence of meningitis, which usually causes a bulging fontanelle and a positive *Brudzinski's sign,* but rarely in this age-group a stiff neck. A positive Brudzinski's sign consists of a rapid flexion of knees and hips in response to an abrupt bending forward of the infant's head when he is lying flat on his back (*Figure 2.15*). The sign corresponds to Kernig's sign and Lasègue's sign which are positive in older children and adults with meningitis (*see* pages 343–345).

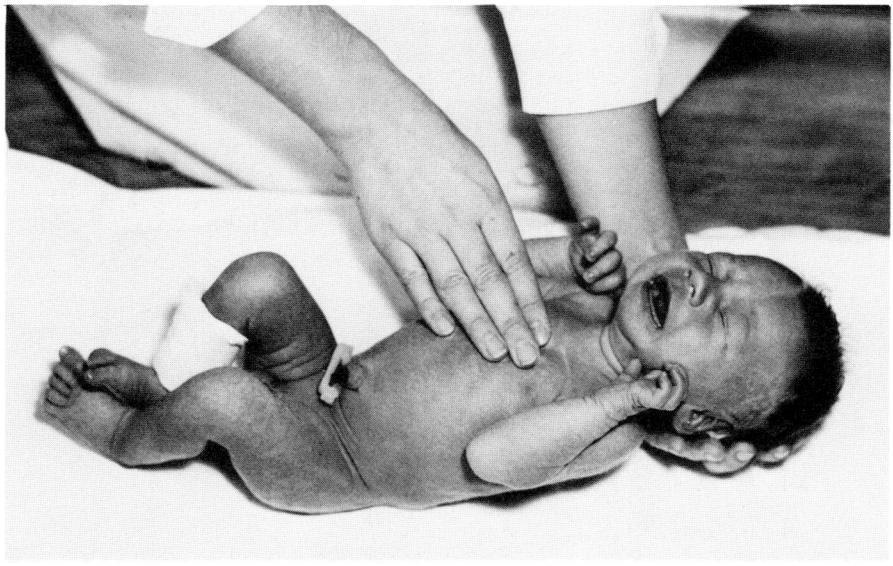

(a)

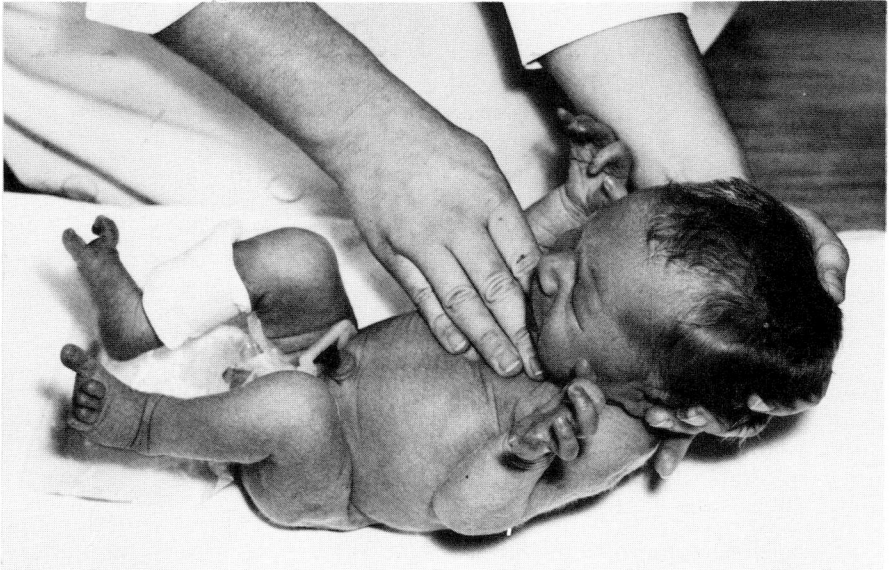

(b)

Figure 2.15a and *b*. A positive Brudzinski sign in a newborn infant with purulent meningitis. Note the marked hip flexion in response to a forward bending of the head

TABLE 2.1. Psychomotor development timetable

Age months	Behaviour and social contact	Motor ability	Reflexes
0–1	None	Can lift head when prone	Moro, sucking, rooting, palmar and plantar grasp, weak tonic neck
1–2	Can fix with eyes, smiles	Some head control	Stronger tonic neck
2–3	Can follow an object, smiles intentionally	Good head control	Neonatal reflexes start to disappear
3–4	Plays with hands, uses voice for pleasure	No head lag, lifts head and shoulders when prone	Tonic neck may be present, other neonatal reflexes have disappeared (except plantar grasp)
4–5	Wants company, plays with feet, localizes sound, may turn eyes and head in response to sound	Can lift head when supine, can grasp objects clumsily but deliberately	
5–6	Aware of new surroundings	Sits with support	Tonic neck may be present, plantar grasp is usually present, but the persistence of other neonatal reflexes is definitely abnormal
6–7	Varied crowing, turns eyes and head in response to sound	Can stand on knees and hands	
7–8	Afraid of new faces	Sits without support, grasps with thumb against radial part of hand (*Figure 2.25*)	Uses arms for protection towards sides (*Figure 2.23*)
8–9	Can play peek-a-boo	Can sit up without help	Remaining tonic neck is abnormal, 'parachute response' present (*Figure 2.24*)
9–10	Understands a few simple words	Pulls to stand, walks holding on to furniture, pinching grasp (*Figure 2.26*)	
10–12	Uses a couple of simple words, understands many more	Walks supported by one hand, can pick up small objects with pinching grasp and transfer them from hand to hand (*Figure 2.27*)	
12–18		Walks unassisted	Plantar grasp, the longest remaining neonatal reflex, disappears

Examination of older infants and children

Psychomotor development

Motor development during infancy and the timetable for the disappearance of neonatal reflexes are briefly summarized in *Table 2.1*. The development never takes place evenly; it occurs in a stepwise manner and the range of normal variability is great. Only obvious deviations from the values given in the table can therefore be taken as evidence of psychomotor retardation. Smaller deviations must be followed-up for some time before definite conclusions can be drawn.

It is apparent from *Table 2.1* that new psychomotor functions develop rapidly during the first year of life. A healthy 4½-month-old infant is shown lying on his back and playing with his feet in *Figure 2.16*; in the prone position, lifting his head and shoulders in *Figure 2.17*; and demonstrating good head control and no head lag when pulled to the sitting position in *Figures 2.18* and *2.19*. *Figure 2.20* shows a 10-month-old infant crawling on his hands and knees and with his belly lifted from the ground. The same infant is shown sitting unsupported with a straight back in *Figure 2.21*, and getting up into the standing position in *Figure 2.22*. The functions described in *Table 2.1*, 'uses arms for protection towards sides' and 'parachute response', are illustrated in *Figures 2.23* and *2.24*. The hand function is shown in *Figure 2.25* (8 months), *Figure 2.26* (10 months), and *Figure 2.27* (10 months). It is also apparent that when the longest remaining neonatal reflex, the plantar grasp, has disappeared at 12–18 months of age, the normal findings on examination of the reflexes are the same in children and adults.

The examination of a child between 6 months and 3 years of age should preferably start with the child sitting on the parent's lap and the examiner on a low stool in front. The examinations requiring the child's active cooperation are done first, provided the child is calm and alert. It is usually wise to start with the hand grasp, offering the child a bright spheric object of appropriate size on the examiner's hand; the older the infant, the smaller is the object he is expected to handle. A child aged 18 months or more should also be tested for his ability to put a peg in a hole, and a child aged 3 years or more for his ability to grasp and use a crayon.

Eye movements can be tested together with the ability to localize sound. In this test the child is shown a silent bright object which he is also enticed to touch or grasp. Before this the examiner must bring his hand with a small bell hidden inside to the child's ear. When the child touches the object, the examiner lets the bell tinkle; a child 7 months or older will then promptly turn his eyes and head towards the sound. The point is that the child must be able to shift his attention from an object stimulating *two* senses in front of him to something new, which is stimulating a third sense and coming in from the side; besides hearing, this test requires both maturation of the central nervous system and a desire for communication.

Part of the following examination may also be performed with the child on the parent's lap, part on the examination table or on a mat on the floor, and part with the child moving freely on the floor.

Examination of the motor system

A unilateral lesion of early onset and long duration will retard the growth of the extremities on one side; the size of the two hands and the two feet should therefore always be compared. The smallest expression of this growth retardation is a

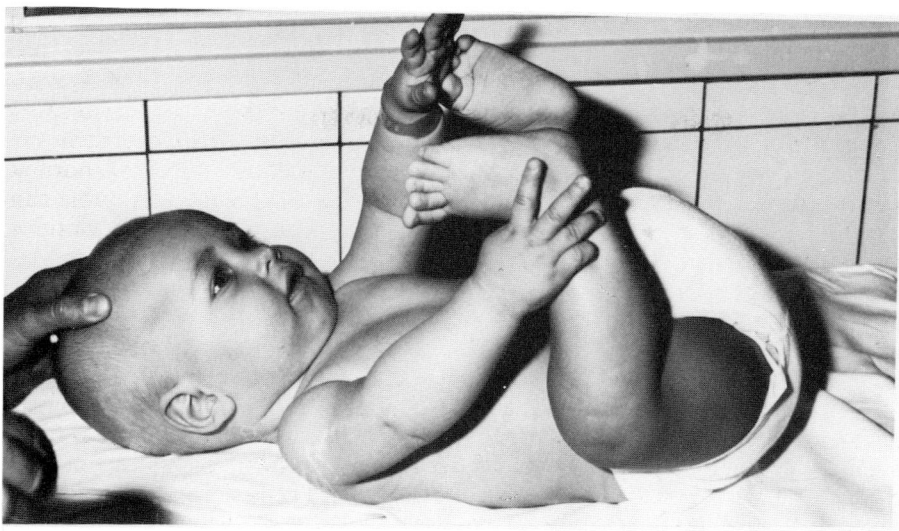

Figure 2.16. A 4½-month-old infant playing with his feet (*see* page 18)

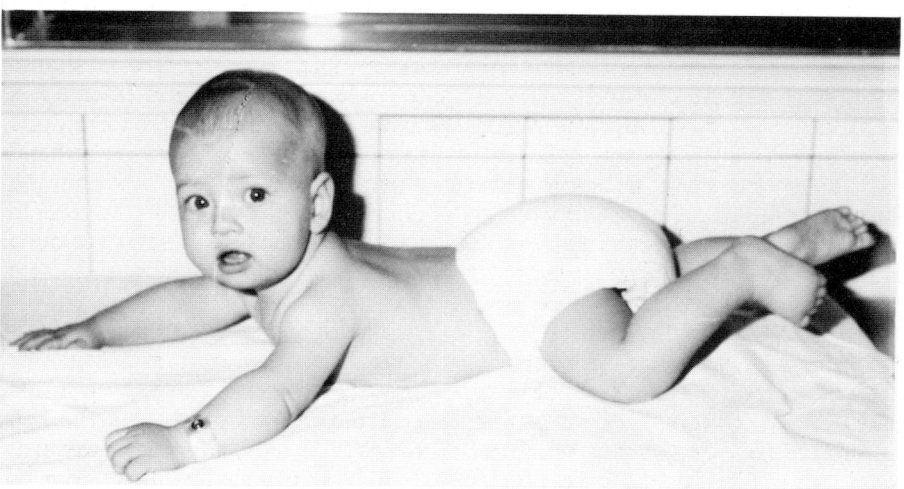

Figure 2.17. A 4½-month-old infant in the prone position, lifting his head and shoulders from the bed, with elbows stretched

difference in nail size between the two hands (*see Figure 12.9*, page 283). A weakness of one arm can usually be found in *Grasset's sign*. The child is asked to hold up both hands with palms parallel, and fingers stretched and kept together, and to sit completely still for a short while with his eyes closed. If one arm is weak, the elbow and fingers will bend and the palm will turn forward (*Figure 2.28*). Increased muscle tone in the arms is best observed as *resistance to supination*; this can be felt as resistance to passive supination. For the test the examiner should preferably use his own dominant hand to examine both hands of the child,

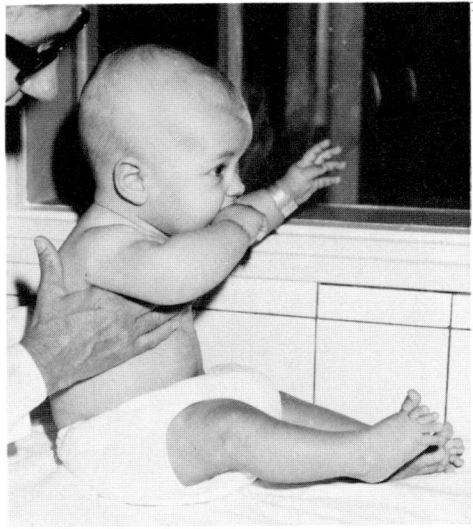

Figure 2.18. A 4½-month-old infant sitting with support and demonstrating good head control

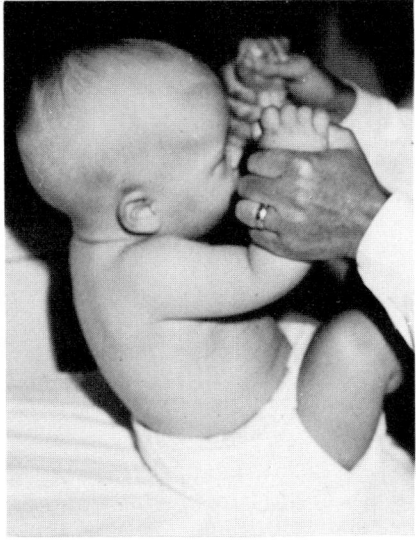

Figure 2.19. A 4½-month-old infant being pulled to a sitting position. Note the flexed elbows and the absence of head lag

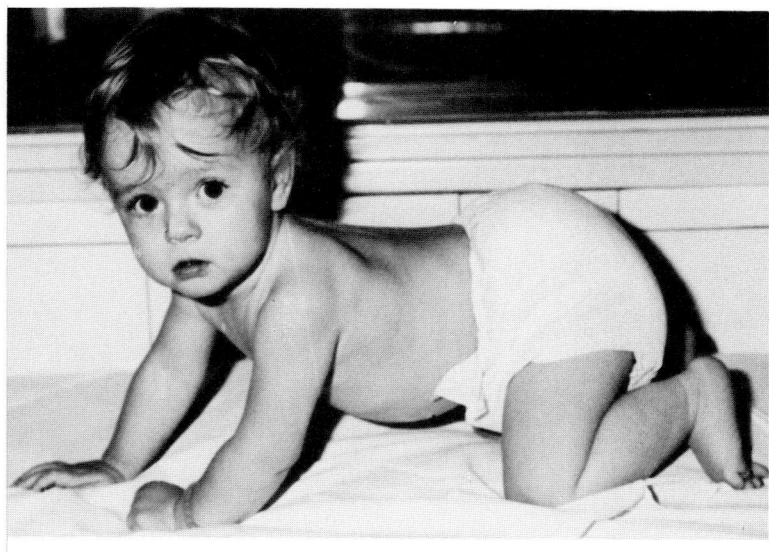

Figure 2.20. A 10-month-old infant crawling on hands and knees with the belly lifted from the bed

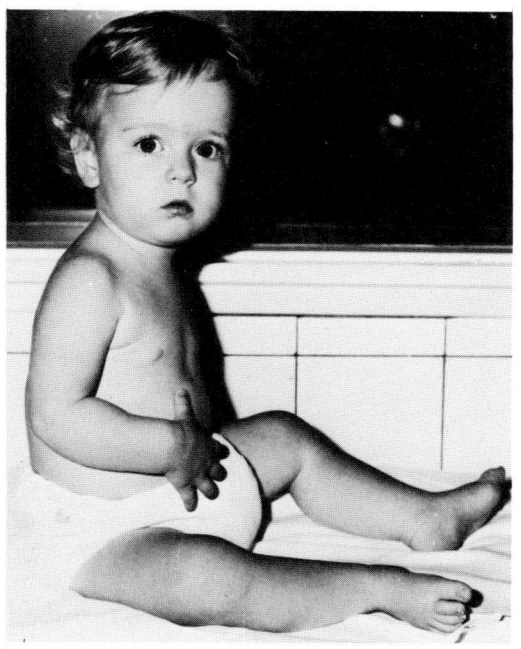

Figure 2.21. A 10-month-old infant sitting unsupported with a straight back and good balance

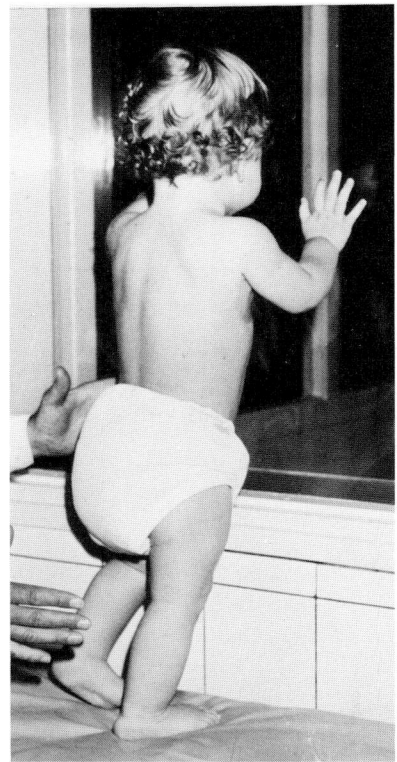

Figure 2.22. A 10-month-old infant getting up into the standing position with only the support of her hands on the wall

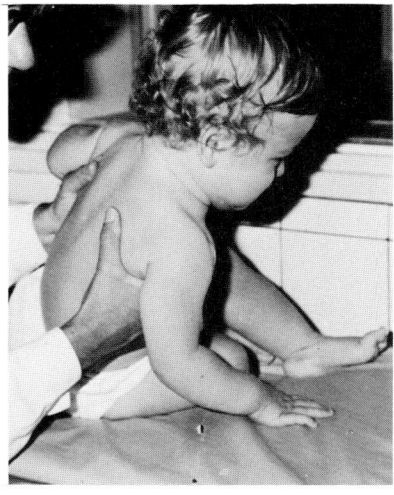

Figure 2.23. 'Uses arms for protection towards sides' (*see Table 2.1*). When the examiner tries to tilt this sitting 10-month-old girl towards one side, she puts out her arm for protection

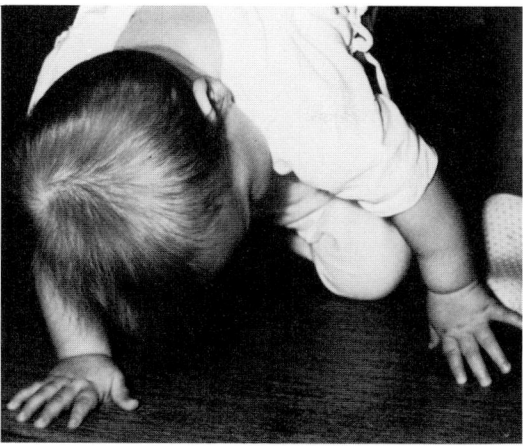

Figure 2.24. 'Parachute response' (*see Table 2.1*). When this 9-month-old boy is moved head first towards the ground, he puts out his hands symmetrically for protection

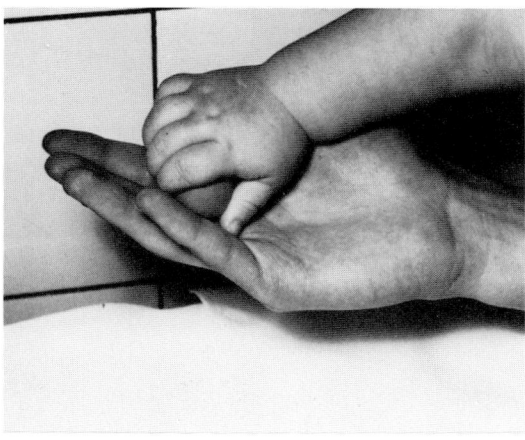

Figure 2.25. The hand grasp of an 8-month-old infant, who uses the thumb clumsily against the radial part of the hand

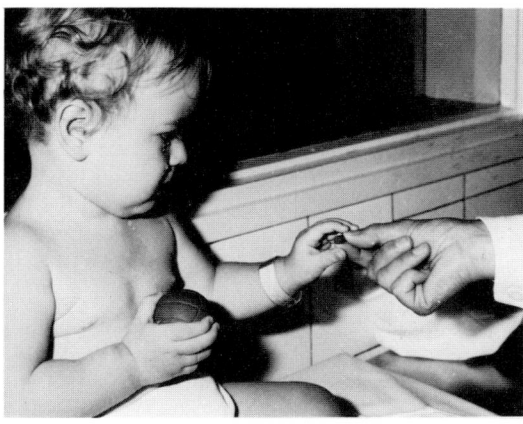

Figure 2.26. The pinching grasp of a 10-month-old infant

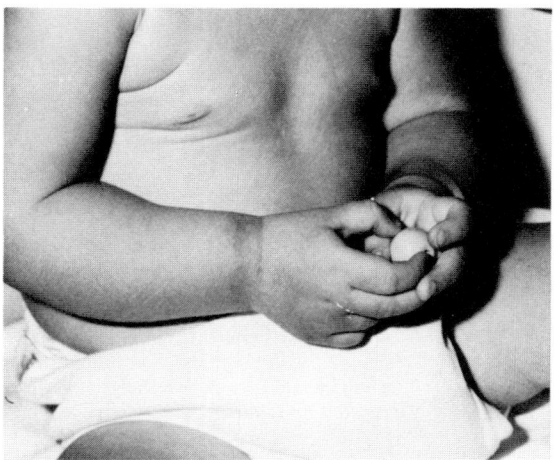

Figure 2.27. A 10-month-old infant transferring an object from one hand to the other

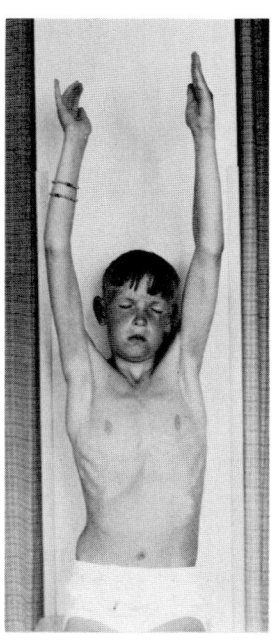

Figure 2.28. A 10-year-old boy with a right-sided hemiparesis demonstrating a positive Grasset sign. Note the flexion of the elbow, the pronation of the hand, and the patient's inability to keep his fingers stretched and together

otherwise a comparison may be difficult. The resistance to supination can also be seen when the child is told to stretch his arms out in front of himself with palms up (*Figure 2.29*). Increased muscle tone in a leg can usually best be felt as *resistance to dorsal extension* of the foot; this may also be seen as difficulty in walking with the heel on the floor (*Figure 2.30*).

Muscle tone can be evaluated only when the child is relaxed; the relaxation can often be facilitated by gentle shaking of the limb. A child with spasticity, attempting to walk on his heels, will often show abnormal co-movements of his

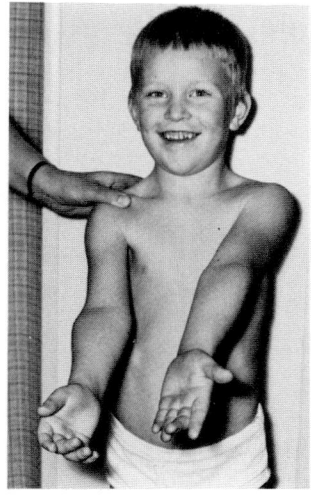

Figure 2.29. A 6-year-old boy with a right-sided hemiparesis demonstrating insufficient supination of his right hand

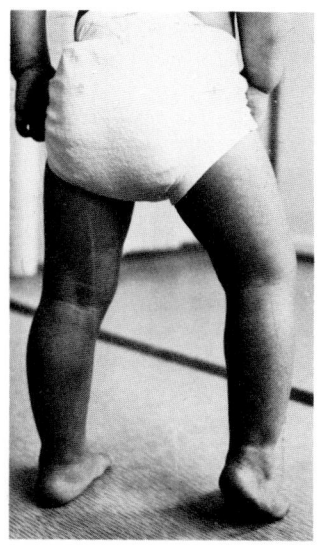

Figure 2.30. A 2-year-old boy with a right-sided hemiparesis demonstrating his inability to get his heel on the floor

arms and hands (*Figure 2.31*). This is even better demonstrated in *Fog's test*; the child is asked to invert his feet and walk on the outside edge of them and to keep his hands at his side. *Figure 2.32* illustrates a normal Fog's test in a healthy 11-year-old girl (*see also* page 282).

Symmetrical associated movements of the type seen in Fog's test are normally seen in young children. They diminish with maturation of the nervous system and disappear at 8–13 years of age. Associated movements of the hands (*Figure 2.31*) when the child walks on his heels are acceptable up to 8 years of age; associated

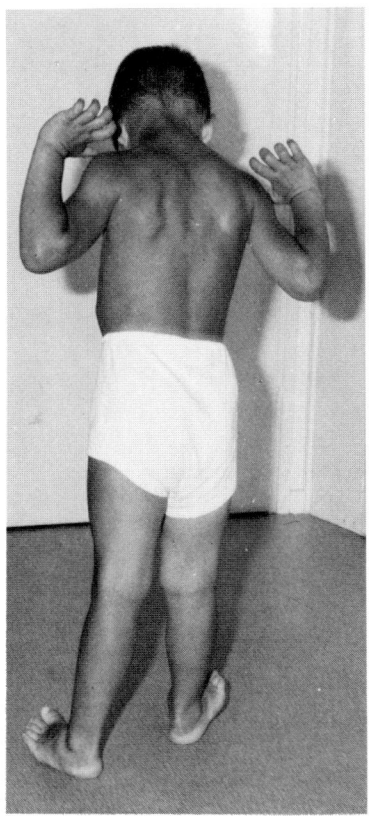

Figure 2.31. A 9-year-old boy with a mild spastic diparesis demonstrating abnormal co-movements of his arms and hands when he tries to walk on his heels

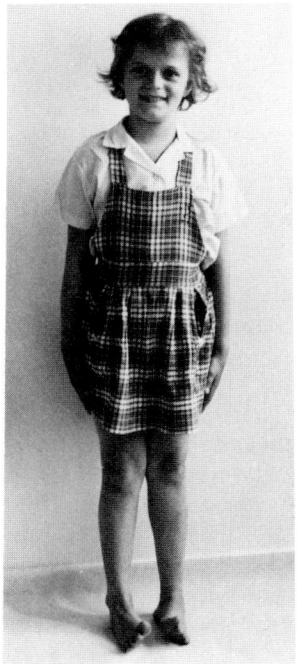

Figure 2.32. A healthy 11-year-old girl demonstrating the absence of co-movements of her arms and hands in Fog's test

movements when the child performs Fog's test are acceptable up to 13 years of age; definite asymmetry of co-movements is unacceptable at all ages. Other associated movements are typically seen in the young child, such as the automatic movements of the tongue when the child is concentrating on a task, or the pendulous movements of the legs in a child working with his hands. If these co-movements are too intense and persist too long they may create a problem of inability to sit still at school. They may also indicate delayed maturation of the nervous system and cerebral dysfunction, which may be the real cause of the child's school problems.

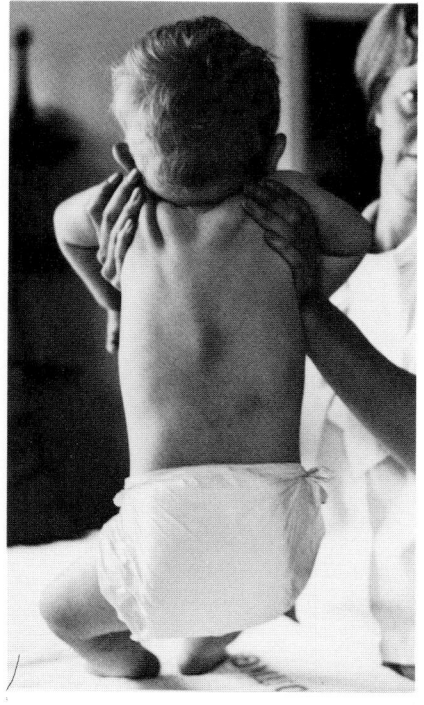

Figure 2.33. Weak shoulder muscles in a 2-year-old child with progressive spinal muscular atrophy. When the examiner tries to lift the child up, the shoulder muscles give way and the child slips between the examiner's hands

The examination of proximal leg muscles and pelvic girdle muscles is best performed by asking the child to squat and get up again without using his hands or by watching the child climb stairs. Shoulder muscles are tested by picking up the child with the examiner's hands around the thorax and in the axillae of the child. A healthy child can easily be lifted in this way, but if the shoulder muscles are weak they give way, and the child slips between the hands of the examiner (*Figure 2.33*). The strength of distal muscles can be evaluated in a young child by watching the way he grasps objects or the examiner's fingers. The strength of distal leg and foot muscles is often better evaluated by watching the way a child walks on his toes and on his heels than by a test of strength with the child lying on his back. In older children the strength of a muscle group is tested in the same way as in adults, i.e. by offering resistance against the movement.

Coordination

Intention tremor can usually be found towards the end of the first year, when the child reaches out his hands for objects, or when a child who does not want to do any tests at all puts his thumb in his mouth. The finger-to-nose test of adult neurology may be replaced by the thumb-in-the-mouth test in the young paediatric group. The precision of small finger movements can be tested by asking the patient to thread pearls on a string or by a competition between examiner and patient to see who can perform the most rapid movements of the forefinger and thumb (*Figure 2.34*), or who can play fastest on a make-believe piano. Simple observation of the way the patient manages buttons when he undresses and dresses himself gives good information about his control of small finger movements. The steadiness of leg movements can be evaluated by asking the child to tap seven times with one heel on a given point on the other shin.

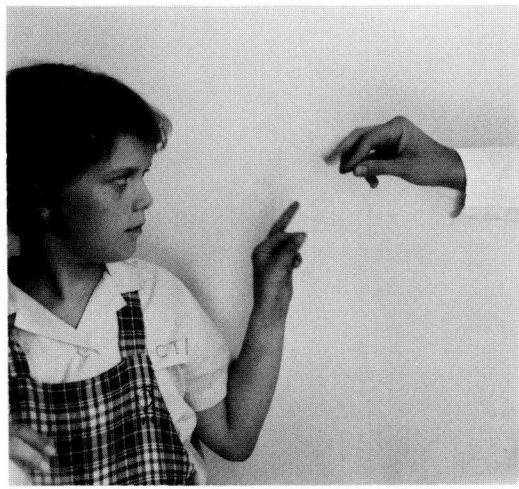

Figure 2.34. Patient and examiner competing in rapid small movements of thumb against forefinger

Diadochokinesis can best be tested by asking the child to tap the palm of one hand with the other hand, alternating as fast as he can between the back and the palm; the tapping hand is the one being tested. The examiner performs the same actions in front of the child, competing in rapid alternation between pronation and supination of the hand (*Figure 2.35*). Examiner and child must always match their best hands against each other. Children perform this test fairly slowly, and only reach adult standard at 10–12 years of age. Associated movements of the tongue, face and feet during the test for diadochokinesis and for rapid small movements of the fingers (*Figure 2.34*) are normally seen in young children; they should be under control at 8 years of age.

Balance and coordination of gross muscle movements can best be studied in a toddler by watching him walk. Older children should always also be asked to run, as running reveals more abnormalities than walking. A normal child learns to hop on one foot at about 4½ years of age. This test should be included in the examination of children above this age. The unsteadiness of movements is particularly brought out if the child is asked to run and then turn round quickly. An

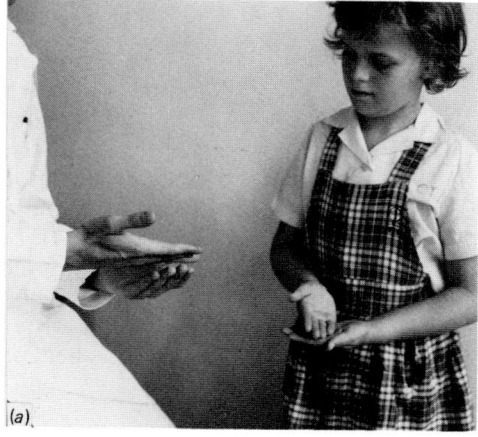

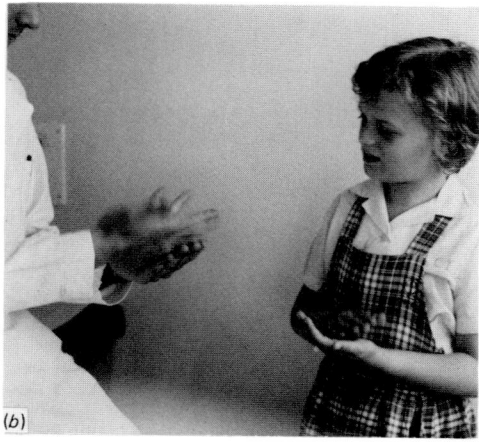

Figure 2.35a and *b*. Diadochokinesis as a competition in rapid alternating movements between patient and examiner

ataxic child cannot hop on one foot. The hemiparetic child may manage his feet fairly well when running, but the affected arm comes up in front of him and is kept there with the elbow bent and no co-movements (*Figure 2.36*); he usually has great difficulty in hopping on the affected foot.

Romberg's test can usually be performed from 3–4 years of age in the same way as in adults, i.e. by asking the patient to stand with feet close together, first with the eyes open and then with eyes closed. A positive Romberg's test means that the patient cannot maintain balance when he closes his eyes. Children reach adult standards of steadiness at about 5–6 years of age and are usually better than adults between 8–10 years of age and puberty. Truncal ataxia can also be observed when the child is sitting unsupported, as during the performance of Grasset's test. The ataxia is more easily elicited if the child puts one leg across the other.

Sensation

Sensation is always difficult to test in children. Active cooperation in testing the response to pinprick cannot be expected below the age of 9–11 years. Vibration sense is usually easier to test; reliable cooperation may be received from 4 years of

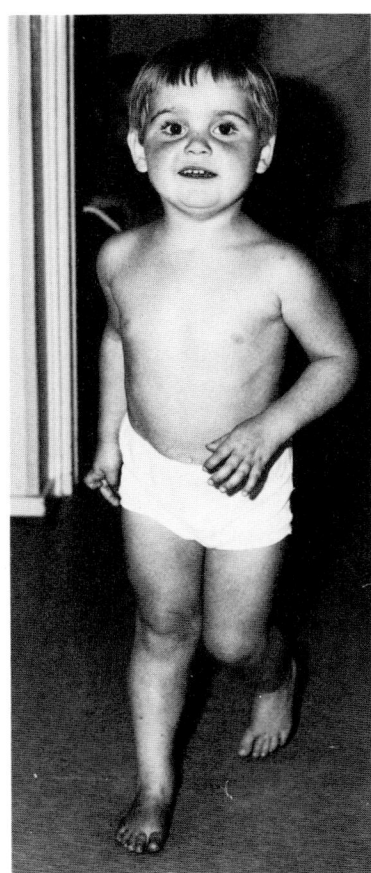

Figure 2.36. A 3½-year-old girl with a mild left-sided hemiparesis. When she is running, her left arm comes up in front of her with the elbow bent. The co-movements, normally seen in both arms of a running child, are absent in this arm. Notice also the mild central facial paresis on the left side

age and can be expected from 6 years. Position sense and two-point-discrimination can often be tested accurately from 6–8 years of age. Children are good at two-point-discrimination and need only 1–3 mm between the points of a divider to appreciate the two points on the fingertips and 5–6 mm on the toes. Stereognosis may, as a rule, be tested from 5–7 years of age.

Vision and hearing

Vision and hearing can usually be tested reliably from 3–4 years of age, and visual fields from 6–7 years. In very young infants one can only test the response to a strong light or a strong sound, both of which cause the infant to close his eyes. An infant, a couple of months old, will follow an object with his eyes, and at 4–5 months of age will turn his eyes and head towards a sound. An infant who loses his sight before 3–4 months of age will show large, nystagmoid, searching eye movements. When testing the visual fields the examiner tries to keep the infant's attention directed straight ahead. An assistant introduces an object from the side, making no sound, and in response to it the infant turns his eyes and head towards the stimulus. A large defect such as hemianopsia can be detected in this way in an infant during the second half-year. The response to sound can be tested in principally the same way.

An optokinetic nystagmus can be elicited in an attentive infant by pulling a striped piece of cloth in front of him. This will normally elicit nystagmoid movements of the eyes. No response from either side will be seen in an inattentive infant, or in a blind infant. Consistent reponses from both eyes when the test is performed from one side, but never when performed from the other side, will be seen in an infant with a visual field defect or a parietal lobe lesion.

Examination of the head

Measurement of head circumference will give a crude estimate of the growth of the brain. The growth of the head is due to pressure from inside the skull, normally caused by the growth of the brain. A mean for the head circumference in the newborn period is 34–36 cm, at 6 months 43–45 cm, at 1 year 48–50 cm, and at 5 years 50–52 cm. The growth of the brain is mainly completed by 2 years of age, and the increase in head size between 2 and 5 years of age is small. Head size remains almost the same from 5 years of age to puberty, when it again increases a few centimetres, mainly due to thickening of the skull bones and the subcutaneous tissue. A single abnormal value is of little significance unless it is grossly outside the normal range. Measurements at regular intervals will give a curve, the slope of which is more significant as an estimate of the growth of the brain.

The growth curve for head circumference would be more accurate if it was related to age from conception rather than to age from birth. However, the former age is seldom known exactly and all standard curves are constructed with the child's age from birth as one variable; in most routine situations this is satisfactory (except for small preterm infants). The growth curve is different for boys and girls; it does not appear to be influenced by race. Possibly, head circumference should be related to height instead of age.

The sutures and fontanelles are evaluated together with the head circumference. In the normal newborn infant the large fontanelle, the sutures, and usually also the small fontanelle are open; the small fontanelle closes within the first few weeks in the full-term baby and later in the premature baby. The large fontanelle is flat in a healthy quiet infant. A bulging fontanelle is a sign of increased intracranial pressure and a sunken one indicates dehydration. The large fontanelle closes when the child is between 8 and 18 months of age. Premature closure of the fontanelle, particularly if the skull circumference is small, should arouse a suspicion of craniostenosis; however, primary microcephaly due to poor development of the brain is more often the explanation (see page 236). If the fontanelle remains open for too long, increased intracranial pressure must be suspected, particularly if the fontanelle is bulging and the head circumference is increasing too rapidly. An abnormally early or late closure of the fontanelle may, however, be seen in normally developing infants; the size of the fontanelle must therefore be evaluated in relation to other findings.

Increased intracranial pressure arising in a child with closed fontanelles causes stretching of the sutures, which may be revealed clinically by *percussion* of the skull; this may produce a typical sound, best described as a 'cracked-pot' sound. *Auscultation* of the skull should also be included in the clinical examination, as this may occasionally reveal a murmur due to an arteriovenous malformation. Transillumination is performed in infants and young children (see page 7).

References

BRAZELTON, T. B. (1973) *Neonatal Behavioral Assessment Scale. Clinics in Developmental Medicine No 50.* London: William Heinemann Medical Books Ltd

FRANKENBURG, W. K. and DODDS, J. B. (1966) Denver Developmental Screening Test. University of Colorado Medical Center, Denver

HYVÄRINEN, L. and LINDSTEDT, E. (Ed) (1983) Early visual development, normal and abnormal. *Acta Ophthalmologica,* suppl. 157

LARGO, R. H. and HOWARD, J. H. (1979) Developmental progression in play behaviour between nine and thirty months. I. Spontaneous play and imitation. *Developmental Medicine and Child Neurology,* **21,** 299–310

LARGO, R. H. and HOWARD, J. H. (1979) Developmental progression in play behaviour between nine and thirty months. II. Spontaneous play and language development. *Developmental Medicine and Child Neurology,* **21,** 492–503

LEIJON, I. (1980) Neurological and behavioral assessments of full-term newborn infants. Linköping University Medical Dissertations No 98, Linköping, Sweden

STENSLAND JUNKER, K. (1972) *Selective Attention in Infants and Consecutive Communicative Behaviour.* Stockholm: Almqvist & Wiksell

TOUWEN, B. C. L. and PRECHTL, H. F. R. (1970) *The Neurological Examination of the Child with Minor Nervous Dysfunction. Clinics in Developmental Medicine No 38.* London: William Heinemann Medical Books Ltd

VOLPE J. J. (1981) *Neurology of the Newborn.* Philadelphia: W. B. Saunders

3

Special examinations

A history and clinical neurological examination must in many cases be supplemented by special studies. Some of them will be mentioned here, particularly the normal findings in infancy and childhood when they deviate from normal adult values. *No values found to be normal in adulthood can, without investigation, be accepted as normal also for infants and children.*

Electroencephalography

In almost all children with a neurological disease, electroencephalography may be helpful in the further management of the child. The active cooperation of the patient is not necessary, and the examination can therefore be performed in children of any age, including those who are mentally retarded. The normal electroencephalogram (EEG) in the newborn infant is flat and slow with a frequency of 1–2 cycles per second. By about 3–4 months of age the frequency has doubled, and the amplitude has increased by about three to four times. Towards the end of the first year the frequency is about 3–5 cycles per second; the amplitude remains at about the same height and the rhythm becomes more regular. At 2–3 years of age short periods of activity within the range of alpha activity (8–13 cycles per second) start to appear, but most of the activity is still irregular with a frequency of 4–6 cycles per second. During the following years the proportion of regular alpha activity increases at the expense of the slower activity. Alpha activity usually appears first and is most marked in the occipital leads. At 7–9 years of age alpha activity is the dominating finding in a normal EEG, but the slower activity is not reduced to the same degree as in a normal adult EEG until 12–14 years of age. Examples of normal EEG tracings in infancy and childhood are given in *Figures 3.1–3.5*. Beta activity (faster than 13 cycles per second), which may be seen in a certain number of normal adult EEGs, is an abnormal finding before puberty, provided the child is not taking medication. Most antiepileptics, particularly barbiturates and benzodiazepines, produce an abundant amount of fast activity on the EEG (*Figure 3.6*).

The changes described above are seen on an EEG recorded in the waking state with no provocations. When the patient opens his eyes and his attention increases, the alpha activity is often blocked. When the patient is exposed to a flickering light of variable frequency, the rhythm in the occipital leads may follow some of the

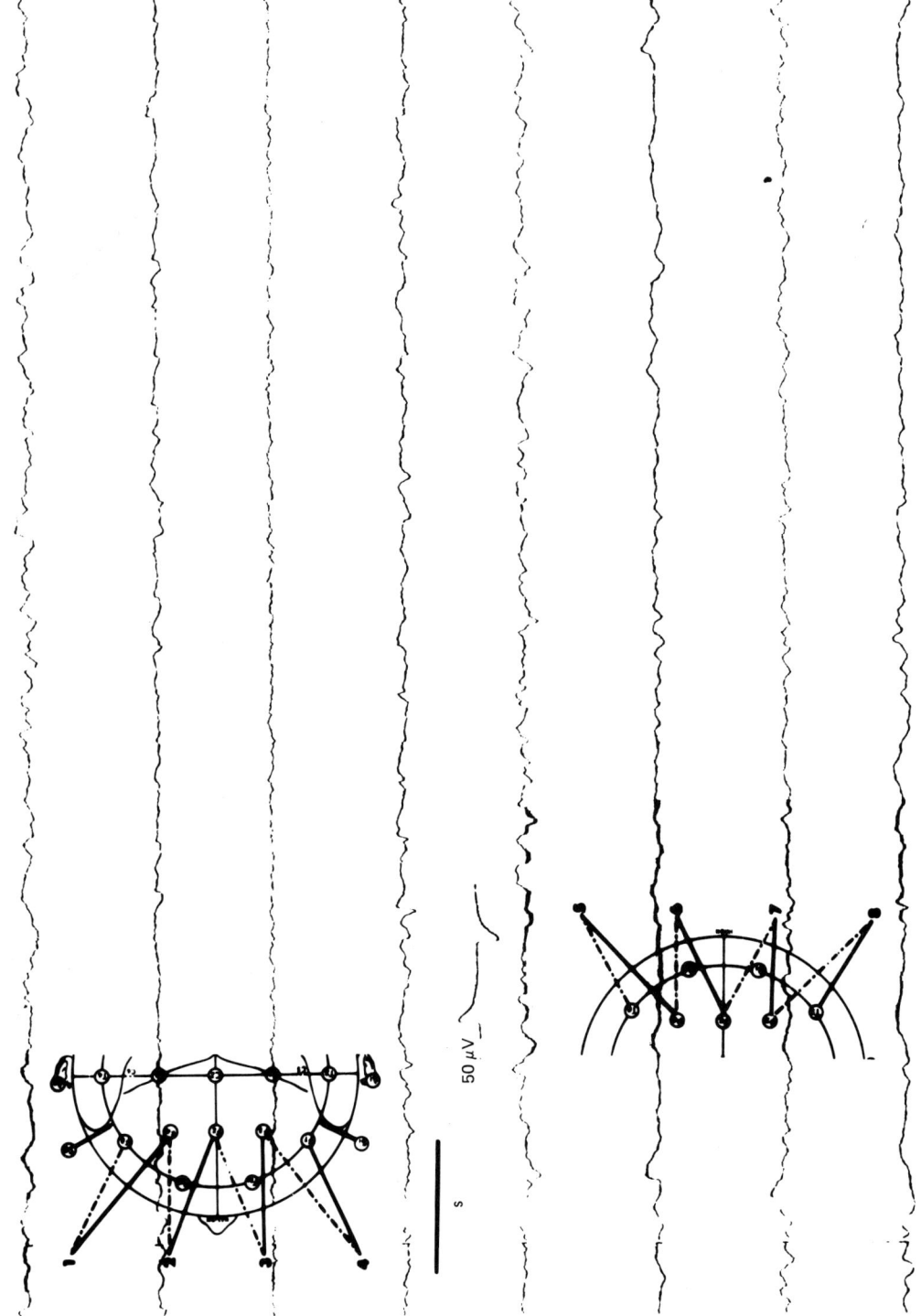

50 µV

s

Figure 3.1. EEG recorded in a healthy full-term 5-month-old infant

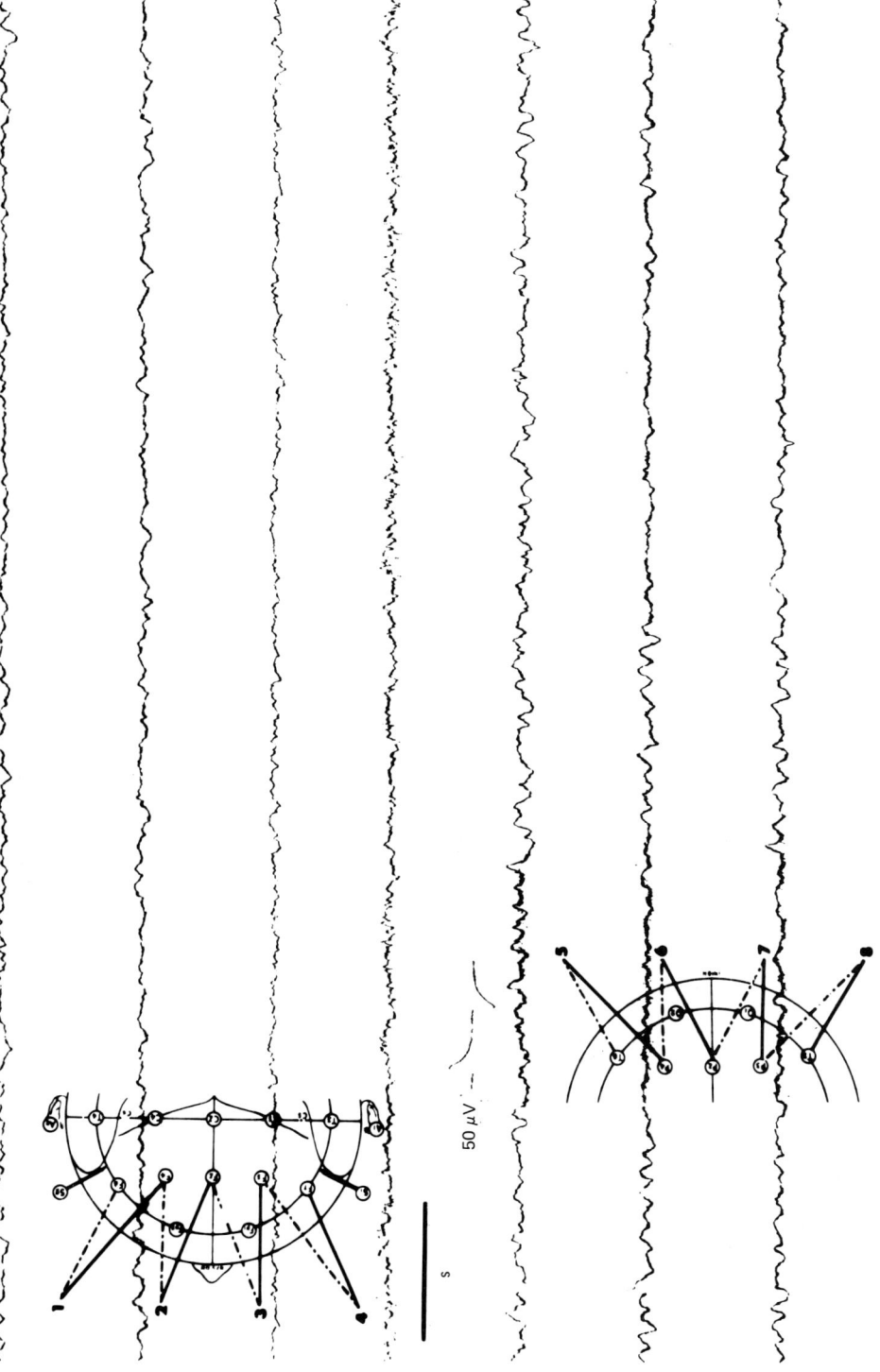

50 μV

s

Figure 3.2. EEG recorded in a healthy 16-month-old child

36

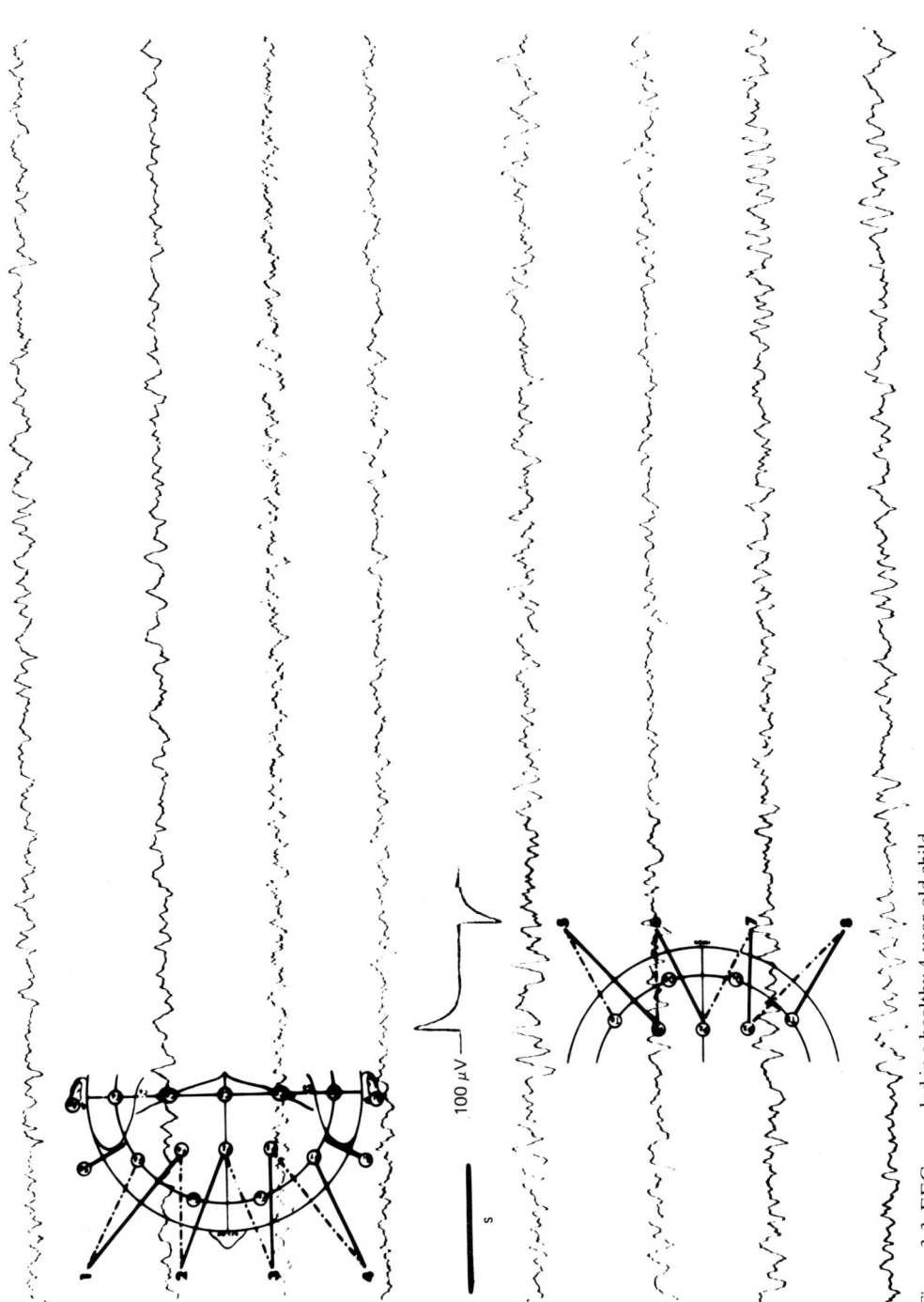

100 µV

s

Figure 3.3. EEG recorded in a healthy 4-year-old child

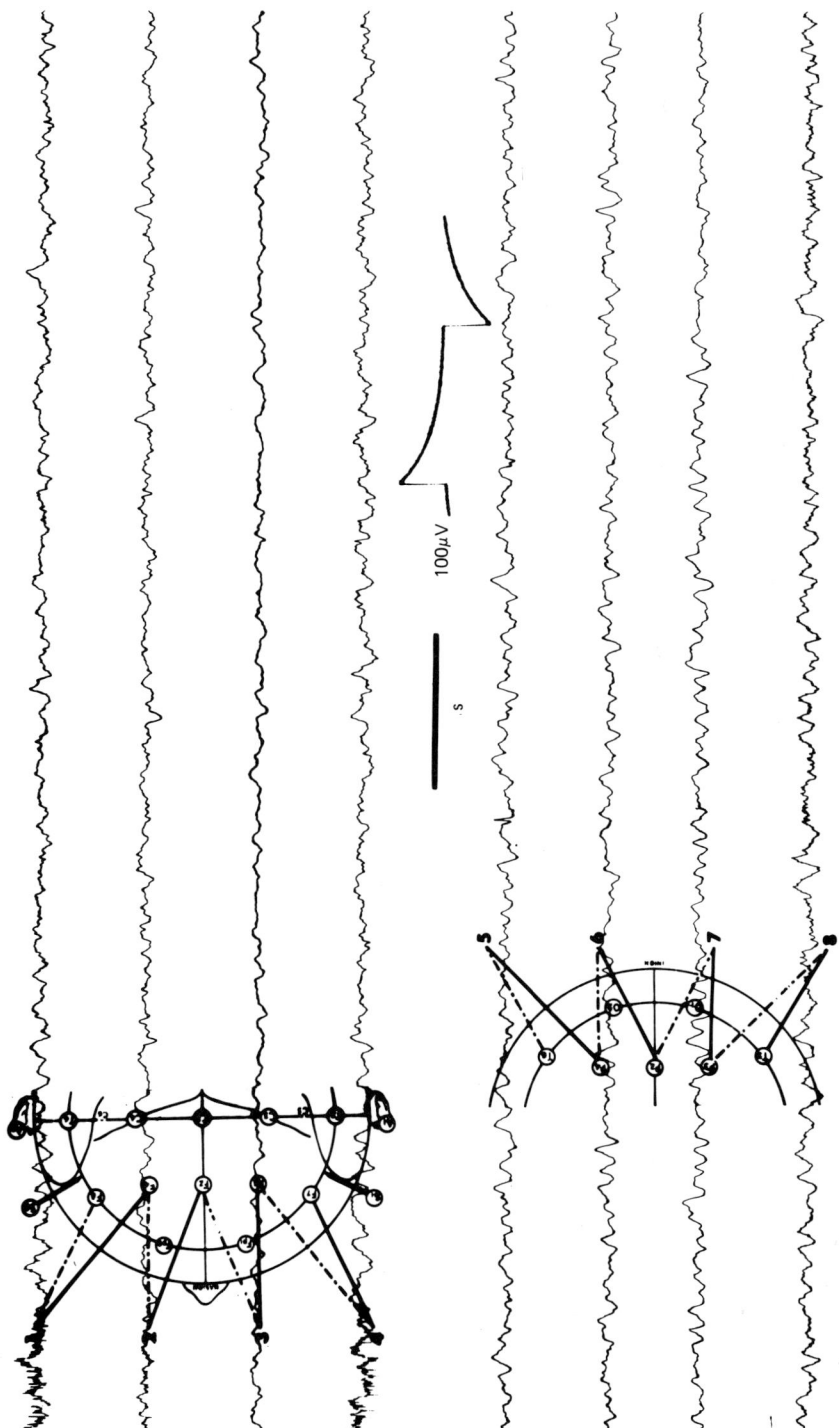

Figure 3.4. EEG recorded in a healthy 5½-year-old child

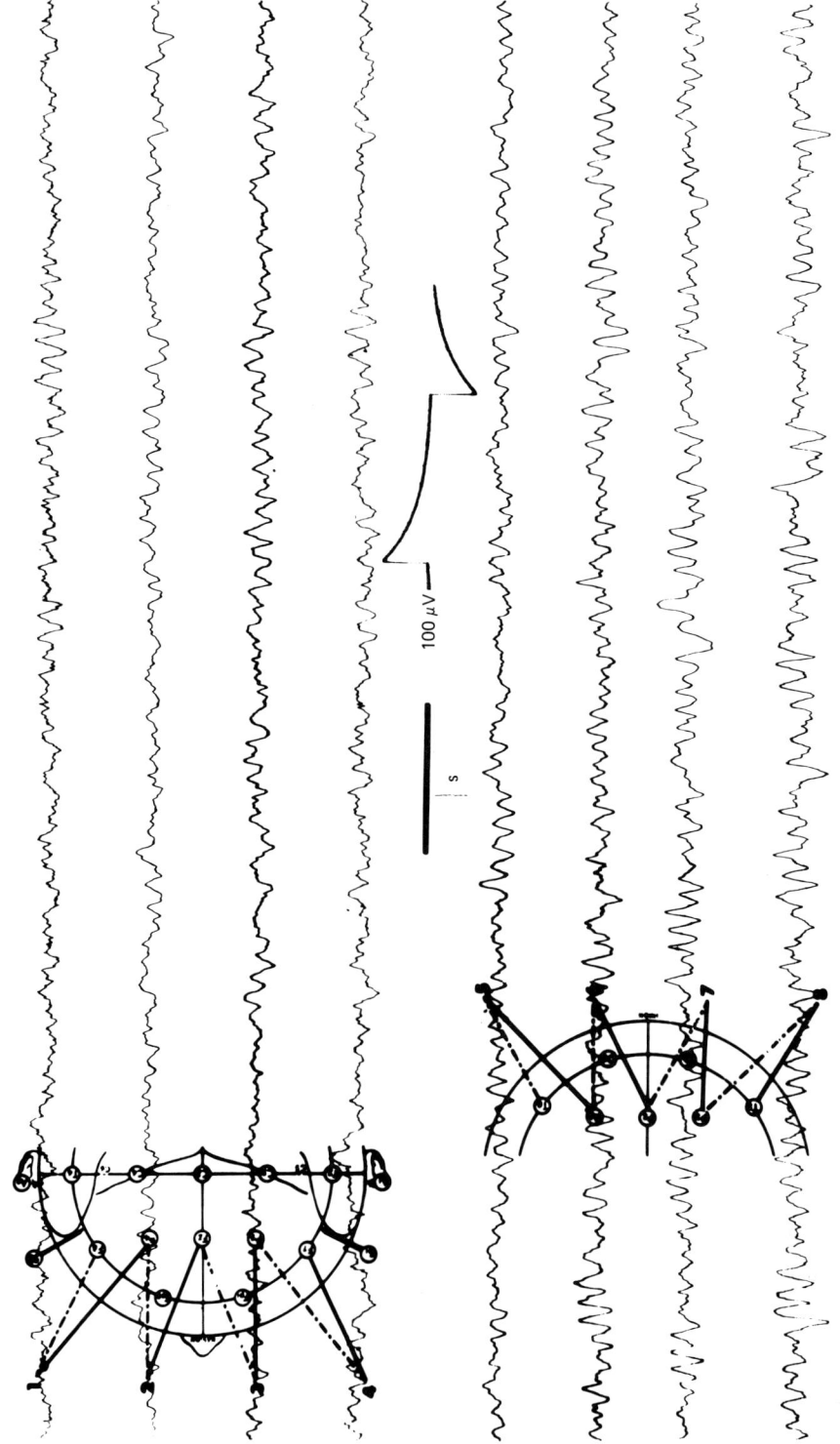

Figure 3.5. EEG recorded in a healthy 9-year-old child

Figure 3.6. EEG recorded in a healthy 12-year-old child with drug-induced (chlordiazepoxide) fast activity

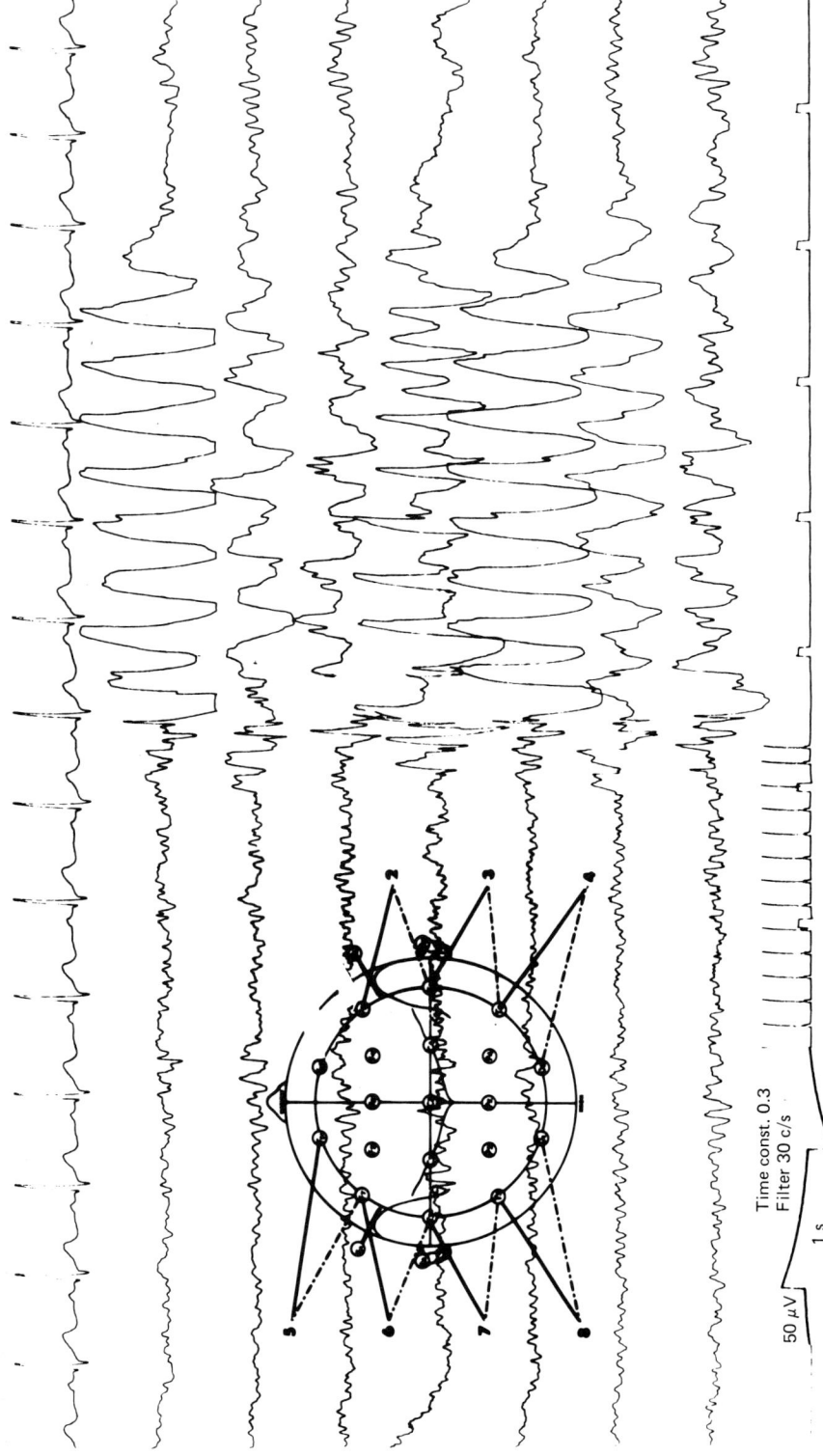

Time const. 0.3
Filter 30 c/s

50 μV

1 s

Figure 3.7. EEG recorded in a 15-year-old boy with spike-wave activity in response to photostimulation

frequencies used. This finding is normal if the change in rhythm is symmetrical; a marked asymmetry may be abnormal. The appearance of spike potentials in response to a flickering light is usually an abnormal finding (*Figure 3.7*). If this occurs, the provocation must be interrupted, as it may otherwise elicit a seizure.

Hyperventilation, which is usually difficult for children below 5 years of age to perform, produces a symmetrical slowing of the activity and an increase in the amplitude. These changes are usually more marked and persist for a longer period after hyperventilation in children than in adults. The intracranial pressure may rise on hyperventilation; this provocation must therefore not be used in a patient in whom increased intracranial pressure is suspected. If spike potentials appear on hyperventilation, the procedure must be interrupted, as it may otherwise elicit a seizure.

Drowsiness and light sleep cause symmetrical slowing of the activity and so-called sleep spindles, which also appear symmetrically in a normal EEG, both in childhood and adulthood. On arousal, the previous faster activity returns. It may be impossible to get a record in the waking state in a restless young child or in a mentally retarded child. A sleeping record can always be obtained with the help of a sedative, which, however, has the disadvantage of introducing some EEG changes. For a small child trimeprazine, 2–4 mg/kg by mouth approximately 2 hours before the recording, is a useful drug. For an older child chlorpromazine 25–50 mg by mouth or by intramuscular injection may be more effective. For all reasonably cooperative children above 1 year of age, *sleep deprivation* during the night before the EEG recording is a better way to obtain an EEG during drowsiness and light sleep. The parents are instructed to restrict the child's sleep during the night before the EEG recording to half the number of hours he usually has; to give him a good breakfast with neither coffee nor tea; and to prevent him falling asleep during transportation to the laboratory. With this preparation it is usually possible to get both waking and sleeping records without the introduction of drugs (*Figure 3.8*).

Within the limitations given in the previous paragraphs, all EEGs should preferably be recorded with all the described provocations. It is particularly important, also, to obtain a sleeping record in all children, since drowsiness and light sleep often provoke abnormalities arising in the temporal lobe, which would often be unrecorded if the recording was performed only in the waking state. For up to 1 week after a grand mal seizure the EEG may show nonspecific postictal abnormalities which may mask significant findings. Fever, regardless of its cause, may also produce nonspecific EEG abnormalities which may last for up to 1 week. Therefore, one should, whenever possible, refrain from taking EEG recordings for 1 week after a grand mal seizure or a period of fever (with or without convulsions).

The EEG is particularly important in children with convulsions and with complaints suspected to be due to epileptic manifestations without convulsions, e.g. migraine-like headache, abrupt and unexplained attacks of bellyache and vomiting, fever, and abnormal behaviour (*see* page 87). In all these situations consistent EEG abnormalities of the paroxysmal type support a diagnosis of epilepsy and facilitate decisions about the further management of the child.

A brain abscess localized in a cerebral hemisphere often causes a typical EEG pattern (*see* page 361). A tumour with the same localization usually also produces EEG abnormalities (*see* page 367). The EEG is rarely of diagnostic help in patients with hydrocephalus or with a space-occupying lesion localized in the midline structures or the posterior fossa. A characteristic EEG pattern is found in patients

42

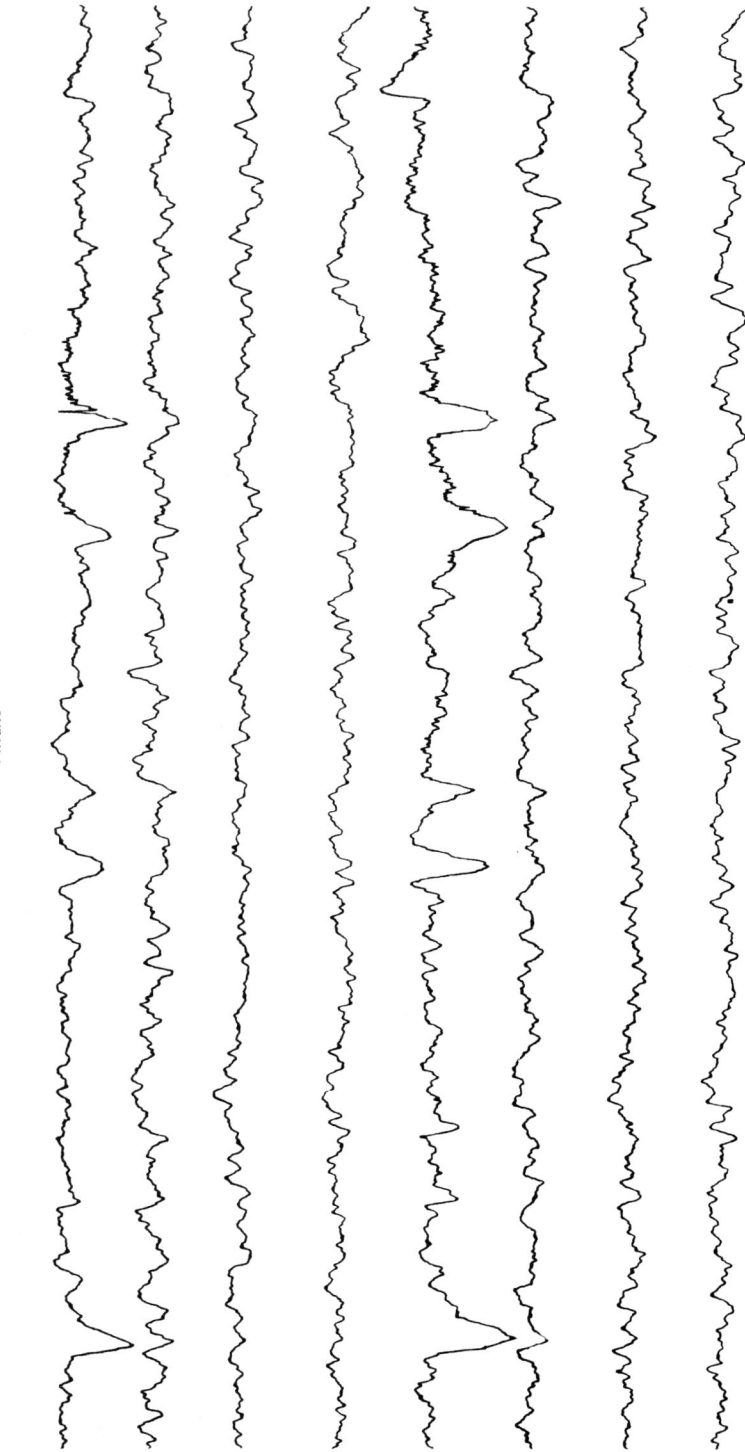

Awake

Figure 3.8. EEG recorded in a healthy 5-year-old girl during wakefulness, drowsiness, and normal (not drug-induced) sleep

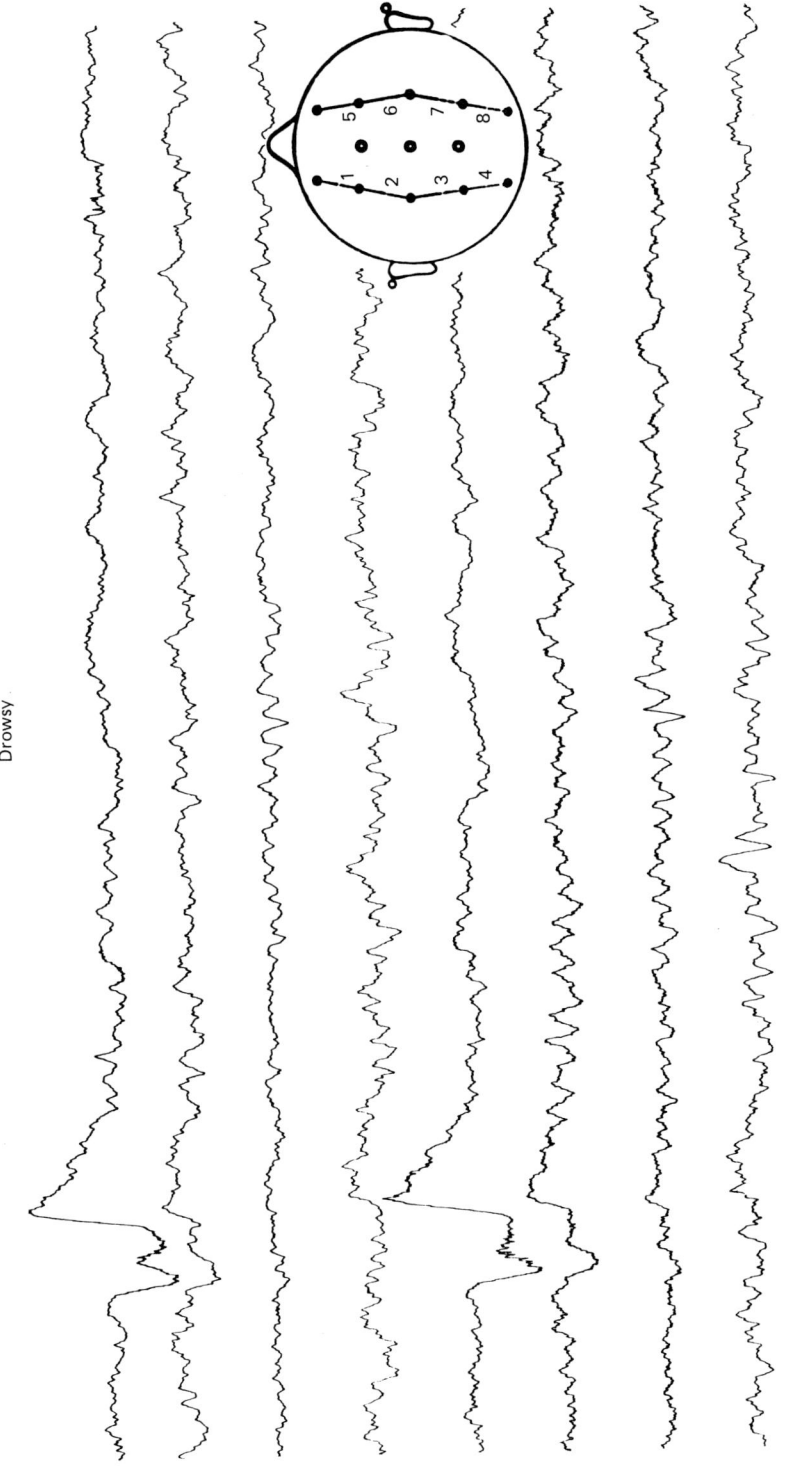

Drowsy

Figure 3.8 (contd)

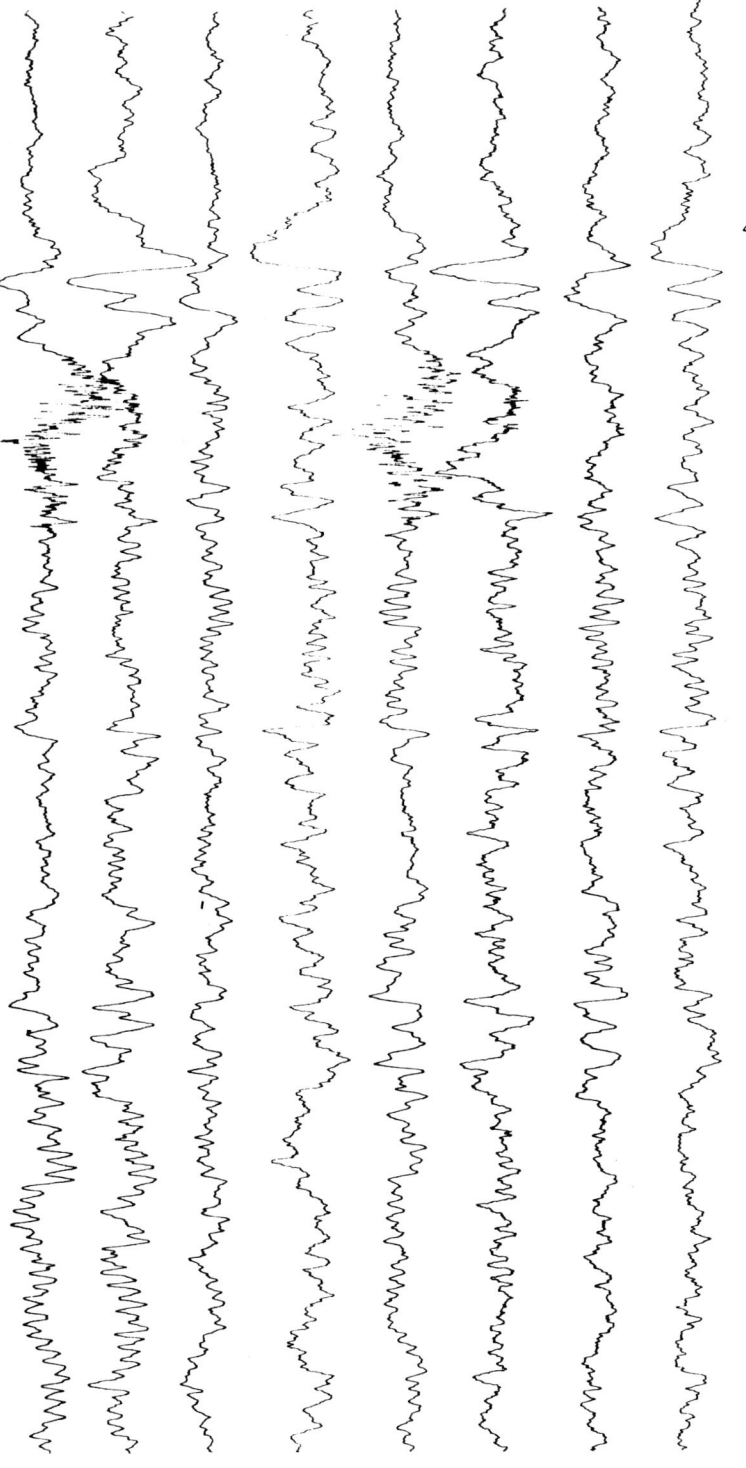

Asleep

Figure 3.8 (contd)

with subacute sclerosing panencephalitis (*see* page 311). The EEG pattern may be of diagnostic help in some of the metabolic disorders (*see* pages 128–137) and degenerative disorders (*see* Chapter 13).

Electromyography and measurement of the conduction velocity of peripheral nerves

These methods are used when the clinical picture suggests a disorder of the lower motor neurones or the muscles. With these techniques the disorder can usually be localized to the anterior horn cells, the peripheral nerve fibres, the end-plates, or the muscle fibres, and the distribution of the abnormality can also be established. Some diseases primarily affecting the central nervous system may also involve the peripheral nerves. Measurement of the conduction velocity of the peripheral nerves may therefore also be a useful procedure when the dominating symptoms are from the central nervous system.

Electromyography

Electromyography is performed by inserting needle electrodes into the muscle and recording the potentials on a cathode-ray oscillograph during relaxation, slight contraction, and intense contraction. The concentric needle electrode, used for conventional electromyography, records the electrical muscle activity between a lead-off surface of 0.15×0.58 mm at the tip of the needle and its shaft. It has been estimated that the spike component recorded by this type of electrode originates from two to twelve muscle fibres adjacent to the electrode tip, provided the recording is obtained from a normal muscle. Several movements of the needles in the muscle are needed for the complete examination of one muscle. An electromyographic examination usually requires the study of at least two muscles. This examination is thus unpleasant, and active cooperation can only rarely be expected in children below 7 years of age. The easiest muscles to examine are usually the anterior tibial on the leg and the biceps muscle on the arm; however, the clinical situation must decide which muscles should be examined. If a biopsy of a particular muscle is planned immediately or within the next few months, electromyography of this muscle should be avoided, as the small injury caused by the electromyographic needle may be found on histological examination of the specimen and confuse the interpretation of the findings. Some of the terms used in electromyography will now be described.

SPONTANEOUS ACTIVITY

This is activity that occurs in the completely relaxed muscle; such activity is abnormal (except fibrillations appearing in young infants, *see below*). Different types of spontaneous activity exist.

Fibrillations
These are mainly positive potentials with a duration of 1–3 msec and a frequency of 2–10/s (*Figure 3.9*). Their origin is considered to be the isolated contraction of a single muscle fibre, a contraction which cannot be seen by direct observation of the muscle, except possibly in the tongue, where the muscle is covered only by a thin

Quadriceps fem.
Fibrillations

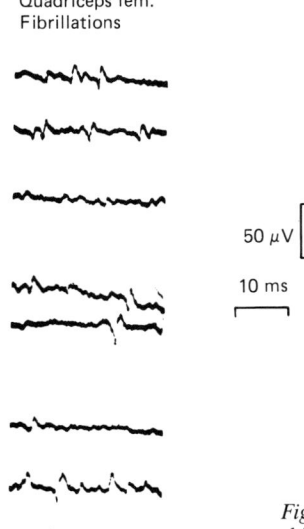

50 μV

10 ms

Figure 3.9. Electromyographic recording of fibrillations in an 18-month-old child with spinal muscular atrophy

mucous membrane. Fibrillations may be seen in the healthy muscles of young infants; they are interpreted as a sign that the child's muscles are not yet completely innervated. In trunk muscles this activity is normally found only in prematurely born infants. In full-term babies it usually disappears within the first month in proximal limb muscles and within 3 months in distal limb muscles. The persistence of fibrillations in any muscle in an individual above 6 months of age must be considered an abnormal finding. Fibrillations may indicate denervation of muscles; they also occur in electrolyte disturbances and in inflammatory primary muscle diseases.

Myotonia
This is a discharge of potentials, starting with a high frequency of 100–200 potentials per second and rapidly decreasing to a few potentials per second; each potential has the same appearance as a fibrillation (*Figure 3.10*). Myotonia is found particularly in myotonic dystrophy (*see* page 194) and myotonia congenita (*see* page 213).

Fasciculations
These are large potentials with a high amplitude and a duration of 10–20 msec. Their origin is considered to be the spontaneous (involuntary) simultaneous contraction of many muscle fibres, constituting a subunit within a motor unit (*see below*). They can be seen directly both in the tongue and in limb and trunk muscles as twitching of part of the muscle with no movement in a joint. They appear particularly in diseases affecting the anterior horn cells, and occasionally in diseases affecting the anterior roots or the peripheral nerves (*see* pages 169–179).

MOTOR UNIT ACTIVITY

During active contraction of a muscle, potentials appear which are caused by activity in the motor unit. A motor unit consists of one anterior horn cell and all its

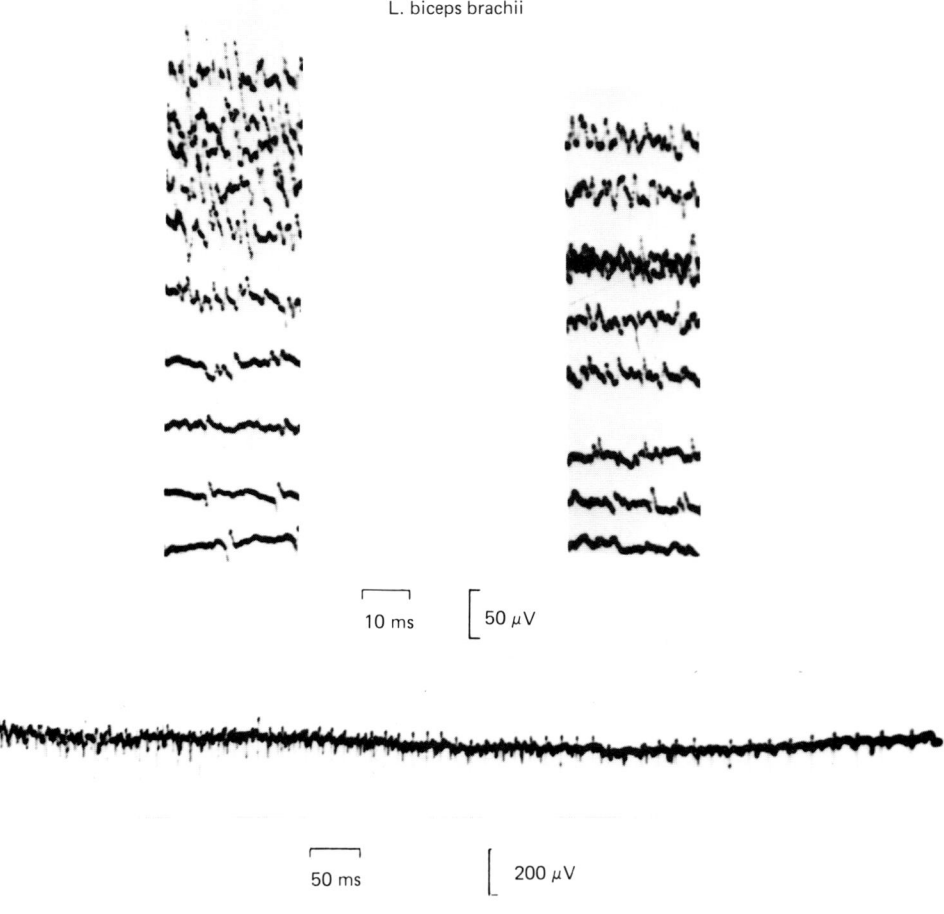

L. biceps brachii

10 ms   50 μV

50 ms   200 μV

Figure 3.10. Electromyographic recording of myotonia in a 5-year-old boy with myotonic dystrophy

branches, including the axon, which is one motor fibre in the mixed peripheral nerve, and all the muscle fibres innervated by this anterior horn cell. When the anterior horn cell is stimulated, all these muscle fibres become active simultaneously; if the anterior horn cell dies, they are denervated. Surviving anterior horn cells often reinnervate denervated muscle fibres; motor units therefore grow in size in partially denervated muscles. The motor unit potentials seen on the EMG can be defined according to number, size and shape. The number of motor unit potentials is estimated during intense, if possible maximal, contraction when the potentials normally cover the baseline completely. Their number is decreased in a partially denervated muscle and normal in a muscle with a primary muscle disease. That the reduced number is due to a partial denervation and not to a submaximal contraction (inability of the patient to cooperate) can be checked by observing the frequency of the potentials; it is high during a maximal contraction of a partially denervated muscle and low if the contraction is submaximal.

Primary muscle disease   Normal muscle   Progressive spinal muscular atrophy

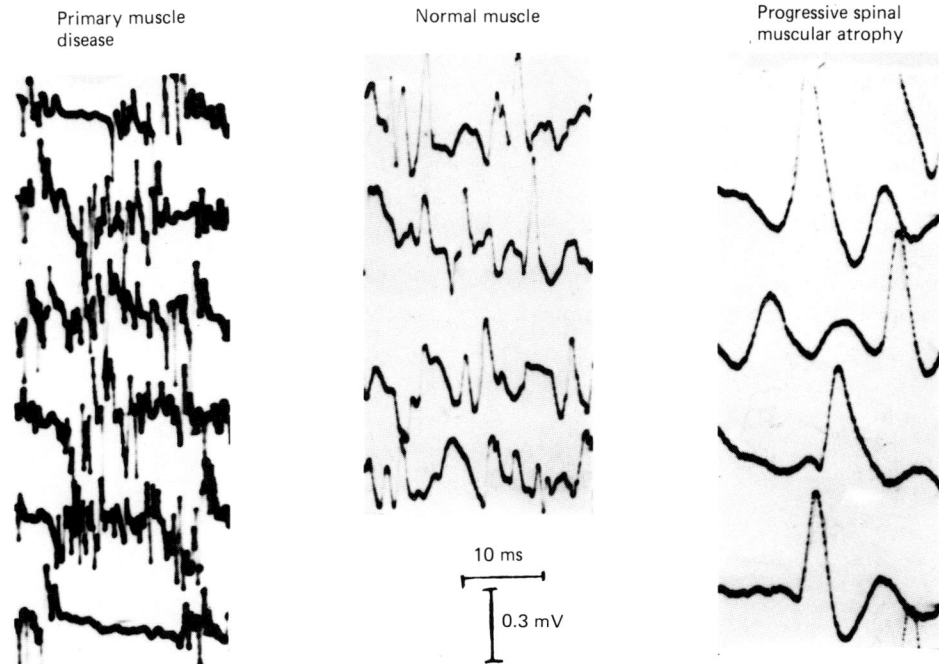

10 ms

0.3 mV

Figure 3.11. Electromyographic recording of normal and abnormal motor unit potentials in children

Size consists of amplitude and duration, the latter parameter being the most important. Twenty different motor unit potentials should be recorded in every muscle examined, their duration measured, and a mean calculated. This *mean duration* varies with the age of the patient and from one muscle to another. Throughout life there is a steady increase in mean duration. The motor unit potentials of muscles with small motor units, e.g., extraocular muscles, have a mean duration of only a couple of milliseconds; in most limb muscles it varies during childhood from about 7 to about 13 msec. The duration varies also with different techniques and different electrodes. In evaluating a mean duration found in a muscle, one must therefore have normal values for various ages and muscles obtained with the same technique. An observed mean must be at least 20 per cent above or below the normal mean duration to be considered abnormal. The mean duration is increased in partially denervated muscles and decreased in muscles afflicted by a primary muscle disease (*Figure 3.11*). Amplitude has a tendency to increase in denervation and to decrease in primary muscle disorders, but as normal variation is great, this parameter is less useful. The shape of the potentials is also taken into account but has less significance than mean duration in evaluation of the EMG findings.

A different type of electrode, consisting of a 0.5 mm cannula inside which a 0.025 mm platinum wire is placed with a recording surface in a side port a few millimetres behind the tip, will permit recording from a single muscle fibre or a few fibres (single fibre EMG). This method allows an estimation of *fibre density,* which reflects the average number of muscle fibres within the uptake area of the electrode. In healthy persons fibre density is 1.3–1.7; the figure varies for different muscles and increases with age; an abnormally high figure is seen in partially denervated muscles with reinnervation. The method may also be used to demonstrate *jitter,* a phenomenon reflecting the neuromuscular transmission in individual end-plates. The electrode is placed in the voluntarily activated muscle to record from two muscle fibres belonging to the same motor unit and thus with time-locked potentials. At consecutive discharges the time interval between the two potentials will vary slightly and this variation, termed jitter, is less than 25–50 μsec in a healthy muscle. In disturbed neuromuscular transmission, particularly myasthenia gravis, jitter is increased and occasionally potentials may disappear entirely, indicating a block of some motor end-plates (*Figure 3.12*). The

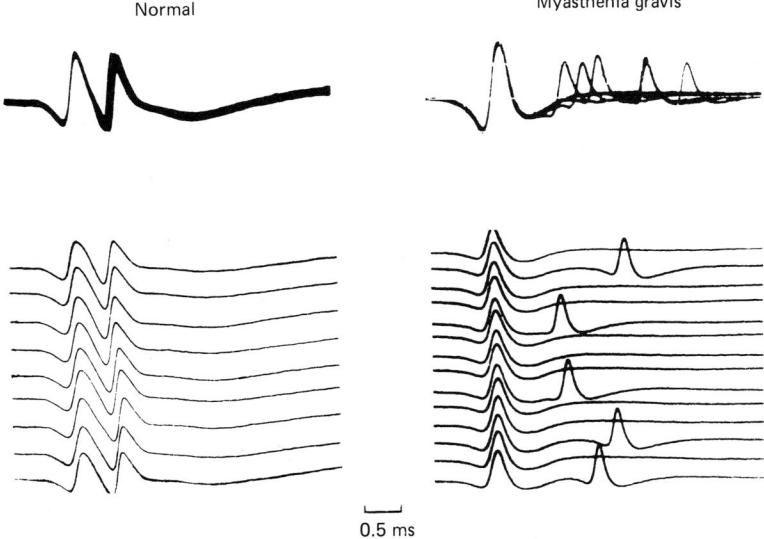

Figure 3.12. Single fibre EMG, showing normal jitter (left) and abnormally increased jitter in a case of myasthenia gravis (right)

use of this type of electrode thus increases the value of an electromyographic examination, particularly in patients with a suspected disturbance of neuromuscular transmission. However, it requires so much active cooperation that the method is seldom useful in children below 10 years of age.

Conduction velocity

MOTOR NERVE FIBRES

The conduction velocity of motor nerve fibres is measured by stimulating the nerve supramaximally at two different points along the nerve and recording from a muscle as distal as possible. The conduction time is obtained by measuring the time from the beginning of the stimulus to the beginning of the response. By subtracting the conduction time obtained at the distal stimulation from that obtained at the proximal stimulation, one can determine the time taken for the impulse to travel in the nerve between the two points. This distance is measured, and the conduction velocity can then be calculated. This method is applied to the ulnar nerve, and is schematically outlined in *Figure 3.13*. The normal value for adults in the ulnar and median nerves is 50–75 m/s, and 5 m/s lower in the peroneal nerve. In the newborn period the normal value is approximately half these values. The values then increase; the increase occurs most rapidly in the peroneal nerve in which the normal adult level is reached at around 1 year of age. In the ulnar nerve the normal adult value is attained at about 3–5 years of age and in the median nerve at 5–8 years. The delay in the maturation of the median nerve appears to be even greater

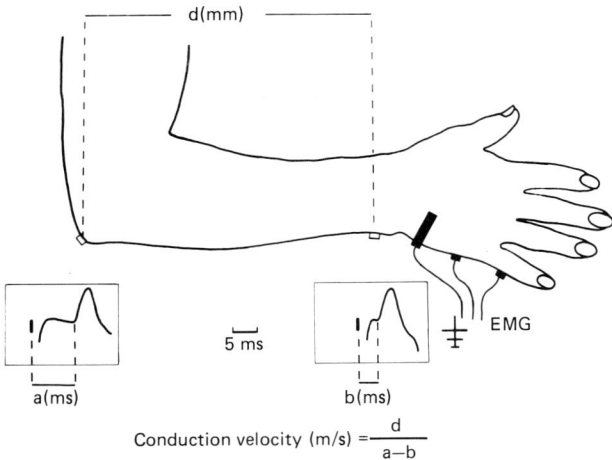

Conduction velocity (m/s) $= \dfrac{d}{a-b}$

Figure 3.13. A schematic outline of the method of measuring the conduction velocity of motor nerve fibres of the ulnar nerve. (Published with the permission of *Acta Paediatrica* (Uppsala))

in mentally retarded children. The values considered *borderline low* (not the normal range) in different age-groups are given in *Table 3.1*. For this method only surface electrodes are used. It is not painless, but few children above the age of 4–6 years object to it.

The *amplitude* of the evoked muscle response is also noted; it is proportional to the number of muscle fibres available for stimulation. If a series of four to eight stimuli is given at a rate of 3–10/s, the amplitude remains the same in a muscle with normal neuromuscular transmission. If neuromuscular transmission is impaired, as

TABLE 3.1. Range of motor conduction velocities considered borderline low in different age-groups*

	Age-group					
	Birth to 1 week	1 week to 4 months	4 to 12 months	1 to 3 years	3 to 8 years	8 to 16 years
Ulnar nerve	20–24	25–29	35–39	40–44	45–49	50–54
Median nerve	15–19	15–19	25–29	35–39	40–44	45–49
Peroneal nerve	15–19	20–24	30–34	40–44	40–44	40–44

* Motor conduction velocity in m/s. Any value below this range is considered definitely abnormal.

in all types of myasthenia gravis and myasthenic syndromes (*see* pages 179–182) for example, the amplitude will show a *decrement* during repetitive stimulation. Thus this test is important if impaired neuromuscular transmission is suspected, particularly in children too young to cooperate in the single fibre EMG (*see* page 48). A decrement may also be observed in healthy young infants, particularly if a higher stimulation frequency is used.

SENSORY NERVE FIBRES

The conduction velocity of sensory nerve fibres can also be recorded. Different methods are available; the best method requires recording of the nerve potential through a needle electrode placed close to the nerve (*neurography*). Not only the conduction velocity but also the amplitude, duration, and shape of the potential in response to various strengths of stimulation can be used to evaluate nerve function. The conduction velocity of sensory nerve fibres recorded by this method is slightly faster than the conduction velocity of motor nerve fibres, but the relationship between the findings in children and in adults is approximately the same. Neurography gives more exact information about nerve function, but it is a more painful and more complicated procedure than recording the conduction velocity of motor nerve fibres.

It is wise to start the examination of a child by recording the motor nerve conduction velocity. If this is abnormally low in several nerves, there is seldom any need for further studies. When further examination can give more diagnostic information, the more unpleasant methods (electromyography and/or neurography) have to be used.

Examination of the spinal fluid

Lumbar puncture is an easy and important procedure which should be performed in most children with neurological symptoms and signs. The technique used in the performance of a lumbar puncture in children is the same as in adults; only in small infants may it cause difficulties. In this age-group the distance to the subarachnoid space is short and the ligaments are so thin and soft that the usual snap is not produced when the needle passes the ligament. It is therefore easy to go through the subarachnoid space and enter the venous plexus on the vertebrae and thus cause a traumatic tap. In young infants, therefore, one should use a short needle and enter the subarachnoid space slowly with the needle open in order to avoid too deep an insertion. During the passage of the needle through the skin the stylet *must* be kept in the needle, otherwise small skin fragments may be deposited in the subarachnoid space; the possibility of a connection between lumbar puncture with an open needle and the later development of an epidermoid tumour in the cauda equina has been suggested.

It is dangerous to perform a lumbar puncture in patients with increased intracranial pressure. The optic fundi must therefore be examined before a lumbar puncture, particularly in children old enough to have closed fontanelles and sutures. In younger children, intracranial pressure can be assessed directly from the tension of the fontanelle. In infants with an open fontanelle a lumbar puncture may usually be performed safely, even when the intracranial pressure is raised. The finding of normal fundi does not exclude the possibility of increased intracranial pressure. The history (*see* page 364), the presence of a 'cracked-pot sound' (*see* page 365) and the findings on skull X-ray (*see* page 365) must also be taken into account. It may be permissible in some cases to perform a lumbar puncture when the intracranial pressure is increased, provided the indication is urgent and the tap is performed in close collaboration with a neurosurgeon who is prepared to intervene immediately if complications arise. It may be wise to do a burr-hole before the puncture so that ventricular puncture can be performed rapidly if necessary.

Routine examinations

CELL COUNT

The cell count is the most important examination whenever an inflammatory reaction is suspected. As acute bacterial meningitis (*see* Chapter 16) is a treatable condition, which in young infants produces vague symptoms, lumbar puncture is urgently indicated in all young infants showing poor general condition, feeding difficulties, colour changes, a tense fontanelle, unexplained fever, or convulsions. An increased cell count is also found in viral meningitis, encephalitis, and during the course of spontaneous subarachnoidal bleeding. In healthy newborn infants the cell count may be as high as 15 cells per cubic millimetre, consisting mainly of mononuclear cells. After the age of 2–3 months the upper limit of normal, i.e. $3/mm^3$, is the same as in adults. The presence of up to a few hundred red cells in the spinal fluid of neonates is common and of no significance.

CYTOLOGICAL EXAMINATION

In young infants it may also be of value to perform a cytological examination for the presence of macrophages containing erythrocytes or iron. Erythrophages appear within 24 hours of subarachnoidal bleeding and disappear after about 1 week; at this time iron-containing macrophages may appear and they may remain for a year or more. This examination is also valuable in older children with a clinically suspected cerebrovascular lesion.

PROTEIN CONTENT

The level of protein in the spinal fluid may be increased in meningitis and encephalitis (*see* Chapter 16). An increased protein level and a normal cell count is seen, for example, in Guillain–Barré syndrome (*see* Chapter 6), in the leucodystrophies (*see* Chapter 13), in expansive lesions of the spinal cord causing spinal block (*see* page 372), occasionally in subdural hygromas (*see* page 240), and in intracranial tumours (*see* page 368). The spinal fluid protein is high in the newborn period; the upper limit of normal is 1.0–1.2 g/ℓ in full-term infants and 1.2–1.5 g/ℓ in preterm infants. It decreases rapidly in the following 3–4 months, the upper limit of normal being about 0.2 g/ℓ in the age-group 3–9 months. It then increases slowly and steadily throughout life. In children below 10 years of age the upper limit of normal is approximately 0.3 g/ℓ and in older children and adolescents 0.4 g/ℓ. Also, the relative proportions of albumin and the different globulins, determined by electrophoresis of the protein, vary with age; the percentage of gamma globulin in the total protein follows roughly the age-curve for the total protein content. Electrophoretic examination of the spinal fluid protein is of particular help in the diagnosis of conditions characterized by progressive neurological symptoms and signs (*see* Chapter 13).

GLUCOSE CONTENT

The glucose content of the spinal fluid is decreased in all types of active bacterial meningitis and in other conditions with a greatly increased cell count, particularly when these cells are malignant, such as leukaemic infiltrations of the meninges (*see* page 317). The glucose content is normal in viral meningitis and encephalitis. The normal glucose content in the spinal fluid remains approximately two-thirds of the blood glucose in all ages. If blood glucose is not determined simultaneously with the spinal fluid glucose, the latter value cannot be evaluated.

IDENTIFICATION OF BACTERIA

In proven or suspected cases of bacterial meningitis the bacteria must be identified as quickly and accurately as possible. The bacteria are cultured, when necessary on special medium, and identified. The spinal fluid used for culturing must be kept at a temperature close to 37°C and neither heated nor refrigerated. Several types of bacteria can now be rapidly identified by the use of tests that demonstrate the presence of fluorescent antibodies (FA test).

CHLORIDE CONTENT

Determination of the chloride content of the spinal fluid is of diagnostic help in cases of suspected tuberculous meningitis, as it is low in this condition.

Other methods

Many more methods are available for the examination of spinal fluid. The type of cells present can be accurately identified, which may be helpful in diagnosing a tumour reaching the meninges, meningeal infiltration with leukaemic cells, lipid storage disorders of the central nervous system, or a haemorrhage in the central nervous system. The level of various enzymes, (e.g. transaminases, creatine kinase, lactic dehydrogenase) may be abnormally high in diseases that cause active degeneration of nervous tissue; in such a situation the pattern of lactic dehydrogenase isoenzymes may also be abnormal. The concentration and distribution of various metabolic products in the spinal fluid may be of diagnostic help in hydrocephalus and in metabolic diseases. However, none of these methods has yet become part of the routine examination of spinal fluid.

Other laboratory studies

The normal range for many laboratory examinations varies with age. Only those examinations of significance in neurological diseases will be mentioned here.

Blood sugar determination must be performed simultaneously with a lumbar puncture (*see* page 52) in all children with suspected meningitis. The blood sugar level in the neonatal period is lower than that found later in life, the lower limit for neonates being about one-third to one-quarter of that for older children and adults.

The activity of serum enzymes (transaminases, creatine kinase, aldolase, and lactic dehydrogenase), which should be determined in muscle disease (*see* Chapter 6), is normally higher in small infants than later in life. The normal level of transaminases (ASAT and ALAT) in neonates is approximately three times that of adults; from about 2–3 months of age it falls to within the normal adult range. The normal level of lactic dehydrogenase, creatine kinase, and aldolase in newborn infants is roughly 1.5–3 times that of adults; it decreases rapidly during the first months of life, but children, at least those up to the age of 5, may have normal values only slightly higher than those of adults. Serum phosphorus and alkaline phosphatase levels, which are determined in some children with convulsions (*see* page 106) and when a metabolic disorder complicated by rickets is suspected (*see* page 134), are higher in children than in adults. The normal range of serum phosphorus in children below 8–10 years of age is approximately 50 per cent higher than the adult range, and the serum alkaline phosphatases may, at least in infants and small children, reach a level double that in adulthood.

The normal range of other electrolytes is essentially the same in children and adults. In some of the metabolic disorders described in Chapter 5, the infant must have received food for some time before the metabolic defect can be diagnosed. An infant with galactosaemia will thus show neither clinical symptoms nor urinary excretion of galactose until he has received milk. An infant with phenylketonuria must have received protein for at least 2–4 days before an elevated phenylalanine blood level can be expected. The demonstration of abnormal urinary metabolites in

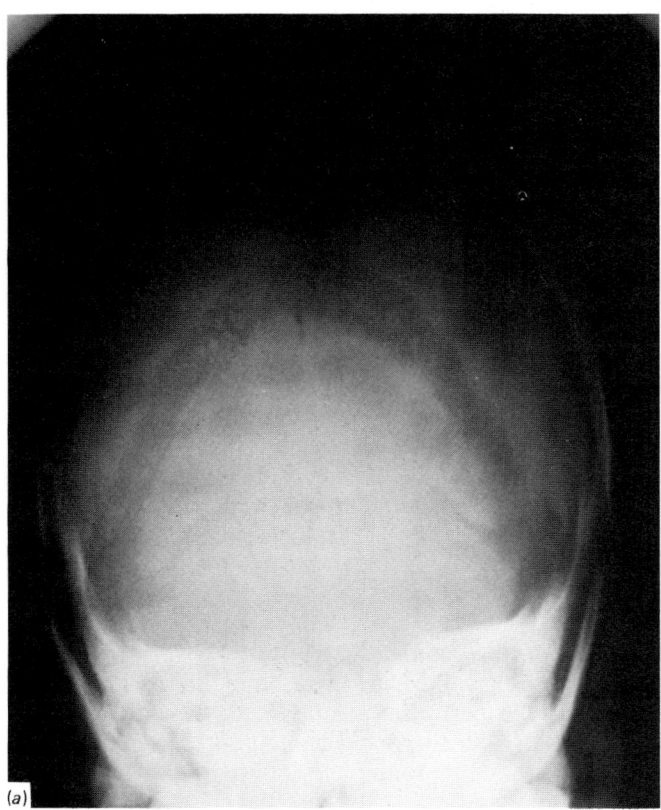

(a)

phenylketonuria takes even longer; a negative Phenistix or negative urinary ferric chloride test does not exclude phenylketonuria in an infant below 2–3 months of age.

Imaging techniques applicable to the neuromuscular system

SKULL X-RAY

Skull X-ray is a simple examination which still has a place in the examination of children with a suspected skull fracture, craniopharyngioma, or craniosynostosis. In an infant with open sutures and fontanelles, intracranial pressure can be better assessed on direct clinical examination than on skull X-ray. In children in whom the fontanelles have closed, skull X-ray is helpful in the demonstration of increased intracranial pressure. This may cause separated sutures (*Figure 3.14*) and a decalcification of the back wall of the sella turcica. A localized thinning of the skull bone may suggest a growing cyst, a subdural hygroma, or a slow-growing brain tumour. The two last-mentioned conditions may also cause irritation and localized thickening of the bone. Premature closure of the sutures may be suspected on clinical grounds (abnormally slow growth of head circumference and/or palpation

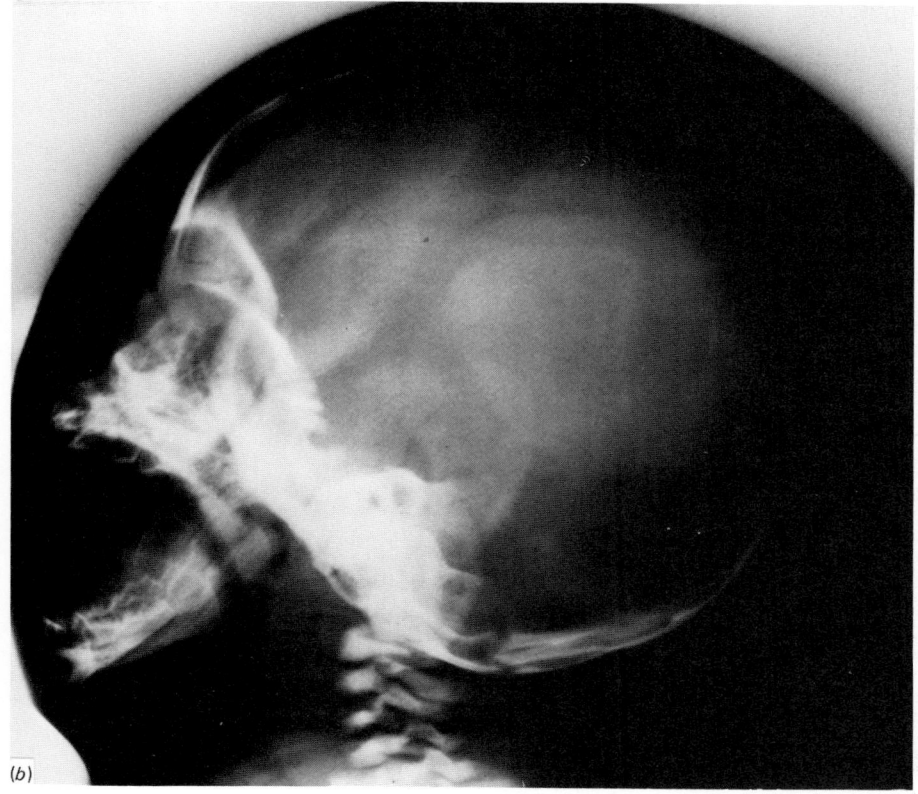

(b)

Figure 3.14. X-ray picture of the skull of a 2-week-old boy with increased intracranial pressure; frontal view (*a*, left) and lateral view (*b*, above). Note the separation of sutures

of sutures and fontanelles closing abnormally early), but should be confirmed on skull X-ray before surgical intervention is considered.

A calcified pineal, localized in the midline, is often found in adults; a displacement of it to one side usually indicates an expansive lesion on one side or an atrophic shrinking process on the other. A calcified pineal is, however, seldom found in healthy individuals before puberty. Minimal calcification in a child above 10 years of age should cause no concern, but a large calcification in a small child is an abnormal finding and suggests a tumour (e.g. teratoma) in the region. Intracranial calcifications in other areas are always an abnormal finding. They are characteristically seen in tuberous sclerosis, Sturge–Weber syndrome, and congenital toxoplasmosis; they may occasionally be found in arteriovenous malformations, hypocalcaemia, and other disorders.

SPINAL X-RAY

X-ray examination of the spine should be performed in all patients with weakness localized to the legs, particularly if this weakness is slowly progressive and combined with sensory disturbances and poor sphincter control. The most important area to examine is the sacrum and the lumbar spine, as malformations, e.g. sacral agenesis, spina bifida (*Figure 3.15*), and diastematomyelia (*see* page

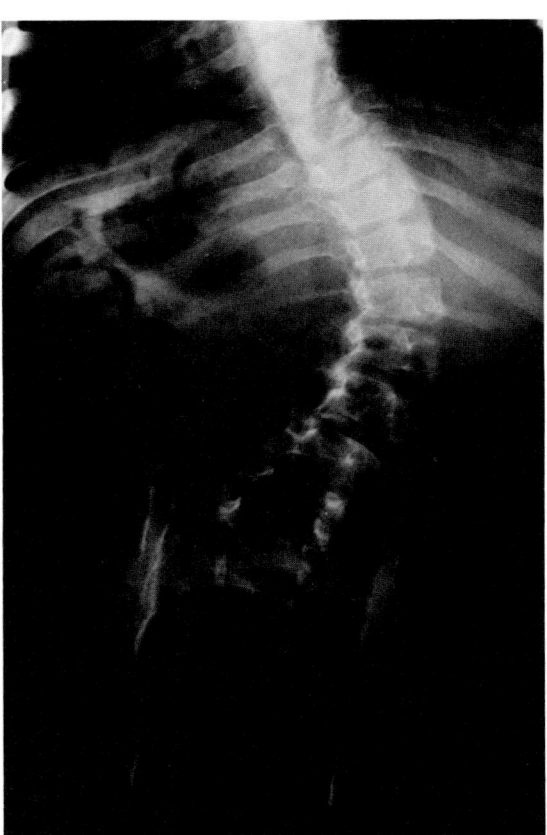

Figure 3.15. X-ray picture of the trunk of a 5-year-old girl with spina bifida cystica

338), are common and may cause stationary or slowly progressive neurological symptoms from the legs and the urinary bladder. An expansively growing lesion may cause the so-called Elsberg's phenomenon, i.e. a widening of the attachment of the vertebral arches on the vertebral bodies at the site of the lesion. A medullary tumour of the same type as seen in adults (*see* page 372) may also occur in children at any level of the spinal cord but is rare. An expansive lesion arising from a primary malformation of the lower part of the spinal cord, e.g. dermoid cysts, lipomyelomeningocele (*see* page 372), is more common in childhood. An expansive lesion may also be an extradural abscess, complicating sepsis or a vertebral infection (*see* page 362), or leukaemic infiltrations; X-ray of the spine may, on these occasions, reveal destruction of one or several vertebrae. If the patient has symptoms from the arms, the cervical spine should be particularly examined for destruction due to infection or malignancy and for malformations of the cervical vertebrae.

SOFT TISSUE X-RAYS

X-ray examination of the soft tissues of the limbs may be useful in the diagnosis of muscle disease (*see* page 165). It may show a decreased muscle mass and an abundant amount of fat in the muscles, proving muscular atrophy; this may be difficult to demonstrate clinically, particularly in young children with a thick fat layer. Intramuscular calcifications are a diagnostic sign which may be helpful in differentiating muscular dystrophy from myositis.

AIR STUDIES

Pneumoencephalography performed via a lumbar puncture or ventriculography performed via a needle inserted in the ventricular system through a burr-hole may only rarely have a place in the examination of a child with a clinical picture that suggests a tumour in the pons or in the hypothalamic region and with no definite findings on ultrasound examination or computerized tomography of the skull (*see* pages 60 and 367).

ARTERIOGRAMS

Carotid and vertebral arteriograms may be needed to complement computerized tomography of the skull if an arteriovenous malformation or an aneurysm is suspected. The technique is the same in children as in adults. As the examination is usually done under general anaesthesia in children, the vessels appear dilated (*Figure 3.16*).

MYELOGRAMS

A contrast study of the spinal cord can be done either with negative contrast, an *air myelogram,* or with positive contrast, an *Amipaque myelogram.* Both are performed through a lumbar puncture. The air myelogram will delineate the cord well all the way up to the foramen magnum but not the nerve roots (*Figure 3.17*); the Amipaque myelogram will give a better picture of cauda equina, conus, and the lower part of the spinal cord (*Figure 3.18*), where most of the abnormalities in childhood are found.

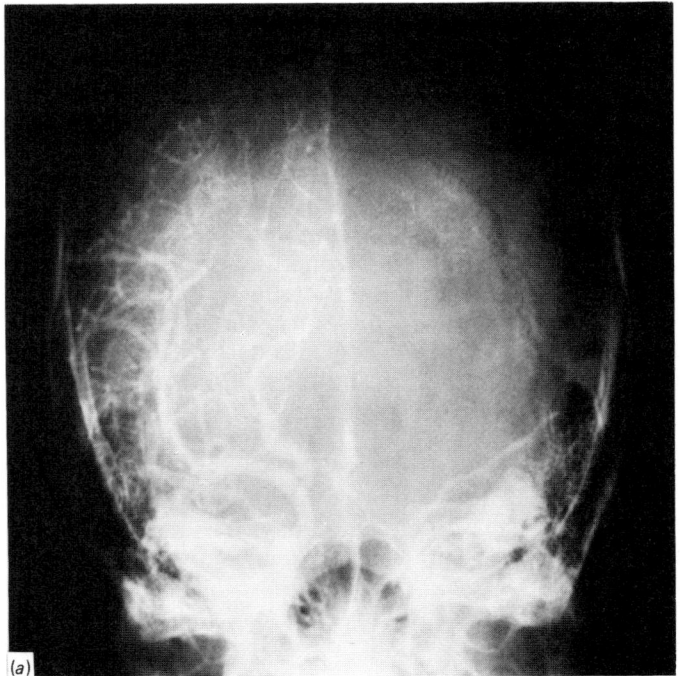

(a)

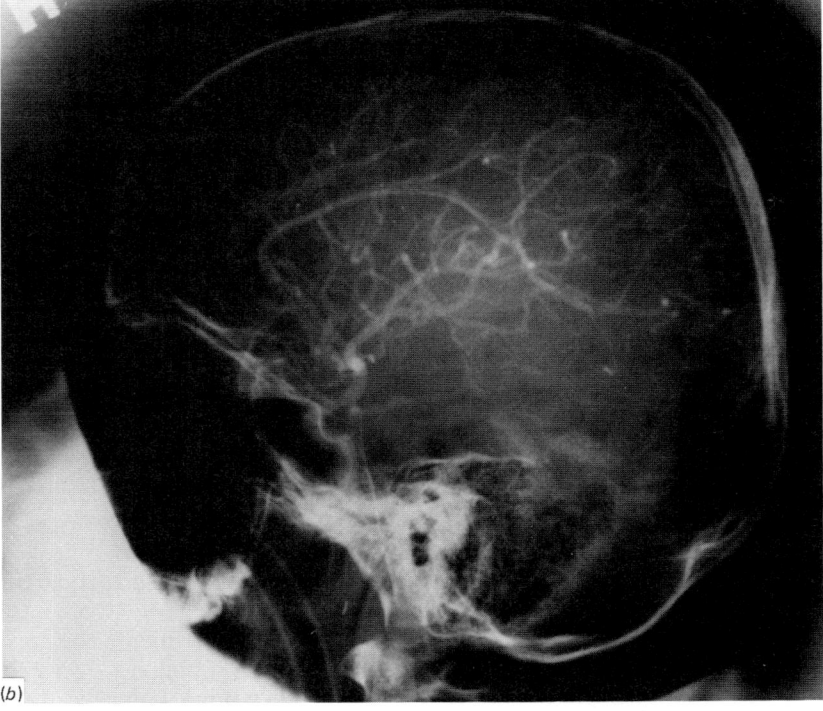

(b)

Figure 3.16. Normal carotid arteriogram from a 13-year-old girl; frontal view (*a*) and lateral view (*b*) (*see* page 57)

COMPUTERIZED TOMOGRAPHY

Cranial computerized tomography was introduced during the 1970s and has rapidly become the most common neuroradiological diagnostic method. The basic principle is to use a narrow collimated X-ray beam, three crystal detectors, and a computer program for analysing the absorption data collected during the scanning procedure; in this way horizontal tomographic sections of the human cranium and

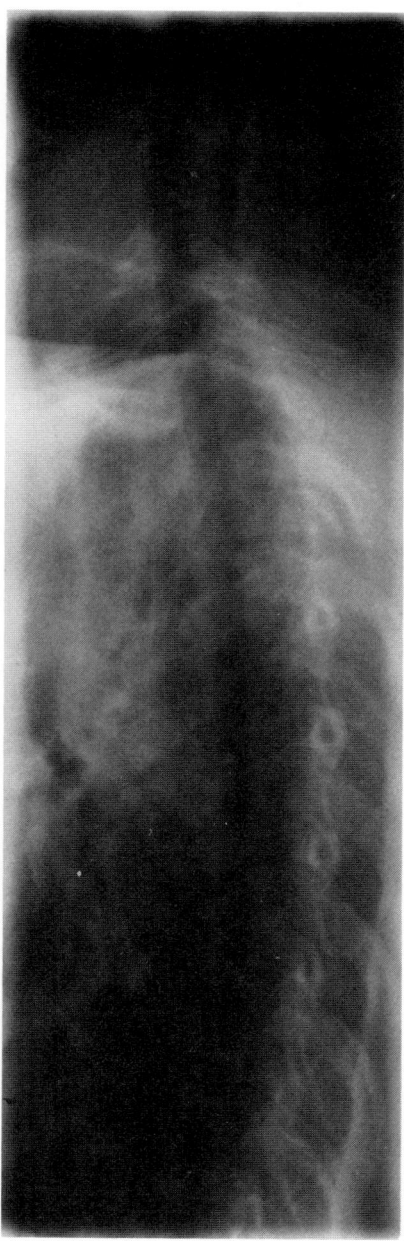

Figure 3.17. Normal air myelogram from a 7-year-old boy

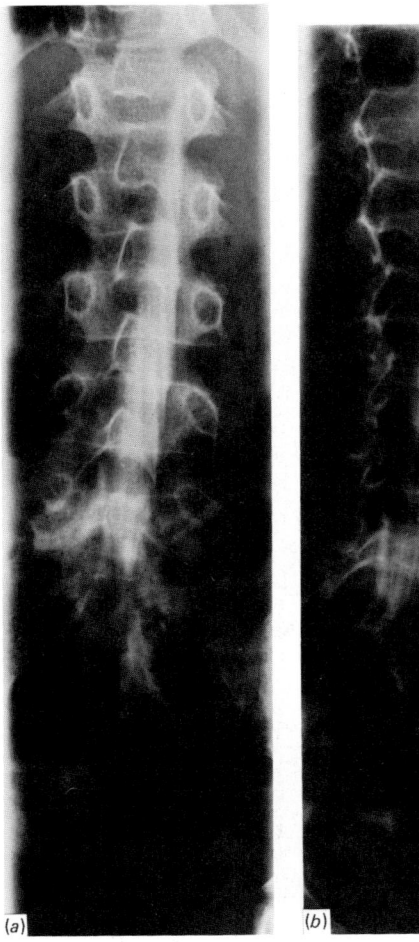

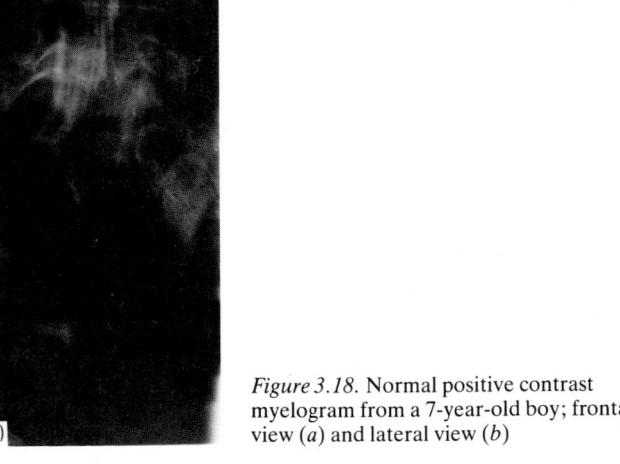

Figure 3.18. Normal positive contrast myelogram from a 7-year-old boy; frontal view (*a*) and lateral view (*b*)

(a)   (b)

its contents are produced. Minimal differences in the radiation absorption of soft tissue can be detected (*Figure 3.19*); thus, in contrast to air studies, oedema of brain tissue, abnormal distribution between grey and white matter, and severe demyelination may also be detected.

A drawback, particularly with the earlier machines, was the time needed for one examination – usually 30–45 minutes – during which complete immobilization of the head was necessary; in small children this could only be achieved by performing the examination under general anaesthesia. With the newer machines the time needed for an examination had been reduced, the thickness of each section has diminished, and sections in the sagittal and frontal planes have also become possible. Thus infants and some young children will require sedation, but only rarely is general anaesthesia necessary. The technical quality has also improved considerably. Intravenous injection of contrast during the examination will enhance the visibility of a tumour, and should be done routinely if this diagnosis is suspected.

The method is useful for diagnosing brain tumours, malformations, brain atrophy, subependymal bleeding (*Figure 3.20*), hydrocephalus, subdural haematoma, intracranial calcifications, and possibly an arteriovenous malformation; in this

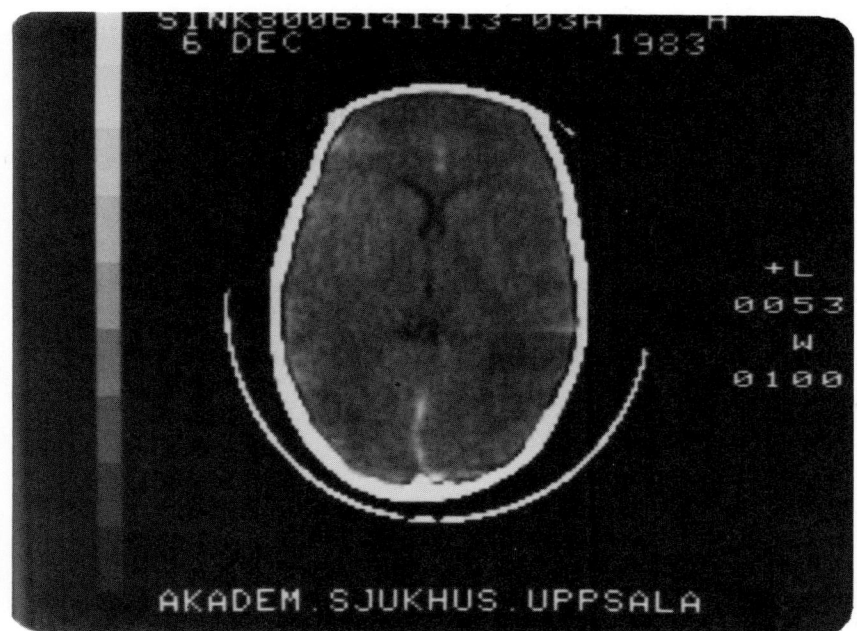

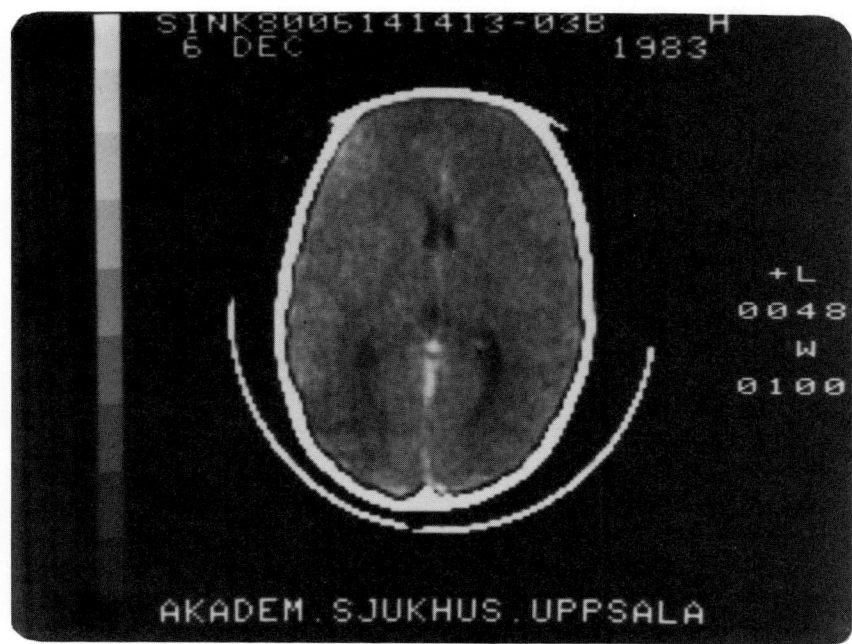

Figure 3.19. Normal computerized tomogram of the skull of a healthy 3-year-old boy

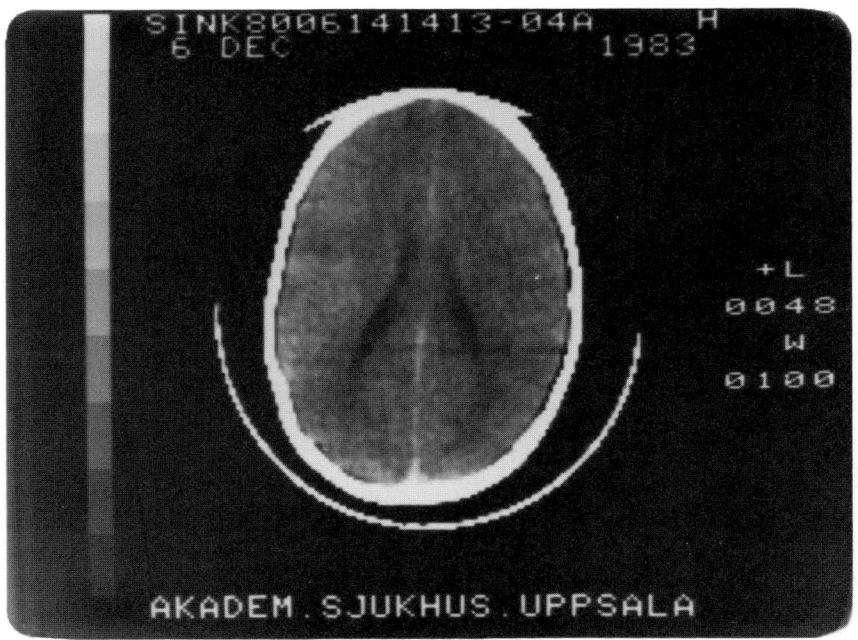

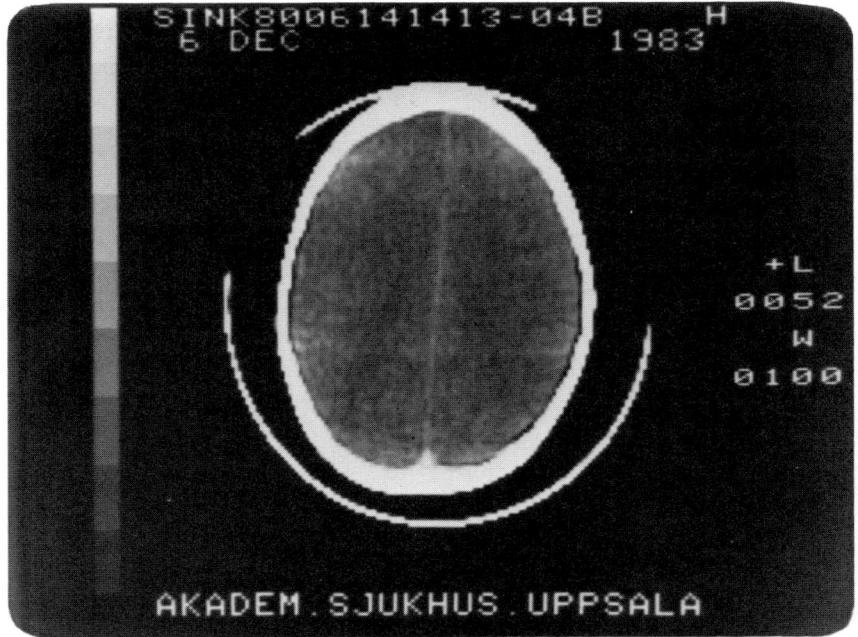

Figure 3.19 (contd)

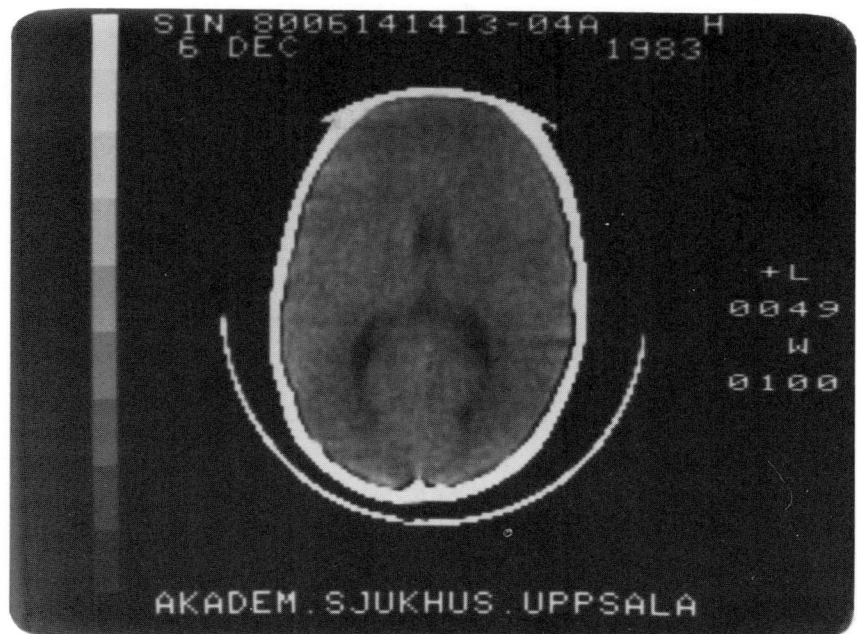

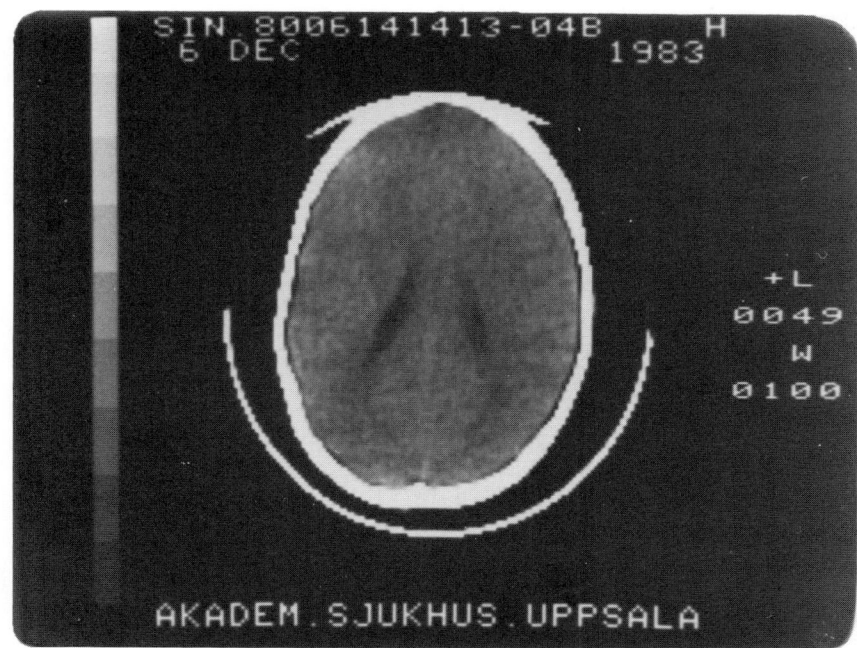

Figure 3.19 (contd)

64

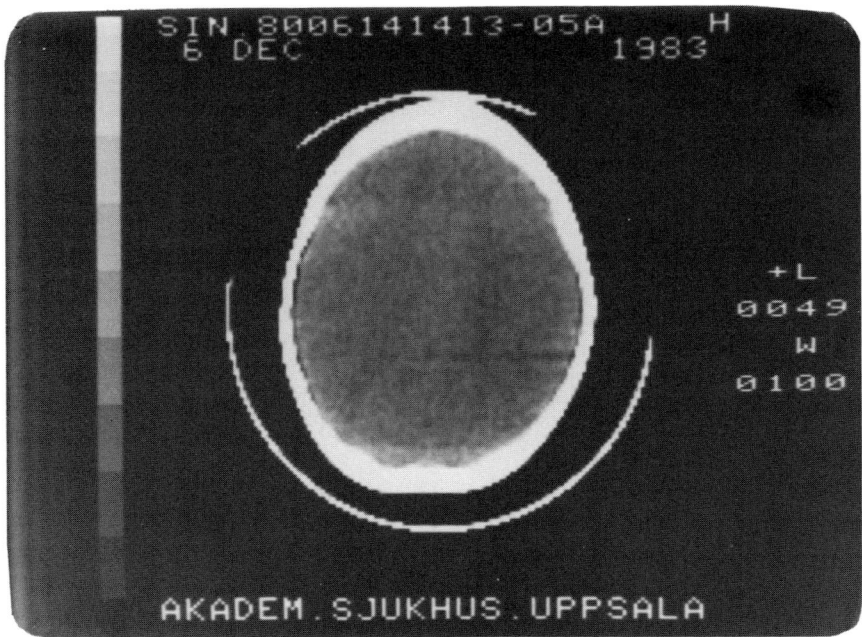

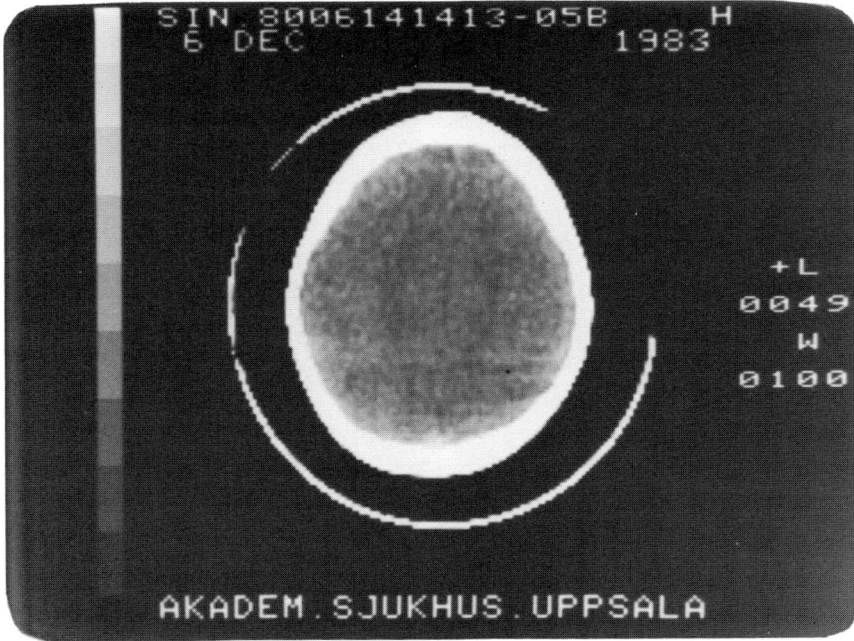

Figure 3.19 (contd)

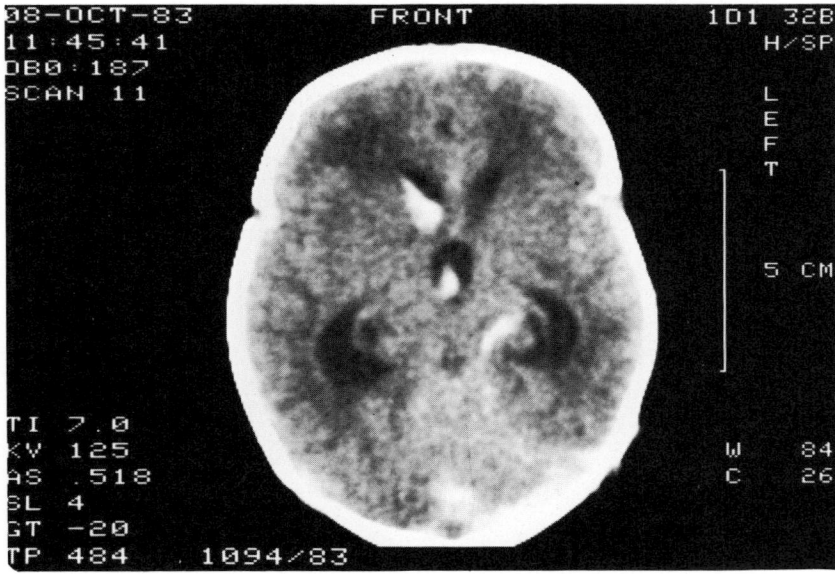

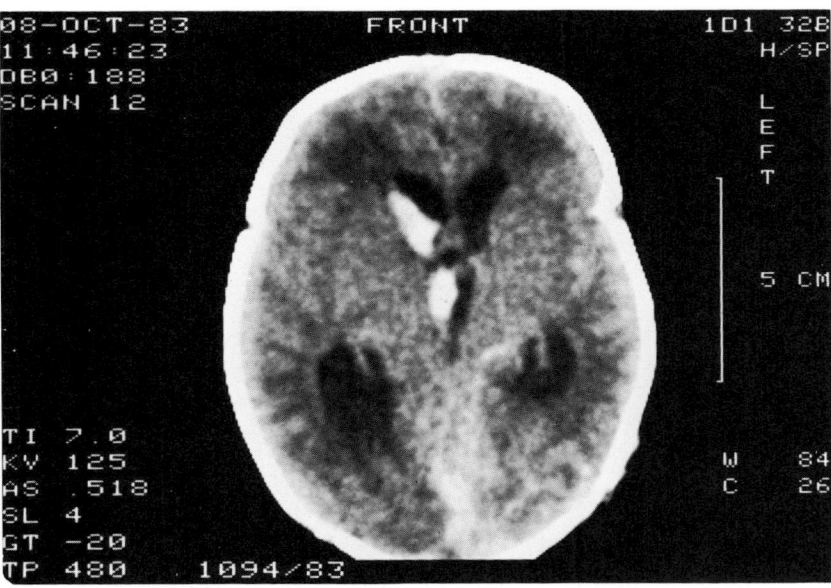

Figure 3.20. Computerized tomogram of the skull of a 1-week-old girl with subependymal bleeding, bleeding in the basal cisterns and around the brain stem, and slightly dilated lateral ventricles

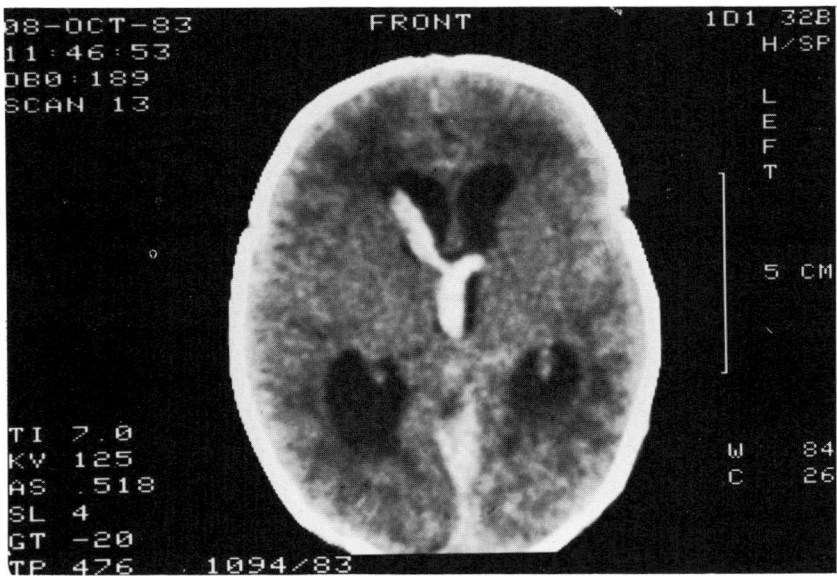

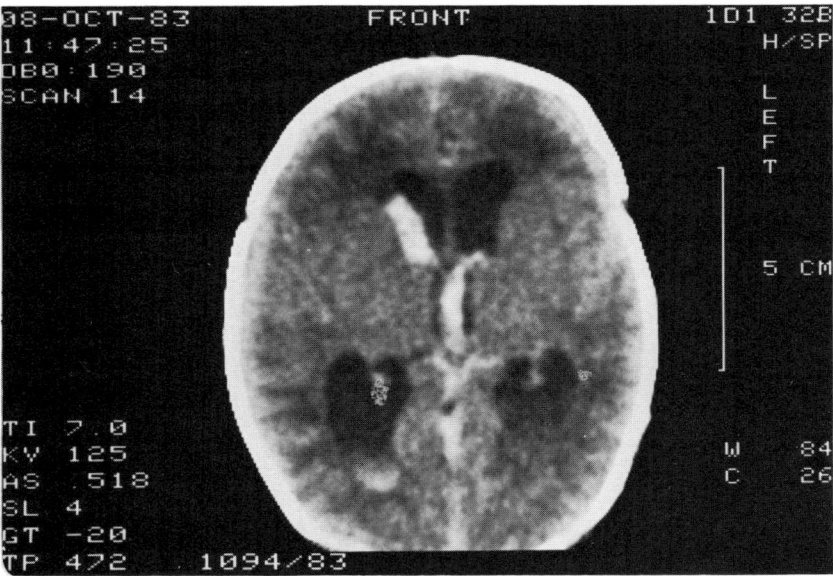

Figure 3.20 (contd)

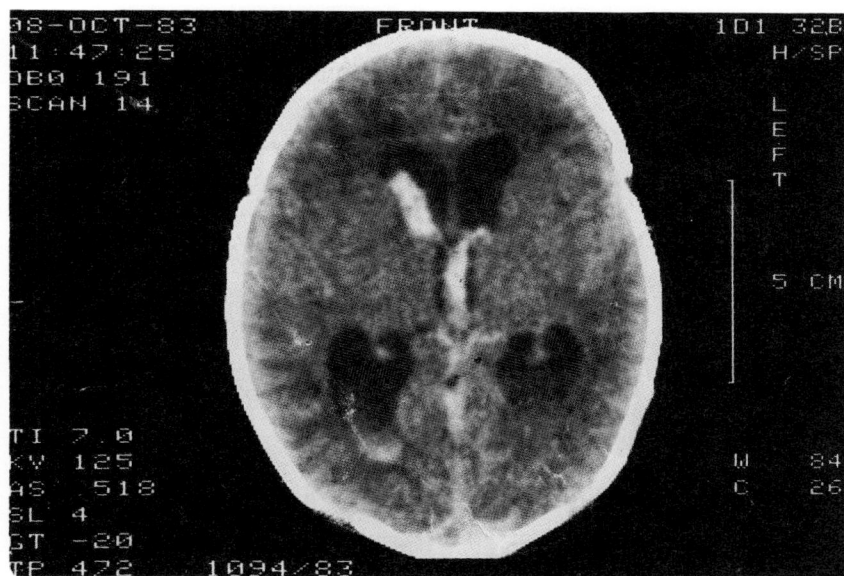

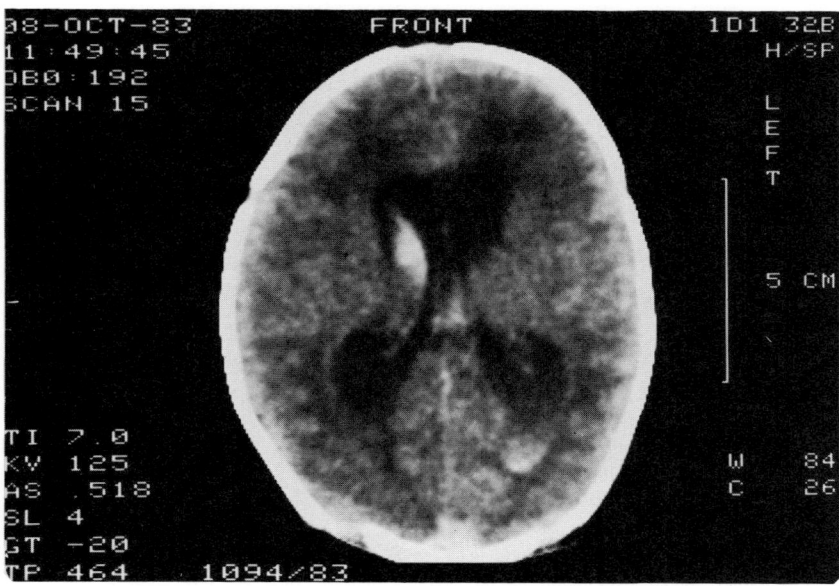

Figure 3.20 (contd)

68

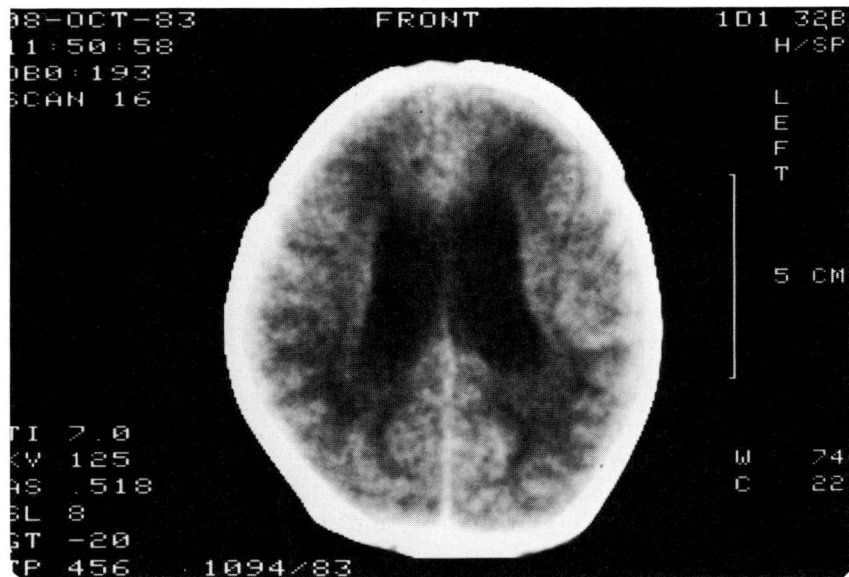

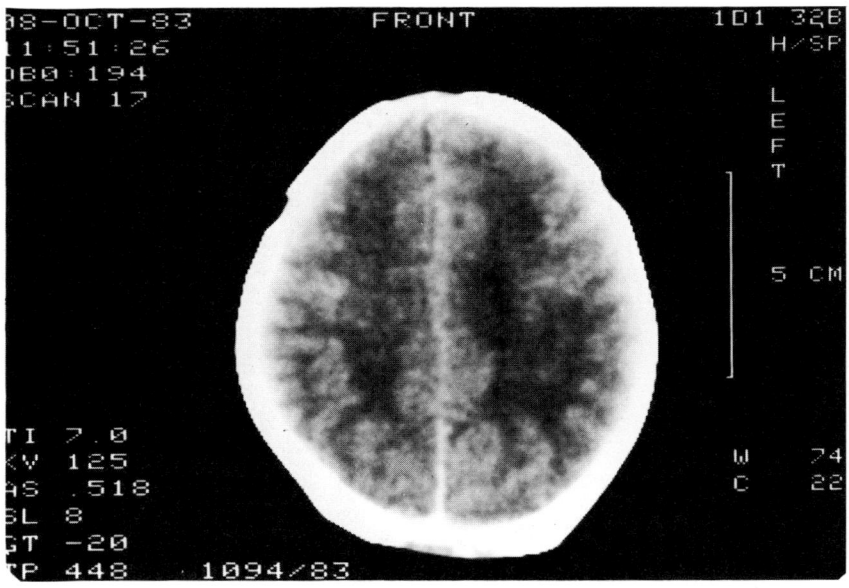

Figure 3.20 (contd)

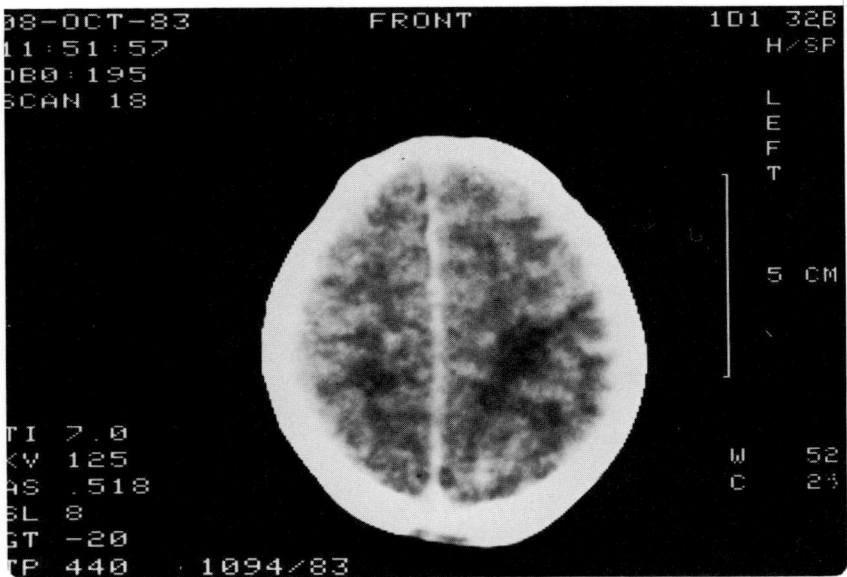

Figure 3.20 (contd)

last situation, however, angiography remains superior. Neither arteriovenous malformation nor tumour can positively be excluded on the basis of a normal computerized tomogram, since both need to reach a definitive size before they can be detected. Besides, the pons and the hypothalamic area are particularly difficult to examine because of disturbances from surrounding bone; a clinical suspicion of a tumour in this region is therefore difficult to dismiss; occasionally a supplementary air study may be necessary and helpful.

Computerized tomography is a technique that can also be applied to other parts of the body. In some situations it is useful for diagnosing tumours and malformations of the spinal cord and cauda equina. The technique is in rapid development and may eventually replace Amipaque and air myelograms in some clinical situations.

Computerized tomography may also be used for the examination of soft tissue. The method allows estimation of the distribution of tissues with varying densities, muscle tissue representing a high density and fat a low density; thus the amount of fat infiltrating a muscle can be evaluated. This method may be helpful in the diagnosis of some muscle diseases and possibly also in the diagnosis of healthy carriers of some of these X-linked disorders.

POSITRON EMISSION TOMOGRAPHY

This can be considered a complement to computerized tomography, providing in addition information on blood flow and metabolism in various parts of the brain. The basic principle is that a tracer, marked with a short-lived radioactive isotope, usually ^{11}C, is injected intravenously and its metabolism followed with the positron camera. The method allows studies of blood flow, blood volume, and protein synthesis in various parts of the brain, the uptake and metabolism of drugs, injuries to the blood–brain barrier, and possibly also the fate of transmitter substances. The method is in rapid development but has not yet become part of routine investigations.

ULTRASOUND SCANNING

Ultrasound scanning of the intracranial structures was originally introduced as the A-scan, which could be performed in one plane only. With this method the midline structures can be defined and a shift to one side is easily detected. In infants and young children with reasonably thin skull bones it is also possible to measure the ventricular size and calculate an index (*see Figure 3.21*). This method still has a place as a rapid screening method for demonstrating increased ventricular size in an infant or midline shift in an older child.

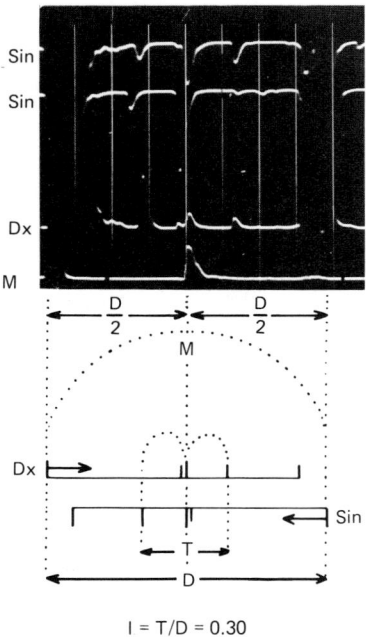

I = T/D = 0.30

Normal newborn baby

Figure 3.21. Echoencephalogram from a healthy newborn infant. The method of calculating the index (I) is also shown

    With modern ultrasound scanning techniques much more information can be obtained. The infantile brain may be examined through the still-open fontanelle with a real-time ultrasound scanner which allows pictures to be taken in two or three planes. With this method the ventricular system can be well delineated (*Figure 3.22*), subependymal, intraventricular, and parenchymal bleeding (*Figure 3.23*) can be demonstrated, and brain malformations can be diagnosed. The recording can be performed in the incubator and on the smallest infant; since it requires no sedation, it is often a better method than computerized tomography in the neonatal period.
    Ultrasound scanning can also be used for the study of other organs. The fetus may be examined through the mother's abdominal wall to estimate its maturation

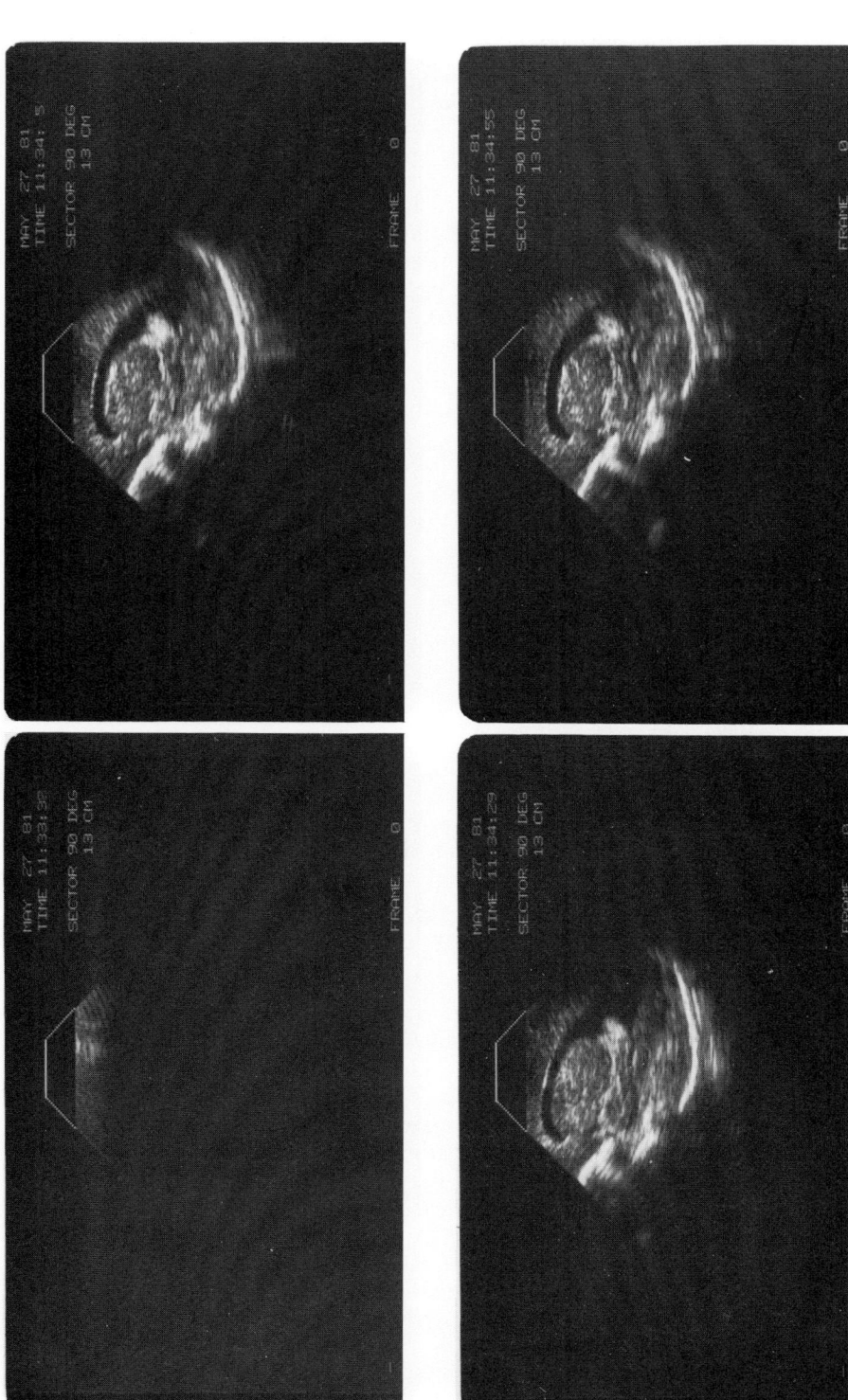

Figure 3.22. Ultrasound examination through the fontanelle of a 1-week-old child showing normal findings

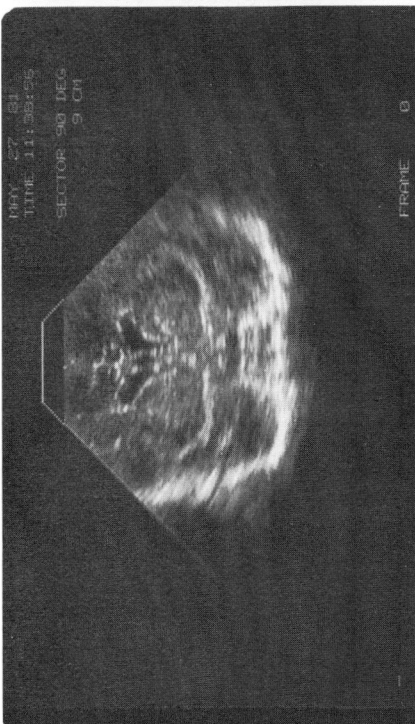

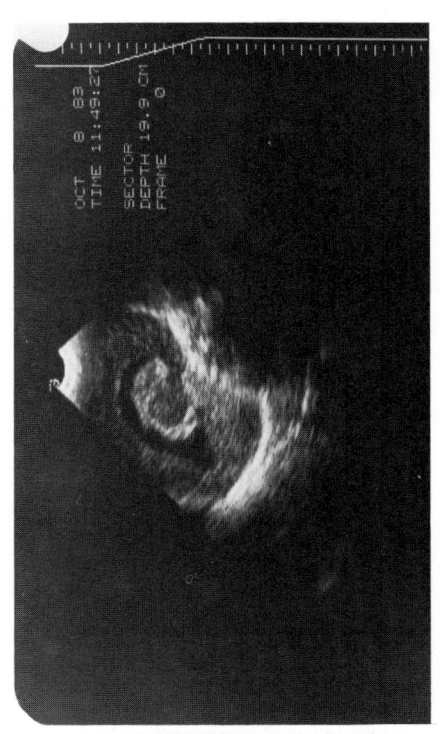

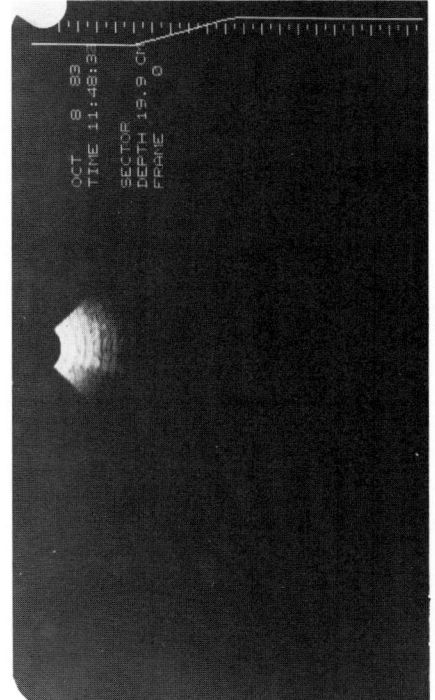

Figure 3.22 (contd)

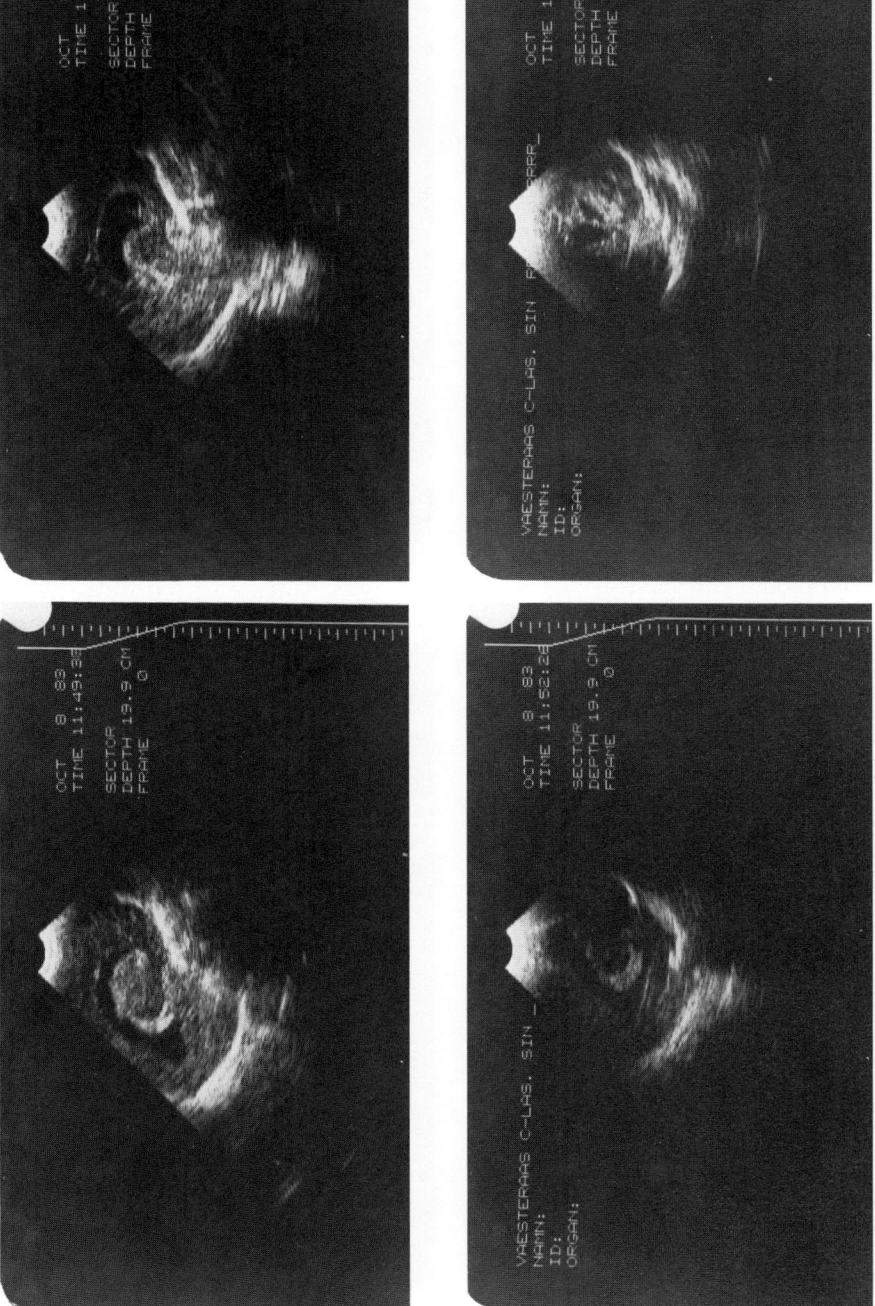

Figure 3.22 (contd)

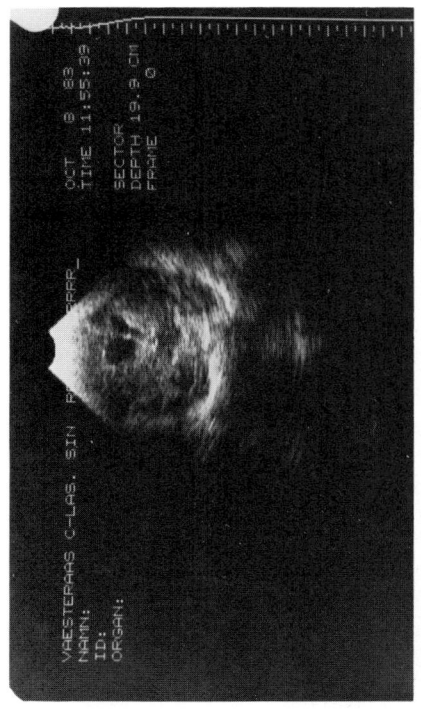
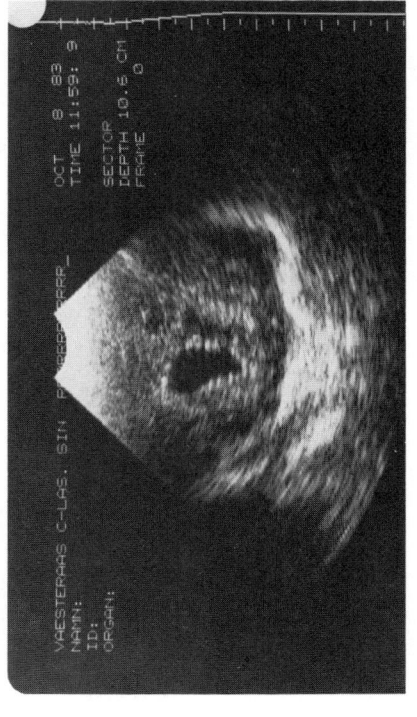
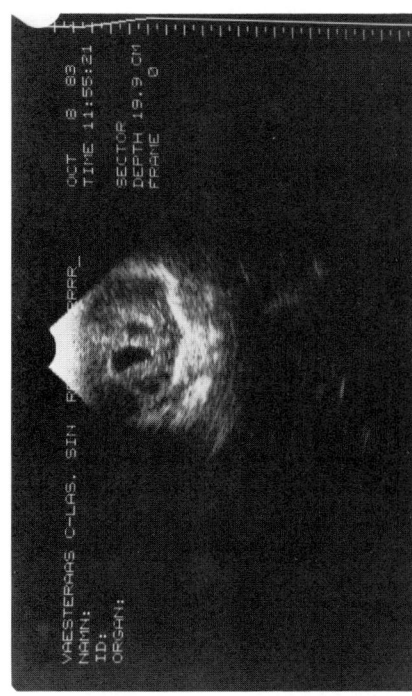
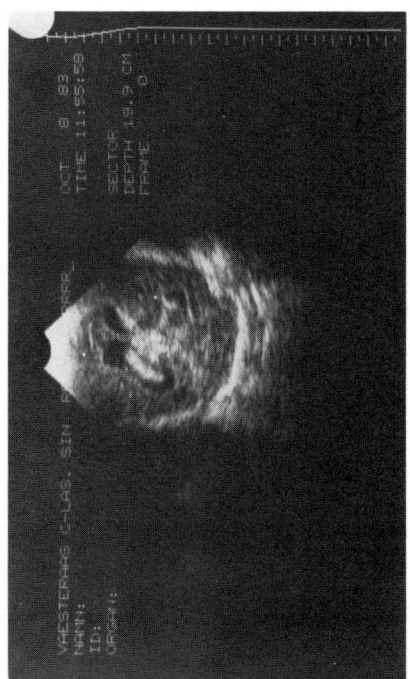

Figure 3.22 (contd)

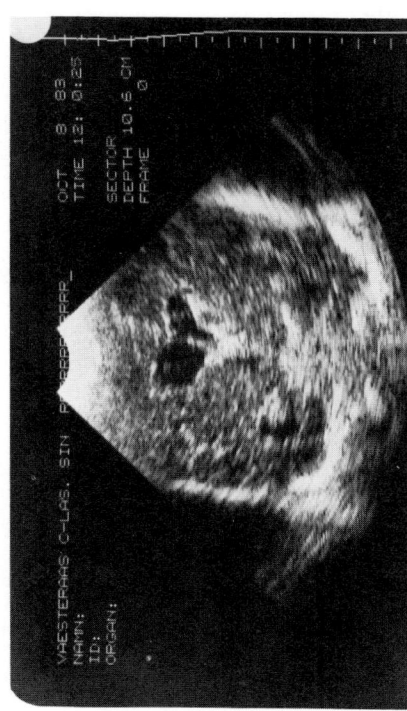

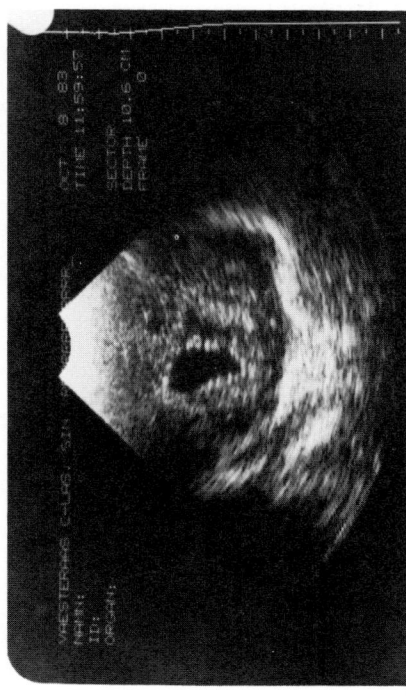

Figure 3.23. Ultrasound examination through the fontanelle of the child with subependymal bleeding whose computerized tomogram is shown in *Figure 3.20*

and to outline its shape and in this way detect malformations, e.g. hydrocephalus and spina bifida aperta (*see* page 334), thus allowing the prenatal diagnosis of these conditions.

The soft tissue of extremities can be examined by ultrasound in order to detect muscular atrophy and abnormalities of gross muscular architecture, which are seen in various muscle disorders (*see* Chapter 6).

NUCLEAR MAGNETIC RESONANCE

This is a new way of picturing various organs of the body, including the central nervous system, without introducing X-rays or isotopes. The method is effective in the investigation of the anatomy of the brain and its metabolism and may in some aspects be superior to computerized tomography. Although this method is undergoing rapid development it is still not a routine medical investigation.

References

BUCHTHAL, F. (1957) *An Introduction to Electromyography*. Copenhagen: Gyldendal

BULCKE, J. A., GROLLA, D., TERMOTE, J.-L., BAERT, A., PALMERS, Y. and VAN DEN BERGH, R. (1981) Computed tomography of muscle. *Muscle & Nerve*, **4**, 67–72

BYDDER, G. M., STEINER, R. E., YOUNG, I. R., HAIL, A. S., THOMAS, D. J., MARSHALL, J. et al. (1982) Clinical NMR imaging of the brain. *American Journal of Nuclear Resonance*, **3**, 459–480

CLAUSSEN, C. D., LOHKAMP, F. W. and V. BAZAN, U. B. (1977) The diagnosis of congenital spinal disorders in computed tomography (CT). *Neuropädiatrie*, **8**, 405–417

CRUMRINE, R. S. and YODLOWSKI, E. H. (1981) Assessment of neuromuscular function in infants. *Anesthesiology*, **54**, 29–32

EEG-OLOFSSON, O. (1970) The development of the electroencephalogram in normal children and adolescents from the age of 1 through 21 years. *Acta Paediatrica Scandinavica*, suppl. 208

GAMSTORP, I. (1963) Normal condition velocity of ulnar, median and peroneal nerves in infancy, childhood and adolescence. *Acta Paediatrica* (Uppsala), suppl. 146, pp. 68–76

GAMSTORP, I. and SHELBURNE JR, S. A. (1965) Peripheral sensory conduction in ulnar and median nerves of normal infants, children and adolescents. *Acta Paediatrica Scandinavica*, **54**, 309–313

HAGNE, I. (1972) Development of the EEG in normal infants during the first year of life. *Acta Paediatrica Scandinavica*, suppl. 232

KAZNER, E., LANKSCH, W. and STEINHOFF, H. (1976) Cranial computerized tomography in the diagnosis of brain disorders in infants and children. *Neuropädiatrie*, **7**, 136–174

PHELPS, M. E., HOFFMAN, E. J., SUNG-CHENG, H. and KUHL, D. E. (1978) A new computerized tomographic imaging system for positron-emitting radiopharmaceuticals. *Journal of Nuclear Medicine*, **19**, 635–647

SITZMANN, F. C. (1968) Kreatinphosphokinase-Aktivität in Serum bei Säuglingen und Kleinkindern. *Zeitschrift für Kinderheilkunde*, **99**, 48–52

STRASSBURG, H.-M., WEBER, S. and SAUER, M. (1981) Diagnosing hydrocephalus in infants by ultrasound sector scanning through the open fontanelles. *Neuropediatrics*, **12**, 254–266

STÅLBERG, E., EKSTEDT, J. and BROMAN, A. (1971) The electromyographic jitter in normal human muscles. *Electroencephalography and Clinical Neurophysiology*, **31**, 429–438

TÖNNIS, D. and FAUPEL, G. (1965) Untersuchungen über das Muskelaktionspotential und das Territorium der motorischen Einheit in den ersten zwei Lebensjahren. *Archiv für orthopädische und Unfall-Chirurgie*, **57**, 339–353

WIDELL, S. (1958) On the cerebrospinal fluid in normal children and in patients with acute abacterial meningo-encephalitis. *Acta Paediatrica* (Uppsala), suppl. 115

4

Convulsions

The management of fits is the main load on any paediatric neurology service, as 7 per cent of all children during their first 7 years have one or more fits, or symptoms which *may* be interpreted as fits and require investigation. In childhood, convulsions are a common symptom with a variable aetiology. The investigation of the child's seizures must proceed along two different and distinct lines to ascertain the answers to the following questions:
1. Which *type* of fit has occurred?
2. What was the *cause* of the fit?

The *type* of fit can be determined through a careful history and direct observation, whenever possible; unfortunately the physician seldom has a chance to see the fit. The type of fit decides to some extent the planning of the diagnostic procedures to determine the cause. The type of fit is the most important factor in the selection of symptomatic anticonvulsant treatment. The aim of the medical investigation, which is indicated in every case of fits in childhood, is to find the cause of the child's convulsions.

Classification according to the type of fit

Generalized grand mal (major generalized epilepsy)

A generalized grand mal attack often starts with some kind of inarticulate sound from the child. The child falls to the ground, if standing or sitting, and becomes stiff – the *tonic* phase of the fit. The eyes usually turn upwards and disappear behind the upper eyelids, leaving only a rim of sclera visible between the half-closed eyelids. The whole body is stiff and stretched at all joints. The jaws are tightly closed; if the inside of the cheek or the tongue is caught between the teeth, the mucous membrane may be injured and bleed. The stiffness also affects the respiratory muscles; respiration stops or becomes severely impaired, and the child usually becomes blue in the face and on the lips. The tonic phase usually lasts for several seconds, and only rarely continues for more than 30 seconds.

It is followed by a *clonic* phase, during which the child has symmetrical jerks in all extremities and in the face, which gives the child a strange grimacing appearance. The jaws move rhythmically, and the chewing on saliva produces foam around the mouth; if the oral mucous membrane has been bitten the foam may become bloody. This all gives the child's face a strange and frightening appearance. During the clonic phase respiration usually starts again but may remain impaired. The clonic phase usually lasts a couple of minutes or less, but can be prolonged which may lead to a dangerous situation, *status epilepticus* (*see* page 109). The jerks gradually abate and the child takes a deep breath with the return of normal colour and appearance. After a grand mal seizure the child usually remains unconscious (unarousable) for a couple of minutes. When he can be aroused, he is tired, usually has a headache, and needs a postictal sleep lasting for at least half an hour.

Occasionally the child will have an *aura* before a grand mal attack. This aura may be some kind of hallucination (for smell, taste, vision, or hearing) or a more diffuse unpleasant feeling. The child may learn to recognize the aura and avoid getting hurt, e.g. by getting off his bicycle, sitting down on the ground, or running to an adult.

Focal grand mal (partial seizures of elementary symptomatology)

An aura, as described above, may be seen in generalized grand mal, but is probably more common in partial seizures, both those of elementary symptomatology and those of complex symptomatology (*see* page 85). In a partial seizure of elementary symptomatology the tonic phase is often absent and the fit starts with jerks in one part of the body, e.g. one side of the face or one hand. The jerks may involve only the area in which they start, or they may progress in a regular way, being repeated stereotypically at every new attack, from face to hand and arm, to foot and leg, and then to the other side, until finally the patient becomes unconscious; this is a description of a Jacksonian attack. A true Jacksonian attack is a rare condition which is always caused by an organic brain lesion. Even rarer is a sensory Jacksonian attack, i.e. paraesthesia moving in the same regular way as described for a motor attack. Occasionally it may be difficult to differentiate a sensory Jacksonian seizure from migraine (*see* page 232). In all types of focal fits involuntary eye movements may also occur so that the eyes and perhaps also the head are turned to one side and fixed there. The child may be conscious and notice the eye and head movements but be unable to resist them. These are called *adhesive movements* or *searching movements*. Rarely, they may be so pronounced that the child is turned round in a circle.

A special type of partial seizure with elementary symptomatology seems to represent a common and benign problem in childhood. This type has several names: it is often called *benign epilepsy of childhood with centrotemporal EEG foci* (or *Rolandic spikes*). Its background is often genetic, as a positive family history is reported in about 40 per cent of cases and typical EEG abnormalities may be found in symptom-free relatives. It always has its onset in childhood (excluding the first year of life), with a maximum age of onset between 5 and 10 years. The attacks usually occur at night, within the first hour after the child has fallen asleep. The attacks may start with a sound from the child which draws his parents' attention to him. At this point the child's face is seen to be twitching, and his hand and perhaps also a foot may also be jerking. The fits are often one-sided, but may also spread to the other side. The whole attack is usually short, perhaps lasting for a couple of minutes or less. When the attack abates the child may wake up, unaware of what has happened, and then go back to normal sleep. This type of epilepsy is associated with typical EEG findings (*see below*), has no organic background, and carries a good prognosis.

Most focal attacks, particularly a Jacksonian attack, should in an older child or adult raise a suspicion of a neurosurgically treatable condition such as a tumour, cyst, or arteriovenous malformation. In younger children (below 3–4 years of age) focal attacks may be due to generalized conditions and neuroradiological examination is less urgent. A clinical and electroencephalographic picture fitting benign epilepsy of childhood is not an indication for neuroradiological investigation.

EEG FINDINGS, CAUSE AND PROGNOSIS

The usual EEG pattern in grand mal seizures consists of spikes and sharp waves which may be generalized or focal. *Figure 4.1a* shows the initial focal phase on an EEG recorded at the onset of a Jacksonian attack, *Figure 4.1b* the unilateral extension of the abnormality, and *Figure 4.1c* the unilateral exhaustion after the attack. The abnormality may be provoked by hyperventilation, drowsiness, or an intermittently flickering light. The typical EEG findings of benign epilepsy of childhood are spikes recorded from one or both Rolandic areas, or adjacent areas, occurring against a *completely normal background* (*Figure 4.2*). The absence of slowing of the background activity is a necessary diagnostic feature, since slowing of the background activity in the same area as the spikes indicates an *organic brain lesion* in need of neuroradiological investigation.

The cause of grand mal seizures varies (*see* pages 92–105); in many cases no cause can be established. The prognosis is also variable; as a rule, however, grand mal seizures with an onset in childhood have an excellent prognosis.

The characteristic symptoms and signs of the kinds of fits that are *not* grand mal are briefly summarized in *Table 4.1* and described in detail below.

Petit mal (primary generalized epilepsy)

This type of fit has its onset in childhood with the peak age of onset between 5 and 9 years. It never starts below 2 years of age. Short attacks starting in children under 2 years of age are never petit mal and are usually more malignant than petit mal. The duration of an attack is usually 5–15 seconds and never more than 30 seconds. The frequency of attacks is high; many, possibly several hundred, a day are usually observed. The typical clinical picture is simply an attack of absence: the patient is out of contact with his surroundings, staring vacantly in front of him (*Figure 4.3*), and doing virtually nothing. All activity, including talking, is thus suddenly cut off and resumed after the attack. The only activity that may occasionally be seen is jerking of the eyelids with a frequency of 3/s. The patient does not fall during a petit mal attack.

EEG FINDINGS, CAUSE AND PROGNOSIS

The typical EEG finding is 3/s spike-wave activity, starting synchronously over all channels on both sides, usually against a normal background (*Figure 4.4*). This classic pattern has the best prognosis and the best response to petit mal drugs (*see* page 117). If each wave is preceded by multiple spikes, the risk of grand mal is increased, and if the frequency is 2–2.5/s or lower, there is a risk that the patient may develop a therapy-resistant epilepsy with various types of short attacks and perhaps also impaired mental function. The 3/s spike–wave pattern occurs

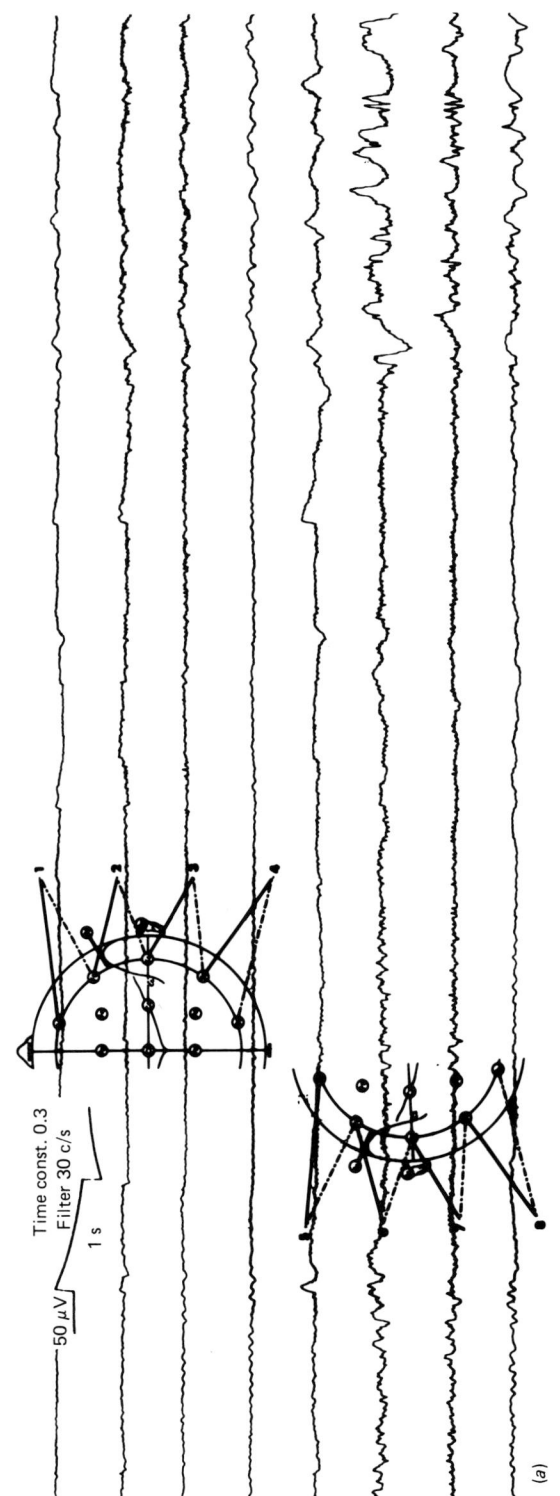

Figure 4.1. The onset (*a*), development (*b*), and after-effect (*c*) of a Jacksonian epileptic attack, recorded electroencephalographically in a 13-year-old boy. The placement of the electrodes is the same in all three pictures

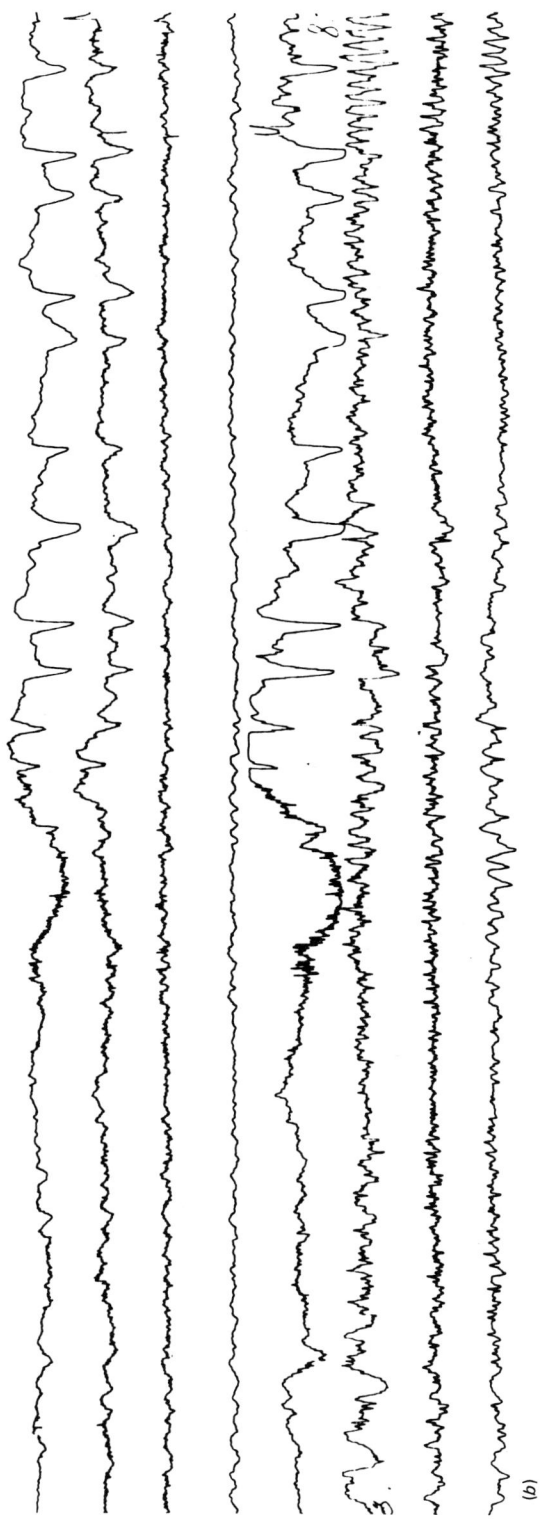

Figure 4.1 (contd)

(b)

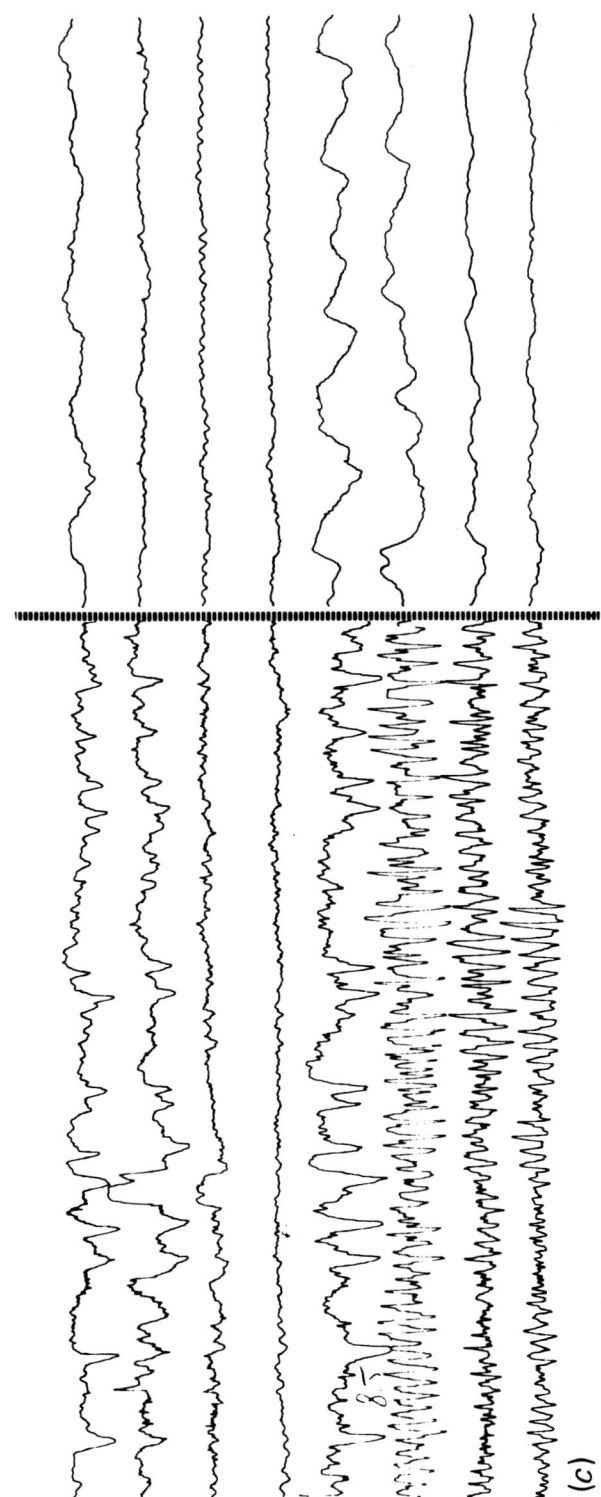

(c)

Figure 4.1 (contd)

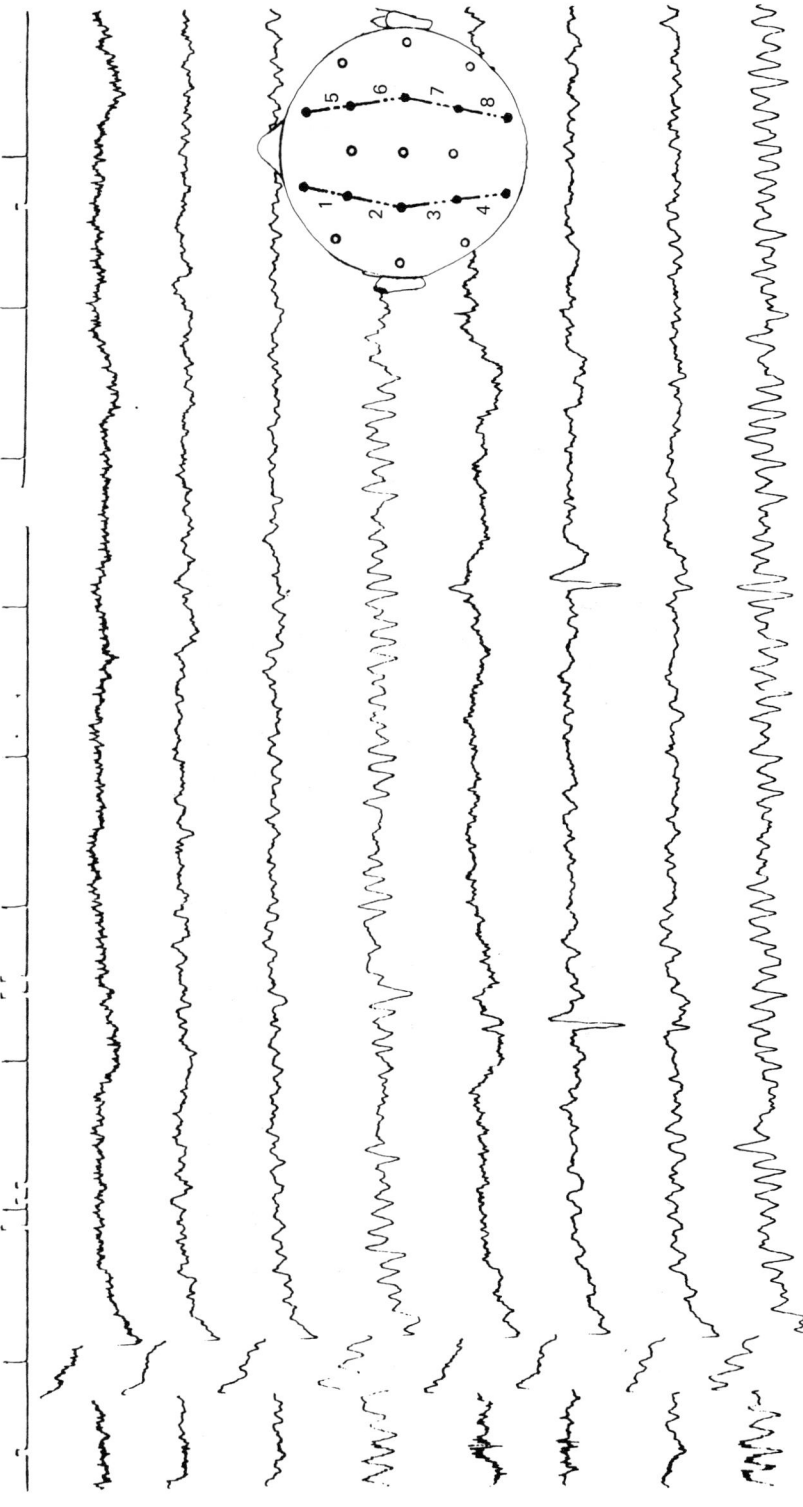

Figure 4.2. Rolandic spikes in a 10-year-old boy with benign epilepsy of childhood. Note the focal spikes occurring against a normal background

TABLE 4.1. Characteristic features of short fits in infancy and childhood

	Petit mal	Psychomotor attacks	Minor motor seizures
Age at onset	Childhood above 2 years of age	Any age	Under 2 years of age
Usual clinical picture	True absences, lapses of consciousness with no activity, except possibly twitching of the eyelids 3/s	Only a lapse of consciousness may occur, but motor activity is the rule. Movements in the oral area: licking, smacking, and swallowing are common. Seemingly purposeful activity, completely uncalled for in the situation, may occur	Abrupt attacks of flexion spasms, nodding spasms, salaam spasms, akinetic spells, massive myoclonic jerks
Frequency	Many a day, occasionally many hundred a day	Variable, from a few a month to many hundred a day	Usually many a day
Duration	Usually a few seconds, never more than 30 seconds	Variable, from a few seconds to hours or days	Usually a few seconds, seldom more than 1 minute
Usual EEG findings	3/s spike–wave pattern starting simultaneously over all channels against a normal background	Temporal lobe focus	Hypsarrhythmia
Method of provoking attacks and typical EEG findings	Hyperventilation	Drowsiness, light sleep	Intermittently flickering light
Effect of petit mal drugs	Good	Usually none	Usually none
Prognosis	Generally good	Variable	Generally poor

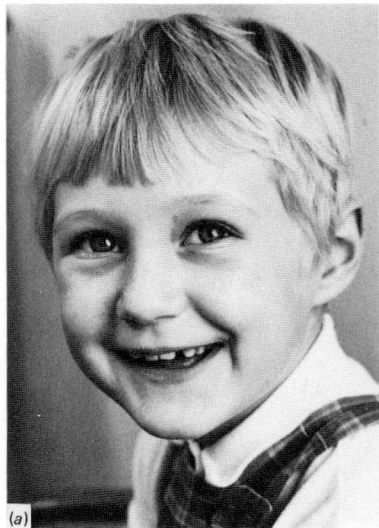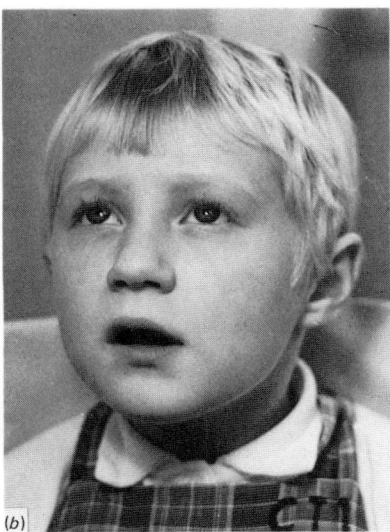

(a)   (b)

Figure 4.3. Petit mal in a 7-year-old girl, before (*a*) and during (*b*) the attack which was provoked by hyperventilation

spontaneously as a rule; it may be provoked by hyperventilation, which may also bring on a clinical attack. If the history suggests petit mal, hyperventilation for 3 minutes should be included in the physical examination, as this may allow the examiner to observe an attack, thus establishing the diagnosis clinically.

Petit mal is usually assumed to originate in the midline structures of the brain stem; a focal brain lesion is not found. The cause of petit mal is unknown. A cerebral reaction to a metabolic disorder is one plausible theory, but nothing has so far been proven.

True petit mal, as defined here, usually responds to petit mal drugs and usually has a good prognosis, at least with regard to mental development and social adaptation. Generalized grand mal and petit mal may occur in the same patient. Grand mal may start when the short attacks are brought under control through petit mal drugs.

Temporal lobe epilepsy (partial seizures of complex symptomatology), also called psychomotor attacks

Although it may be difficult to establish a firm diagnosis in young children, psychomotor attacks or temporal lobe epilepsy may start at any age. The usual duration of an attack is a few minutes but can vary from a few seconds to several hours. The usual frequency is at least several attacks a month, although many patients have several short attacks daily. Spontaneous variation is common, as periods with daily attacks may be followed by attack-free intervals lasting for weeks or months.

The clinical picture varies considerably. The attack may consist of a short period of absence during which the patient stares vacantly and does virtually nothing; the duration of such a period may be less than 30 seconds, in which case the attack cannot be distinguished clinically from a petit mal seizure. It is, however, more

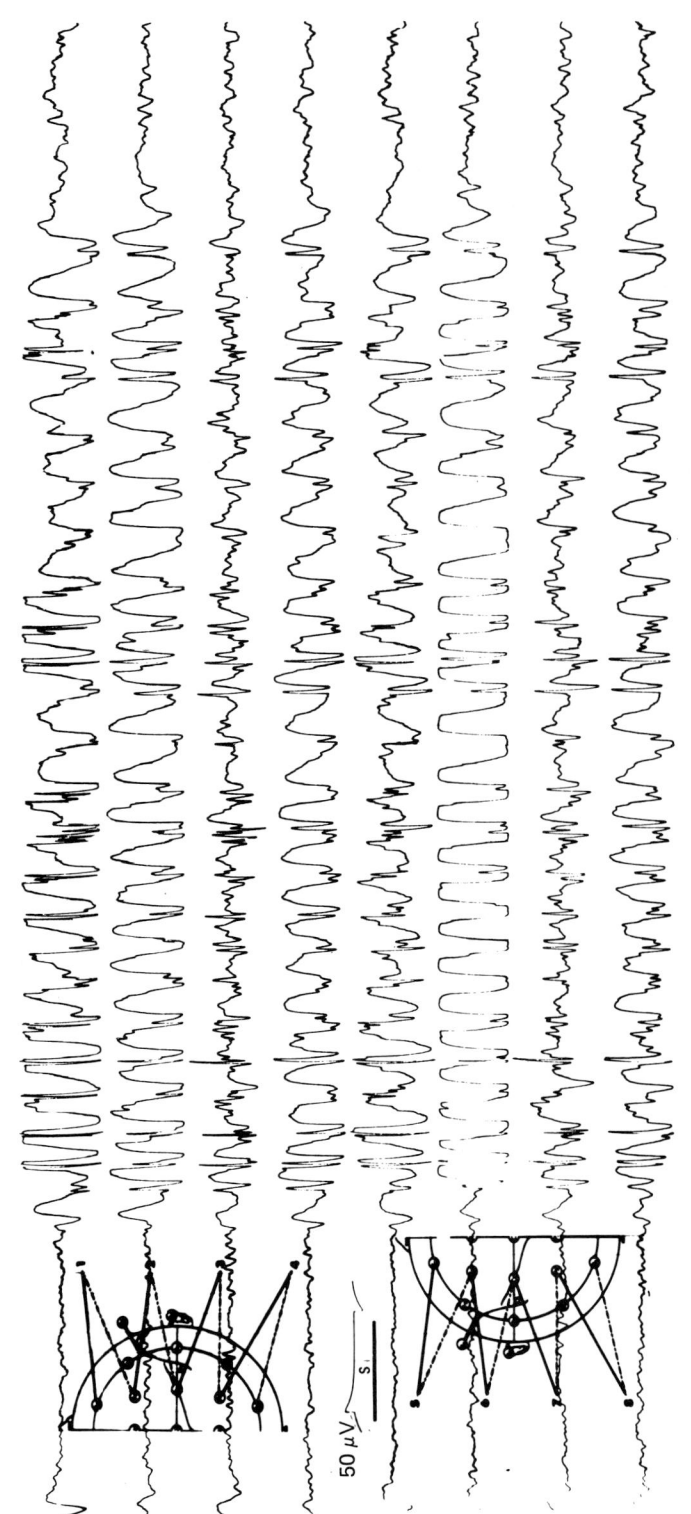

Figure 4.4. EEG recorded in a 13-year-old girl with petit mal

50 μV

S₁

common for the duration to be longer and for the patient to be in some way active during the attack. The activity may consist of movements in one part of the body, such as stretching out an arm or turning the head and eyes towards one side. Movements in the oral area such as grimacing, licking, lip smacking, swallowing, and other movements of the tongue are particularly common. The patient may also perform a series of complicated movements such as getting up and running to and fro on the floor, or picking up things and turning them round – movements which may appear purposeful but are completely uncalled for in the situation. This type of attack may also occur at night, and the patient may be found walking in his sleep.

Sudden spells of peculiar behaviour, e.g. uncontrollable laughter, may be psychomotor attacks. During an attack the patient is usually unable to answer questions but he is seldom completely unaware of what is happening, he does not fall, and as a rule he remembers what he has experienced, what he has been doing, and frequently the reactions of those around him. It is typical for an attack of temporal lobe epilepsy to start abruptly; it may end abruptly but can also abate gradually. The common denominator in fits of temporal lobe epilepsy is a sudden and completely unprovoked change in the child's mood and behaviour. To the child, a correct diagnosis means that he is relieved of responsibility for bad behaviour that he cannot control; also, pharmacological treatment may be available to resolve the situation (*see* page 117).

As is apparent from the name, a psychomotor attack also contains a psychic component, i.e. a subjective experience. This may be a hallucination: the patient may see, hear, smell, or taste something that does not exist. Most of these hallucinations are vague and the patient cannot describe any details. Only rarely are the hallucinations distinct: the patient may report that he hears voices and also what they say; visual hallucinations, may be vivid pictures. Occasionally the patient is indifferent to his hallucinations, but usually they are intensely unpleasant and often alarming to him. Several patients describe their experience as 'a lump coming from the belly up through the chest and clutching at the throat and giving a feeling of suffocation and intense indefinable horror'. A vague feeling of alarm, without hallucinations, may also constitute the psychic component of a psychomotor attack. These attacks may occur at night: the child suddenly starts to scream, is apparently in panic, and cannot be roused for a while; such attacks may be combined with sleep-walking. A child may find it difficult to describe what he has felt during an attack. It often takes patient and understanding questioning to get the child to verbalize his experience.

Vegetative symptoms are often part of a psychomotor attack. The patient may develop vertigo, nausea, headache, or bellyache before or during the attack. He may suddenly turn red or pale, perspire, or have tachycardia or increased salivation.

Temporal lobe epilepsy may also manifest itself as longer attacks of vegetative symptoms without disturbed consciousness. Thus, an occasional patient with attacks of migraine-like headache, unexplained bellyache, or unexplained fever may have a temporal lobe focus (often appearing only when the EEG record is obtained during drowsiness and light sleep, *see* page 41) and may respond favourably to drugs used for grand mal or psychomotor epilepsy (*see* page 117). These symptoms are often called *epileptic equivalents*.

Psychomotor attacks may occur as the only manifestation of epilepsy. However, in many patients they are combined with grand mal, generalized or focal. If so, psychomotor attacks may either alternate with grand mal or occur as the aura of grand mal. Treatment with grand mal drugs may then abolish the large attacks and leave the patient with the aura as isolated psychomotor attacks.

Many though not all children with psychomotor epilepsy also have mental symptoms between the attacks, e.g. short attention span, lack of concentration, or hot temper. If the fits are overlooked, the patient may be misjudged as a spoilt, difficult, ill-behaved child. These mental symptoms may be due to the localization of the brain injury causing the psychomotor attacks, and are probably aggravated by the unpleasantness the child experiences during the fits and his fear of them.

EEG FINDINGS, CAUSE AND PROGNOSIS

Common EEG findings in psychomotor epilepsy are focal temporal lobe abnormalities (*Figure 4.5*). These abnormalities, as well as the attacks, are usually provoked by drowsiness and light sleep. *Every EEG in a child must therefore include a record obtained during sleep.* Such a record may be obtained by giving the child a sleeping pill or, preferably, by keeping him awake for half of the night before the EEG is to be recorded; in this way the possibility of the EEG being influenced by a drug is avoided. Various other types of EEG abnormalities may also be recorded in temporal lobe epilepsy. The EEG abnormalities in young children (4 years of age or younger) are often bilateral and nonspecific, or possibly focal with localization to the occipital lobe. During maturation they tend to move forward and some years later may be fixed in the anterior part of the temporal lobe. A normal EEG does not exclude temporal lobe epilepsy, as the lesion may have a localization in the temporal lobe such that it cannot be recorded through ordinary scalp electrodes.

A glial scar in the temporal lobe is the usual cause of temporal lobe epilepsy. In many cases the likely explanation for this scar is a perinatal brain injury; in some cases trauma or encephalitis may be the cause. A genetic background has been suggested in some families.

The abnormal behaviour in temporal lobe epilepsy may respond to adequate antiepileptic treatment. Both the psychomotor fits and the mental symptoms may be difficult to treat, and the prognosis concerning social adaptation varies.

Minor motor seizures

Minor motor seizures start in infancy, usually during the first year of life, only rarely after the second. These attacks have many names: a few of them, describing the type of fit, will be mentioned here. In a young infant lying on his back, the attack may be a massive flexor movement, called *flexion spasm*. If the infant is sitting up, he may suddenly lose muscle tone and head control; this is termed *nodding spasm*. If the child is walking the abrupt loss of tone may make him fall suddenly forward in a position mimicking a salaam greeting, *salaam spasm,* or in a limp heap on the floor, *akinetic spell.* The attack may also have the character of *massive myoclonic jerks.* A complete list of all the names used for this type of attack would contain several hundred names. Here, the term minor motor seizures will be used for all of them.

The attacks have an abrupt onset and the sitting or standing child may fall with no opportunity to protect himself with his hands. Each fit may last for only a few seconds, and seldom for more than 1 minute. After the fit the child regains consciousness immediately and seems not to need postictal sleep. The jerks may come in series, each jerk lasting for a second or less and the whole series containing

89

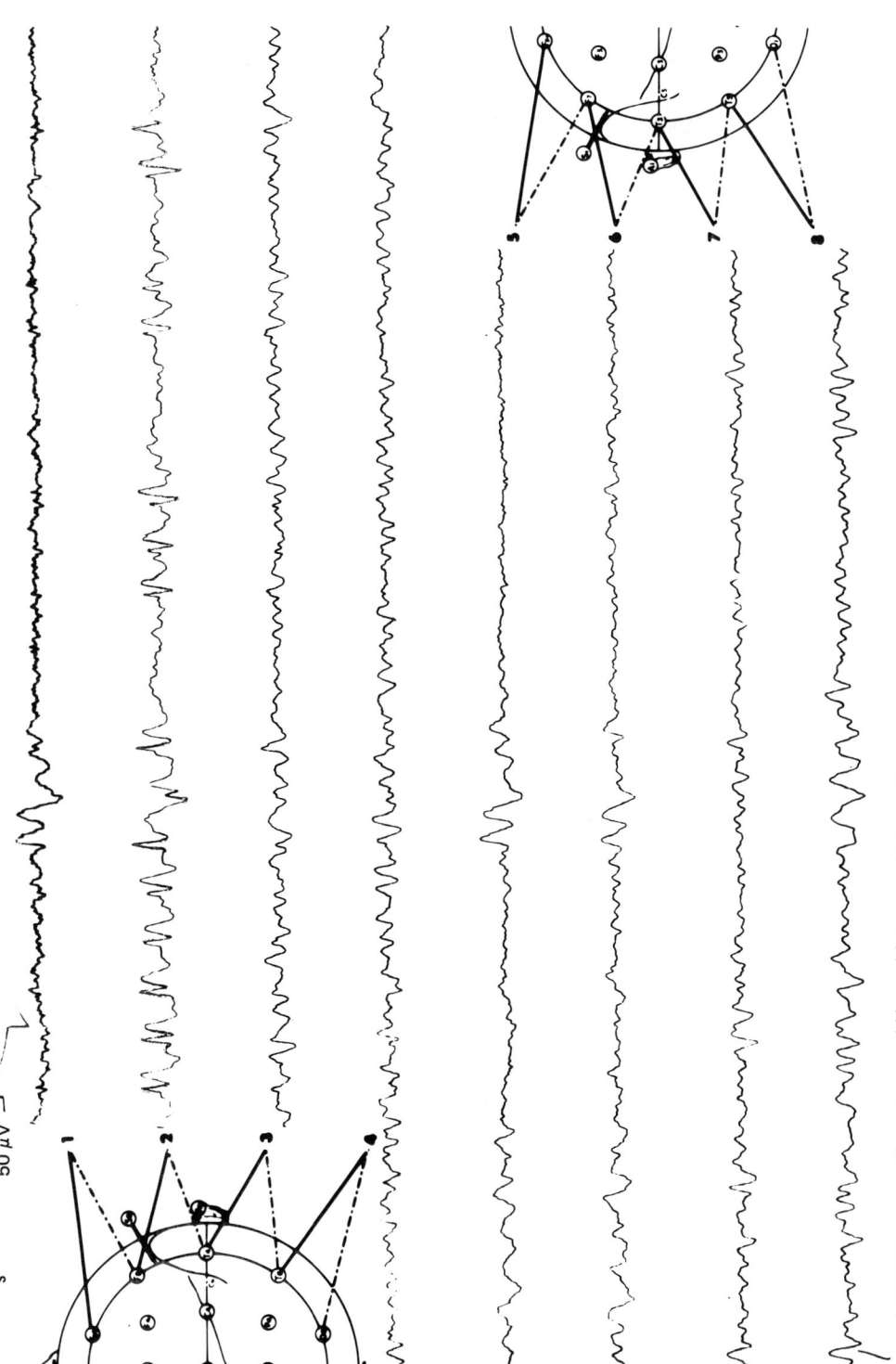

Figure 4.5. EEG recorded in an 8-year-old boy with temporal lobe epilepsy

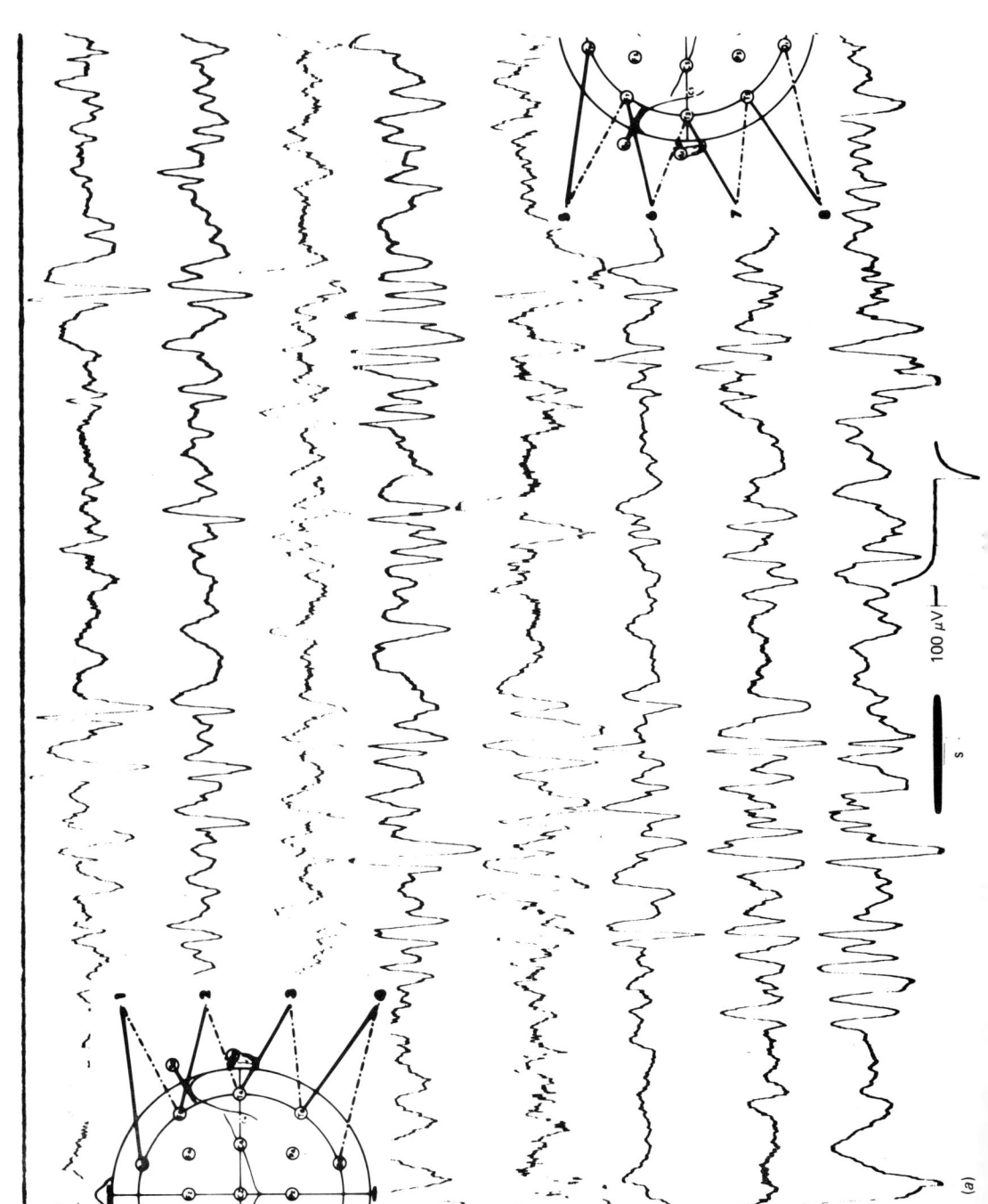

(a)

100 µV

s

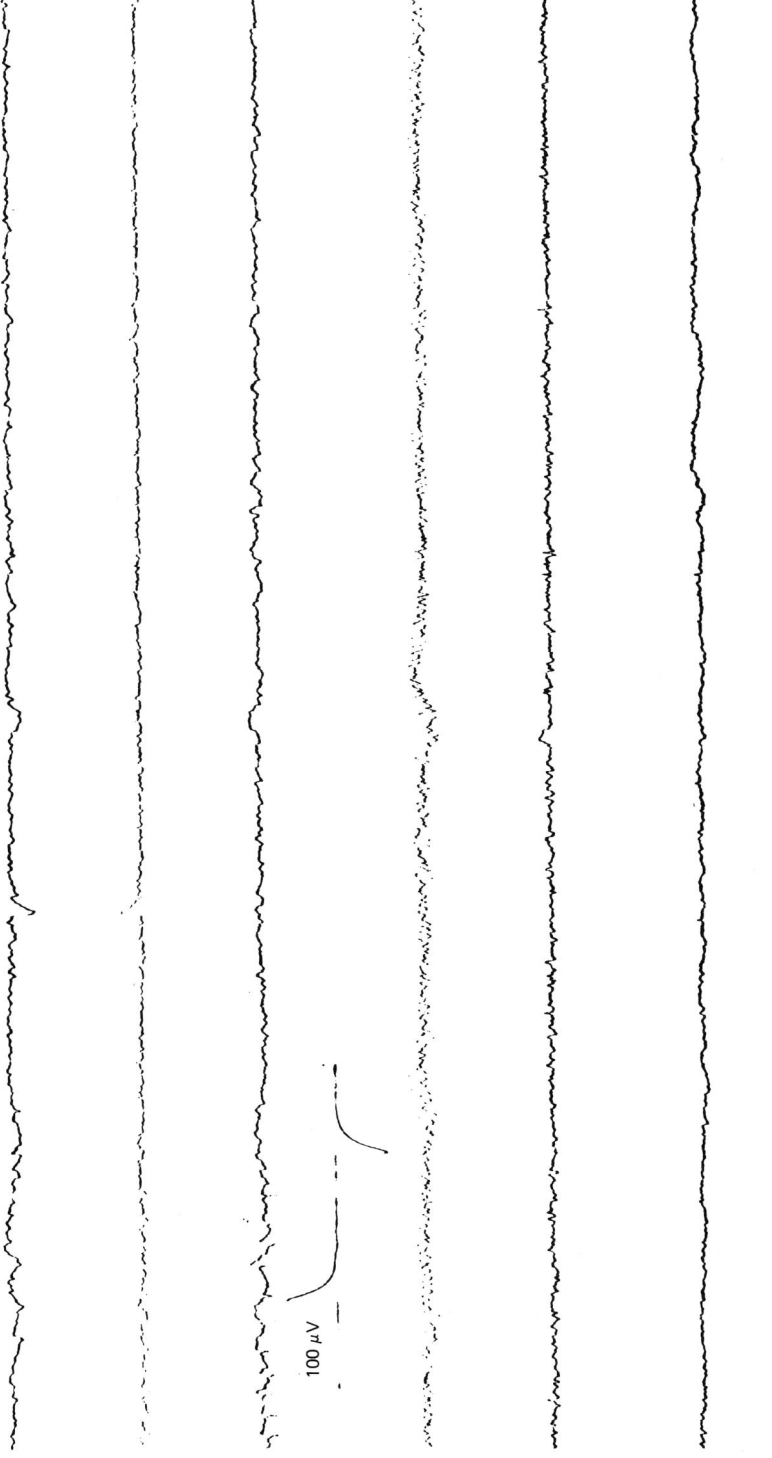

100 μV

(b)
and shortly after (b) treatment with ACTH. The placement of the electrodes is the same in both recordings

10–50 jerks. The flexion spasms seem to be particularly unpleasant, as the infant so often cries after them. The frequency is variable, ranging from at least several fits per day to, occasionally, several hundred a day. They may also come in periods so that the child may have several seizures daily for a few weeks and then be free of fits for a couple of weeks.

EEG FINDINGS, CAUSE AND PROGNOSIS

The typical EEG finding is a gravely disordered pattern with high amplitude and low frequency and multifocal spikes arising completely at random. This pattern is termed *hypsarrhythmia* (*Figures 4.6a* and *4.6b,* respectively before and after treatment with ACTH – *see* page 116). In some cases this pattern is interrupted by short periods of complete electrical silence, a finding that is considered a poor prognostic sign. Hypsarrhythmia is usually seen without any provocation, and it may be worsened by an intermittently flickering light.

Most children with minor motor seizures are or become severely retarded. The whole triad, minor motor seizures, hypsarrhythmia, and mental retardation, is often termed *infantile spasms.*

Both the clinical type of attack and the EEG pattern appear to be an *age-dependent* reaction of the infantile brain to various noxious influences. Minor motor seizures may therefore be caused by perinatal trauma or anoxia, metabolic disorders, tuberous sclerosis, inflammation, or other types of cerebral injury. As a rule, they decrease in frequency as the child grows older; they are then replaced by grand mal seizures and often psychomotor attacks. The hypsarrhythmia also disappears and is succeeded by other EEG abnormalities.

In a few cases the cause of minor motor seizures can be established and removed; if so, the prognosis may be good. The prognosis may also be good when minor motor seizures occur in a normally developing infant of at least several months of age, provided no cause can be established and treatment (*see* page 117) starts within a few weeks of the onset of fits. On the whole, however, minor motor seizures carry a poor prognosis, as the fits are often hard to control and the child's mental development is or becomes retarded.

Classification according to the cause of the fit

Conditions in which fits constitute a main part of the clinical picture are included here. In some of the diseases discussed in Chapters 5 and 13 and not mentioned here, fits may occasionally be seen. The first three groups, i.e. seizures due to fever, or to a scar after brain injury or disease, and idiopathic epilepsy, contain by far the largest proportion of children with convulsions.

Fever

Fever decreases the threshold for fits in all children. This is apparent in those who have an underlying cause for convulsions, i.e. children with afebrile convulsions in whom fever may temporarily increase the frequency of fits. However, in young children a high body temperature alone may cause a seizure in an otherwise healthy child. This is called a *benign febrile convulsion* and is seen in about 3.5 per cent of all children. The conditions necessary to establish the diagnosis are summarized in *Table 4.2.*

TABLE 4.2. Benign febrile convulsions

Age of onset	6 months to 4 (possibly 6) years
Body temperature	Fever (always enquire about previous episodes of higher temperature without convulsions)
Type of seizure or seizures	Generalized grand mal
Duration	Usually a couple of minutes; never more than 10 minutes, unless complications have occurred
Neurological signs	None, except possibly in the immediate postictal period

The liability to febrile convulsions is a genetic disposition inherited as an autosomal dominant trait with decreased penetrance and variable manifestation; no increased incidence of afebrile convulsions, i.e. epilepsy, is found in the family. The family history may be negative because the affected parent does not know that he has had a febrile convulsion, because of the decreased penetrance of the gene, or because the affected parent has not had a sufficiently high temperature during the optimal age-period for the gene to manifest itself. A child who is the offspring or sib of an individual known to have had febrile convulsions has about a 50 per cent risk of having a febrile convulsion. The precautions recommended for children known to have had febrile convulsions should therefore also be applied to their sibs and their offspring.

The first febrile convulsion usually occurs between 10 and 20 months of age. A convulsion that occurs before the age of 6 months is very likely to be something more serious, even if the patient has a high fever. The upper age limit, 4 years, is the age at the time of the *first* febrile convulsion. Although febrile convulsions may occasionally have an onset between 4 and 6 years of age, the onset of convulsions in this age-group is generally due to something other than fever, particularly if the child has previously had higher fever without convulsions. Fever is a necessary condition. It is not the infection but the fever, caused by the infection, that provokes the fit. A child often has a given threshold of temperature at which a convulsion is elicited and this threshold increases with increasing age of the child. Previous periods of higher fever without convulsions therefore imply a more serious background to the fit. Most febrile convulsions occur during the phase of increasing fever, when the parents have perhaps not yet noticed that something is wrong with the child and have not measured the temperature. Convulsions involve intense physical work which may cause fever; occasionally it may be difficult to decide whether fever was present before the convulsion or occurred after it.

The type of seizure is always grand mal; it is usually generalized and seldom focal. The usual duration is between half a minute and a couple of minutes. A seizure that lasts for more than 10 minutes indicates either a more serious condition than a benign febrile convulsion or a complication. The presence of reversible neurological signs in the immediate postictal period is rare but still compatible with the diagnosis of benign febrile convulsion; a child with this diagnosis is otherwise healthy and has no abnormal findings.

The prognosis for children with benign febrile convulsions is good. If no complications occur, they will outgrow their tendency to react to fever with convulsions and show no sequelae. The risk of recurrence of febrile convulsions, however, is high, particularly before 3 years of age. The risk of a further convulsion occurring during the same period of fever is about 20–30 per cent. The risk of recurrence during a subsequent period of fever depends on the age of the child at the time of the first febrile convulsion. If the child was below 13 months, the risk is 60–70 per cent; if the child was aged between 13 and 32 months, the risk is about 30 per cent; and if the child was more than 32 months of age, the risk is 10–15 per cent. The risk is always highest during the first 6–12 months following a fit. A completely uncomplicated febrile convulsion carries a slightly increased risk of the later development of temporal lobe epilepsy. Features that are considered complications include a duration of more than 10 minutes (particularly if prolonged to more than 30 minutes) and a definite focal character to the fit; the danger increases if these two features are combined, as they are in the syndrome of *acute infantile hemiplegia*. This syndrome is characterized by a prolonged, severe, one-sided, febrile convulsion, and usually occurs in a child who also has gastrointestinal symptoms and electrolyte disturbances. When the child eventually comes round from the fit, he will have a permanent hemiparesis, delayed mental development, and afebrile epileptic fits that are hard to control. Less severe sequelae may also occur after febrile convulsions with complications. If any complication at all has occurred, the risk of epilepsy is about 4 per cent; the type of epilepsy is mainly temporal lope epilepsy, and is probably due to scarring caused by anoxia during the fit.

The management of the acute situation, when the child is still convulsing, is the same regardless of whether the child is febrile or afebrile (*see* page 109–111).

A child's first convulsion is always a terrifying experience for the parents. The immediate emotion they *all* feel is 'I thought my child died in my arms'. Their natural reaction is to rush to the nearest place where they can get medical attention. On their arrival the convulsion has usually stopped and the child is well again except for a fever, which is usually caused by a viral infection and does not affect his general condition. The parents need time and understanding to be able to talk about and overcome their upsetting experience before they are able to receive and comprehend explanations about their child's condition and instructions for the future care of their child. It is important that physicians and nurses are aware of the strong emotional reaction that the first convulsion arouses. If the parent has brought the child acutely to a hospital, it is wise to admit child and parent for 1–2 days. The main reason is this strong reaction which may otherwise block the parent's ability to listen to explanations and instructions from the physician; another reason is the high risk of a second convulsion occurring during the same febrile episode (*see above*), and a third the difficulty of excluding meningitis or encephalitis in a young child without a lumbar puncture, which should therefore be done during the child's stay in hospital. Any behaviour of the shocked parent must be accepted as natural in the situation (the physician knows that febrile convulsions are benign but the parent does not). The parents must be encouraged to talk about the shock before they can be reached with realistic information. They must be patiently informed about the benign nature of the condition – not only that it is benign but also how we know that it is so. Thereafter, practical instructions and prescriptions are given:

1. Don't measure your child's temperature when he appears well, but if you happen to notice that an infection is starting, keep him cool by removing woollen clothes and blankets, lower the room temperature, and give him a coolish shower. If his temperature is high give him paracetamol or salicylate in a dose appropriate for his body-weight. In this situation it is also advisable to give diazepam *suppositories,* 5 mg every 8 hours, until the fever has disappeared.

2. As a rule the convulsion is the first symptom of a febrile illness; the parents thus seldom have a chance to observe the fever before the convulsion. If a convulsion has started, cooling is very important: remove all clothes, open windows, give the child a coolish shower or sponging. Give him also diazepam *rectal solution,* 5–10 mg for a child in the age-group in which febrile convulsions are common. If the convulsion is not clearly abating within 5 minutes, bring the child to the nearest place where he can get medical help. Do not put anything in his mouth until he has completely regained consciousness.

The message that must reach the parents is: 'A febrile convulsion is unpleasant and frightening but not dangerous unless it is prolonged. It is best prevented, but if this is not possible the aim should be to make it as short as possible. Follow the instructions you have received, and you will have a good chance to do so on your own'.

The value of daily prophylactic anticonvulsant treatment of febrile convulsions is controversial. Two drugs, phenobarbitone and sodium valproate (*see* page 114), have proved effective in reducing the number of relapses of febrile convulsions, provided they are given regularly in an adequate dose. A regimen of irregular doses is more dangerous than no medication. The introduction of diazepam rectal solutions has made available to lay people a method for the immediate treatment of a febrile convulsion, which considerably reduces the risk of a prolonged seizure; this has diminished the need for daily prophylactic treatment. However, a few indications for prophylactic treatment remain:

1. If one family member has had a prolonged febrile seizure that has left a permanent sequela, prophylactic treatment of the next child in the family with febrile convulsions is indicated and is usually requested by the parents.
2. Prophylaxis is indicated if the child has had a prolonged, focal, febrile convulsion that carries a definite risk of a permanent injury next time.
3. If the child has his first febrile convulsion before 13 months of age and has several relapses, prophylaxis must be considered. If prophylactic treatment is started, it must follow the same principles as for the treatment of epilepsy. It should continue until the child is at least 3 years of age (longer, if family members are known to have had later febrile convulsions) provided no side effects occur, otherwise the indications must be reconsidered. Before stopping the treatment, an EEG should be recorded. It is probably unwise to stop treatment if the EEG shows definite epileptic abnormalities; in this case the treatment is continued for another year and the EEG again recorded.

Sequelae after traumatic brain lesions or diseases such as encephalitis or meningitis

This is another large group which contains, in particular, all children who have had a perinatal traumatic or anoxic brain injury that has healed with a glial scar, which eventually has become the starting-point of epileptic fits. Children in this group may have neurological signs such as cerebral palsy; children with hemiparesis and with tetraparesis are particularly liable to have seizures (*see* pages 281 and 286). They may have mental symptoms such as mental retardation, short attention span, or concentration difficulties. However, most of these children have no neurological or mental symptoms or signs; the injury has therefore caused only an epileptic scar and no other damage. The perinatal period is the time when a small brain injury is most likely to occur; a short period of anoxia may have occurred without any obvious symptoms in the newborn baby. The onset of fits due to a small perinatal injury has its peak incidence around 3–4 years of age. If the seizures are due to a postnatal injury, such as trauma or encephalitis, the time of its occurrence is usually well established; the peak incidence of onset of epilepsy is then 9–18 months after the injury. Severe febrile convulsions may also cause a brain scar which may become epileptic and thus cause afebrile epileptic fits. If the fits start in early infancy and are due to a severe brain lesion, they may be of the minor motor type. As a rule, however, they are grand mal or temporal lobe seizures. Since they are caused by a non-progressive injury, they have a tendency to improve.

So-called idiopathic epilepsy

This is the group that remains when all known causes of seizures have been excluded. It is still a large group, probably the third largest group of convulsive disorders in childhood. It is not a homogeneous group but probably contains several, as yet unknown, metabolic disorders. A genetic factor is known to play a role in petit mal, in benign epilepsy of childhood with Rolandic spikes, and in some cases of temporal lobe epilepsy, but because of the heterogeneity of the group its importance is hard to evaluate. Idiopathic epilepsy includes all cases of petit mal, many cases of generalized grand mal, and several cases of minor motor seizures. With the exception of the last-named group, which has a poor prognosis (*see* page 88), the prognosis is good in idiopathic epilepsy with an onset in childhood. The seizures can usually be controlled, and mental development and social adaptation are generally good.

Epilepsy caused by fever, or by a scar after brain injury or disease, and idiopathic epilepsy comprise the majority of convulsive disorders in infancy and childhood. No attempt has been made to arrange the conditions to be discussed below according to their order of incidence.

Acute conditions affecting the brain or meninges

Acute meningitis or encephalitis may start with a convulsion or a series of convulsions. It is particularly important to consider this possibility when a febrile child has convulsions; in this situation meningitis and encephalitis must be excluded before benign febrile convulsions can be diagnosed.

A focal or generalized grand mal seizure may occur, particularly in a child aged 1½–5 years, from about one to several hours after a head trauma and be followed by unconsciousness which lasts for a few minutes or less. Such a fit is caused by reversible brain oedema and lasts for only a few minutes; there are no further seizures and no neurological or mental symptoms. The prognosis is thus excellent, and surgery is not required. In the acute situation, however, it is difficult to establish a diagnosis, and these patients must therefore be carefully watched for signs of intracranial bleeding or brain swelling severe enough to require neurosurgical intervention.

Progressive degenerative brain diseases (*see* Chapter 13)

During some phase of their course all progressive degenerative brain diseases can produce convulsions, usually grand mal seizures, but occasionally minor motor seizures. These conditions are rare and therefore an unusual cause of epileptic fits in a child.

Phacomatosis

Two conditions within this group, Sturge–Weber syndrome (cerebral angiomatosis) and tuberous sclerosis (epiloia), cause epileptic fits.

STURGE–WEBER SYNDROME

The typical symptoms and signs in Sturge–Weber syndrome are: naevus flammeus of the face following the distribution of one or more branches of the trigeminal nerve (*see Figure 4.7,* between pp. 100–101), usually on one side only, but occasionally on both sides (*see Figure 4.8,* between pp. 100–101); angiomatosis of the choroid with increased intraocular pressure on the side of the naevus; hemiparesis of the side opposite the naevus; and grand mal seizures, occasionally generalized but often focal and localized to the paretic side. Mental development is usually retarded. The origin of the neurological symptoms and signs is angiomatosis also of the cerebral cortex, often with calcification of the convolutions, which may be seen on a skull X-ray or, even better, on a computerized tomogram. The disturbed circulation in the cortex may lead to progressive symptoms. It is possible to remove the affected area of the brain surgically; this procedure may be considered in early cases with intractable convulsions.

TUBEROUS SCLEROSIS

Tuberous sclerosis is a genetically determined disease, usually inherited as an autosomal dominant trait with variable penetrance and manifestation. Many cases seem to be sporadic; most of these are probably new mutations. The complete picture consists of severe convulsions, severe mental retardation, and the typical skin lesion, adenoma sebaceum. This is the best known clinical picture but probably not the most common one. The diagnosis may easily be overlooked in individuals who show only a few skin abnormalities, possibly combined with a few easily controlled seizures and normal mental development. Mild and severe cases may occur in the same family in an unpredictable way. In all patients with tuberous sclerosis there is an increased incidence of tumours, particularly in the nervous system but also in the heart and kidneys. The convulsions often start in infancy as infantile spasms, later developing into other types of minor motor seizures and grand mal.

Skin lesions, which may already be visible in the newborn period, consist of leaf-shaped depigmented spots. Such spots may be easy to see in a tanned child but difficult in a blond infant. Whenever tuberous sclerosis is suspected it is important to investigate the whole skin carefully in ultraviolet light in order to detect spots that would otherwise be invisible (*Figure 4.9*). Before genetic counselling is given to a family, its apparently healthy members must also be examined in this way. Other skin lesions are adenoma sebaceum which may appear first in a butterfly distribution on the face when the child is between 2 and 5 years of age (*see Figure 4.10,* between pp. 100–101), 'shagreen patches', and periungual and subungual fibromas which may cause pain in the fingers and toes. Intracranial calcifications are common and best seen on computerized tomography of the skull; their localization, like a string of pearls, in the wall of the lateral ventricles is a helpful diagnostic sign, but their absence does not exclude the diagnosis, particularly in a young child. Occasionally phacomas may be seen on fundoscopy. Seizures are treated symptomatically, tumours are operated on according to the same principles as in other tumour patients, but nothing specifically can be done for the disease *per se.*

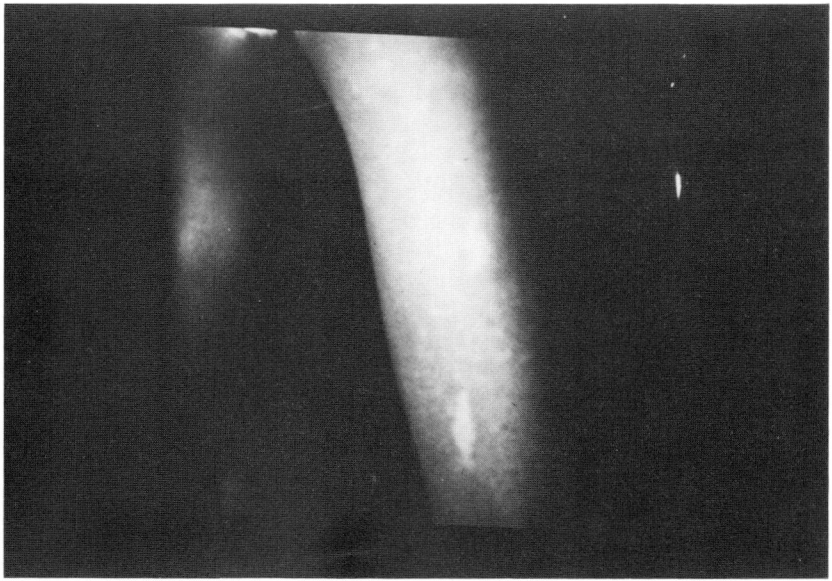

Figure 4.9. The skin on the leg of a patient with tuberous sclerosis. The skin is illuminated with ultraviolet light (Wood's light), which brings out the typical depigmented spots

Expansively growing intracranial lesions

Intracranial tumours are seldom the cause of convulsions in children. The incidence of brain tumours in children with convulsions is less than 1 in 1000. The brain tumours that produce convulsions as a dominating symptom are the slow-growing astrocytomas of the cerebral cortex. The diagnosis is difficult to establish in these cases. It should be particularly suspected in children with therapy-resistant convulsions and progressive mental deterioration. Because of the localization of the tumour, symptoms and signs of increased intracranial pressure (*see* page 364) cannot be expected. Benign cysts (*Figure 4.11*) and brain abscesses (*see* page 361) can produce convulsions. The latter usually have a fairly rapid course, over days or weeks, with an increasing incidence of convulsions which are usually focal.

Intracranial arteriovenous malformations

Such malformations may cause fits (usually focal grand mal seizures) because the shunting of blood from the arterial to the venous side produces local brain atrophy with a glial scar; bleeding from the malformation may also cause local brain damage and diffuse subarachnoidal bleeding. An arteriovenous malformation should be strongly suspected in a patient with a history of focal grand mal fits and subarachnoidal haemorrhages (which may be misinterpreted as 'meningitis'). An intracranial bruit may occasionally be heard. Brain atrophy may be demonstrated on computerized tomography (*see* page 60); this examination may also reveal the arteriovenous malformation, provided it is large enough. Arteriography (*see* page 57) is a better technique for demonstrating vascular malformations, but even this investigation may miss a small malformation, particularly if the examination is performed shortly after a haemorrhage when a thrombosis may obscure the

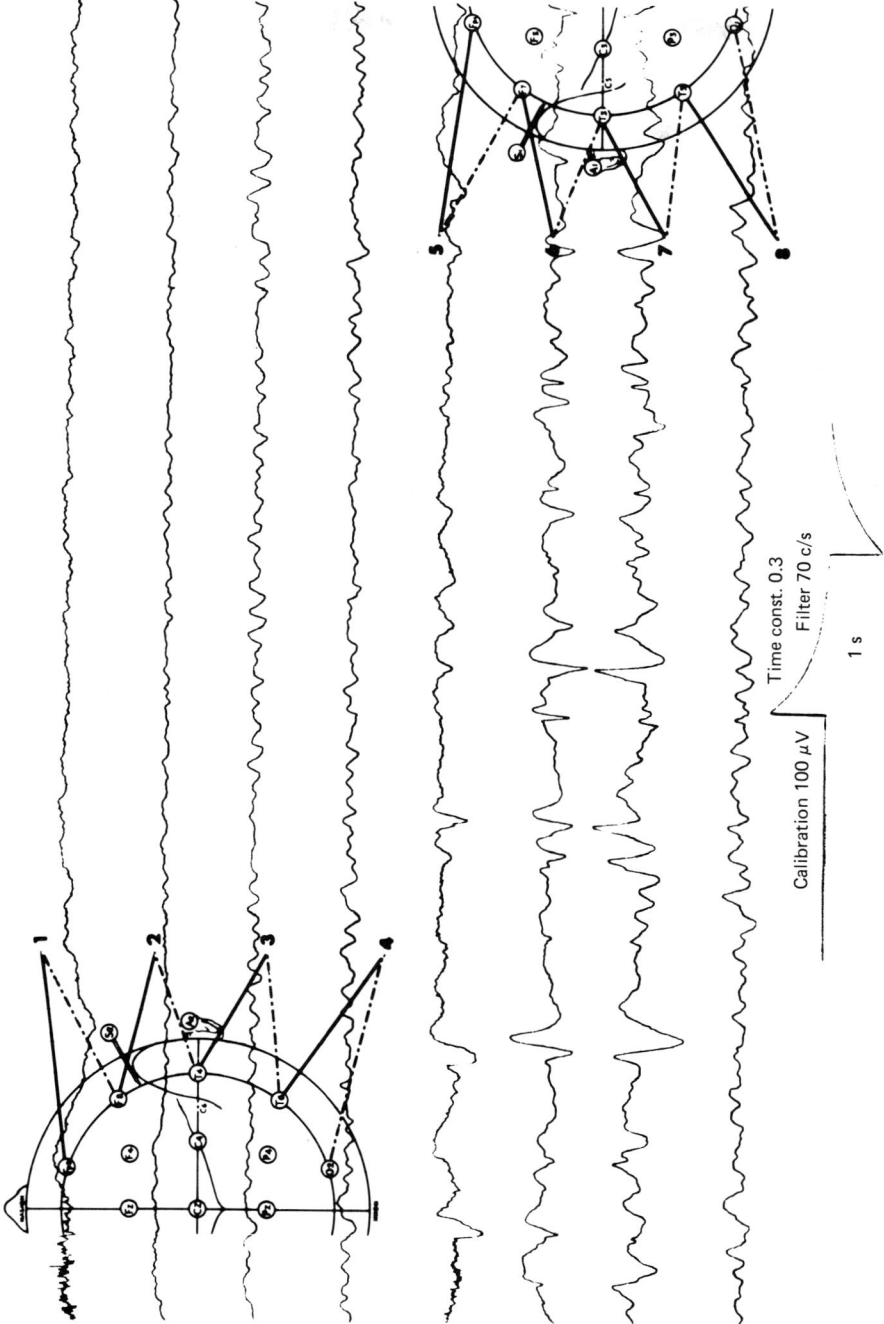

Figure 4.11. EEG recorded in a 4-year-old boy with psychomotor attacks and a large cyst in the left temporal lobe

Calibration 100 μV

Time const. 0.3

Filter 70 c/s

1 s

picture. If the condition is untreated, the prognosis is poor in these cases. Neurosurgical therapy must therefore always be discussed, but its success will depend on the localization of the malformation.

Hypocalcaemia

Hypocalcaemia causes convulsions which may be clinically indistinguishable from ordinary grand mal seizures. Some symptoms and signs may suggest hypocalcaemia, but their absence does not exclude this possibility. Such symptoms are a painful spasmodic position of the hands and feet (carpopedal spasm) and laryngospasm with hoarseness and stridor. A febrile convulsion in a child with stridor (false croup) should particularly raise a suspicion of hypocalcaemia.

Neuromuscular hyperirritability can be demonstrated by tapping a superficial nerve with the reflex hammer; this usually has no effect in a healthy person, but in a hypocalcaemic patient provokes a contraction of the muscle group innervated by the nerve. A positive Chvostek sign, i.e. contraction of facial muscles in response to a tap on the facial nerve in front of the auditory canal, may occasionally be found in a healthy person but usually suggests hypocalcaemia. Chvostek's sign may, however, be difficult to evaluate in a crying infant. One may then tap the fibular nerve where it goes around the fibular head, which produces a contraction of the peroneal muscles – Lust's sign. A positive Lust's sign, however, is found in many healthy infants.

The best way to prove a clinically significant hypocalcaemia is by electrocardiography; the characteristic finding on the electrocardiogram (ECG) is a prolonged Q-T interval. An ECG is better for this purpose than measurement of the serum calcium level, as the former relates to the *free* calcium level, which is more important than the *total* concentration (which includes the protein-bound portion), measured chemically as the serum calcium level. Children with long-standing hypocalcaemia may eventually develop opacities of the lens.

Hypocalcaemia is not considered to be a diagnosis. When hypocalcaemia has been found, the patient must be examined further to establish the cause of the disorder. Lack of or malabsorption of vitamin D, disease or removal of the parathyroid glands, and renal disease are among the common causes of hypocalcaemia.

Hypomagnesaemia

Hypomagnesaemia may cause convulsions and tremor, particularly in the newborn period. The clinical picture is similar to that seen in hypocalcaemia, which may also be present and may not respond to treatment with calcium before the low serum magnesium has been corrected by the administration of magnesium (1 ml of a 50 per cent magnesium sulphate solution can be given intramuscularly to a neonate).

Hypoglycaemia

Glucose is important for the metabolism of the ganglion cells of the central nervous system; lack of glucose will therefore quickly produce neurological symptoms. Hypoglycaemia is often found in newborn infants with various symptoms, such as cyanotic spells, hyperexcitability, abnormal respiration, or convulsions. The blood glucose is normally low in the newborn period; only values below 1.0–1.6 mmol/ℓ

Colour plate section

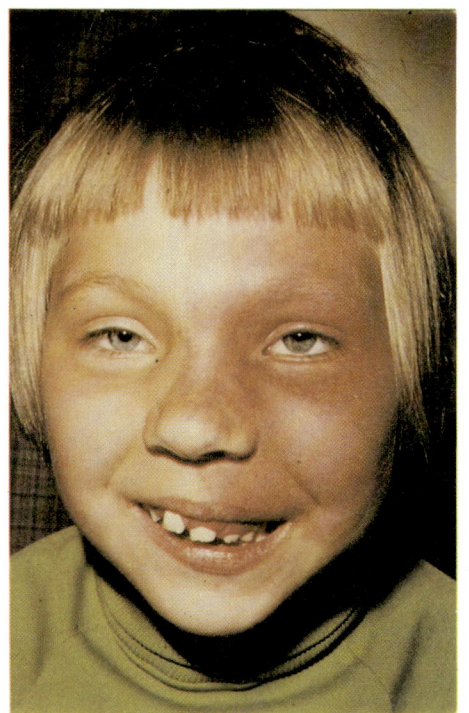

Figure 4.7

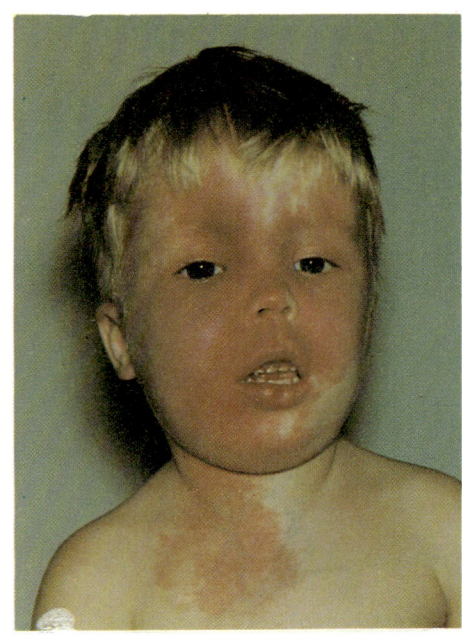

Figure 4.8

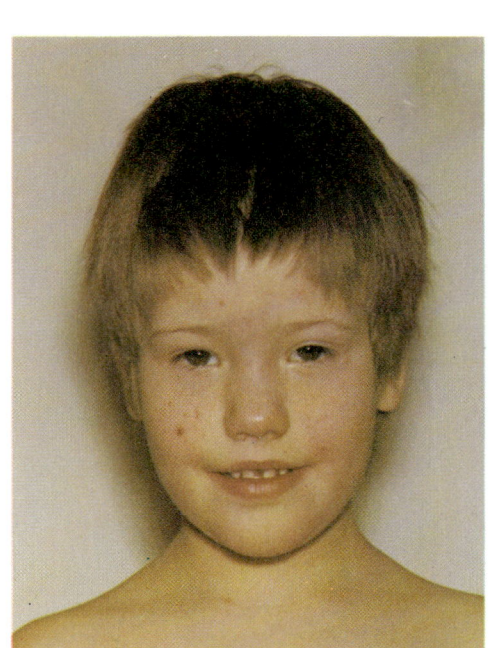

Figure 4.10

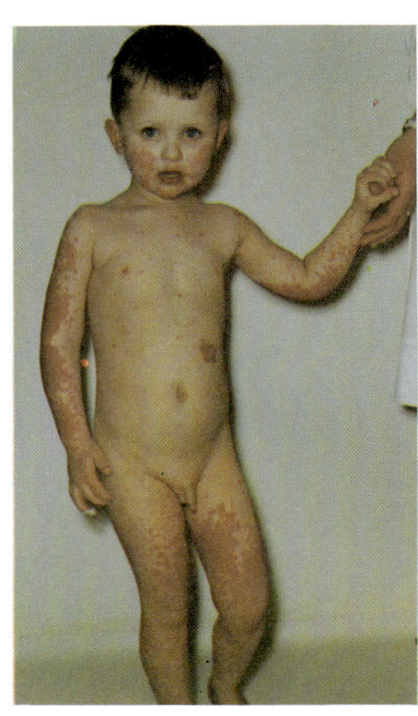

Figure 4.12

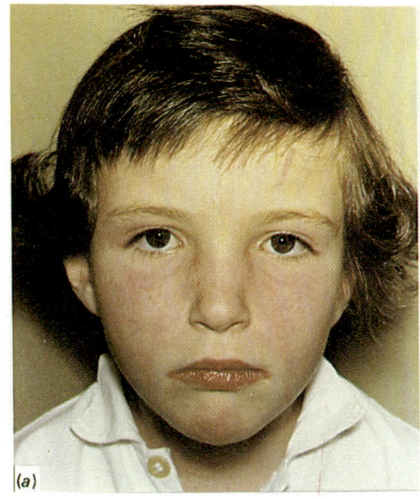

Figure 6.43a

Figure 4.7. An 8-year-old girl with Sturge–Weber syndrome. Note also the increased vascularity of the left conjunctiva (*see also Figure 12.8,* page 283)

Figure 4.8. A 3-year-old boy with Sturge–Weber syndrome and extension of the haemangioma over both sides of the face, one side of the neck, and upper part of the chest

Figure 4.10. A 5-year-old girl with tuberous sclerosis and typical adenoma sebaceum on her face

Figure 4.12. A 4-year-old boy with fever and a severe skin reaction due to phenytoin

▶

Figure 6.43. An 8-year-old girl with dermatomyositis. Note the rash in a butterfly distribution on her face (*a*) and the rash on her knuckles (*b*). She also had a rash on her elbows and knees

Figure 6.44. An 11-year-old boy with dermatomyositis. Note the bluish discoloration of the lower part of his upper eyelids. In this case the dermatomyositis occurred as a side effect of phenytoin treatment

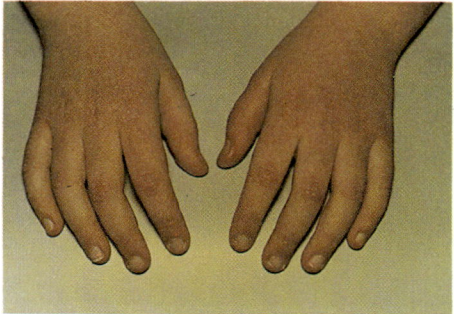

Figure 6.43b

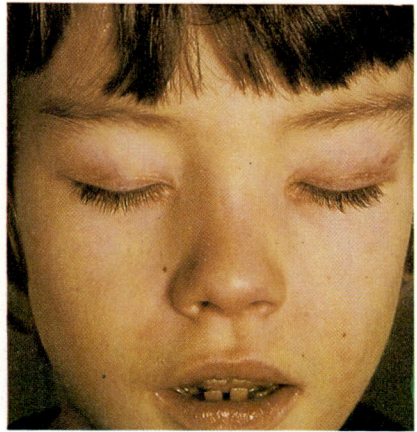

Figure 6.44

▶

Figure 9.3. A 4-year-old boy with porencephalic cyst under pressure, causing asymmetry of the skull

Figure 9.14. An 8-month-old child with hydrocephalus due to an aneurysm of the vein of Galen (*see Figure 9.9*). Note the pronounced engorgement of the superficial veins, compared with only mild enlargement of the head

Figure 13.2. The optic fundus of a girl with juvenile neuronal ceroid lipofuscinosis (Batten-Spielmeyer–Vogt-Sjögren disease)

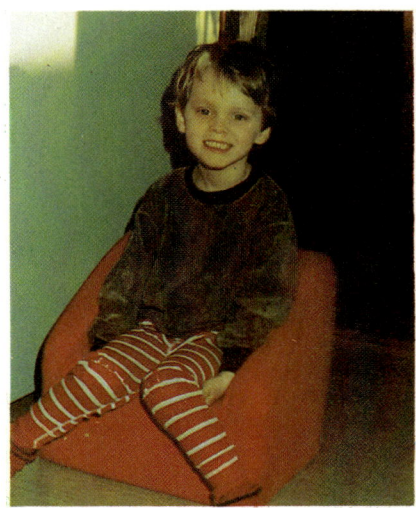

Figure 9.3

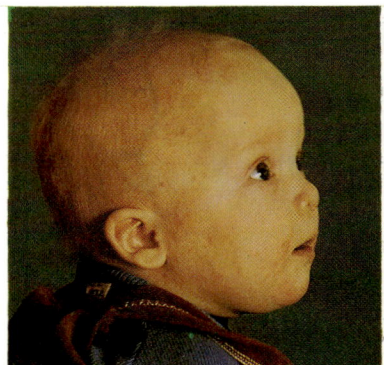

Figure 9.14

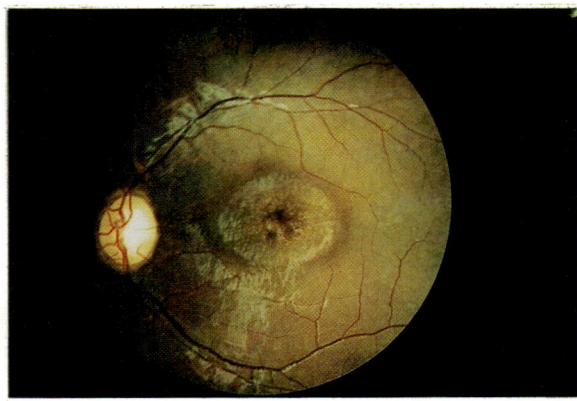

Figure 13.2

(20–30 mg/100 ml) can be considered definitely abnormal. In older infants and children hypoglycaemia may produce convulsions indistinguishable from ordinary grand mal seizures; it may also cause attacks of unconsciousness, pallor, and flaccidity without convulsions. During hypoglycaemic attacks, tachycardia, increased blood pressure, pallor, and clammy perspiration may be observed due to the increased production of adrenaline which is the normal response to hypoglycaemia. If, as may happen, hypoglycaemia is caused by the lack of this normal adrenal response, these symptoms are absent.

The relationship between hypoglycaemia and fits is complicated. Low blood glucose may cause convulsions, but in some cases it may also be interpreted as being equivalent to an epileptic fit, i.e. secondary to epileptic activity in the brain. Thus, hypoglycaemia must be diagnosed and corrected when found, as a low supply of glucose is always harmful to the brain, although correction of this deficiency will not always prevent further seizures; symptomatic antiepileptic therapy may also be necessary.

During a seizure caused by hypoglycaemia, the blood sugar usually increases and may therefore be normal or even high after the seizure. The blood sugar is often normal between hypoglycaemic spells. To establish a diagnosis of hypoglycaemia one must therefore either try to obtain a blood sample for glucose determination in the early phase of the fit or in different ways provoke an abnormal decrease of the blood sugar. *The opportunity offered by a child convulsing in the hospital should always be used for the immediate sampling of blood for sugar determination.* A normal result in this situation will avoid having to make repeated determinations during attempts to provoke hypoglycaemia.

Hypoglycaemia is not a diagnosis; when found, its cause must be established. The various possible causes belong to general paediatrics, metabolism, and endocrinology; some of these causes are discussed in Chapter 20. A convulsing child with hypoglycaemia is immediately given glucose intravenously, occasionally supplemented with or replaced by glucagon 0.3–0.5 mg subcutaneously. The long-term treatment of hypoglycaemia will depend on its cause.

Intoxications

Practically all poisons and drugs may produce convulsions in overdose (for details see textbooks of toxicology). Some drugs may also in pharmacological doses decrease the threshold of convulsions and should therefore be avoided or used with caution in patients liable to fits. All antihistaminic drugs, chlorpromazine and its derivatives, and antidepressant drugs carry some risk of lowering the threshold of convulsions. These drugs may be of great value in the treatment of behaviour disorders in epileptic patients but they should be used only after due consideration has been given to their possible side effects.

Other metabolic disorders

The relevant disorders of lipid metabolism are described in Chapter 13. Hypocalcaemia, hypomagnesaemia, and hypoglycaemia have been discussed earlier in this chapter. Other disorders of carbohydrate metabolism that may produce convulsions are fructose intolerance and galactosaemia. Both are inherited enzyme defects.

FRUCTOSE INTOLERANCE

The usual symptoms of fructose intolerance are intestinal disturbances, poor weight gain, and attacks of hypoglycaemia – occasionally with convulsions; transient icterus with hepatic enlargment, fructosuria, albuminuria, and aminoaciduria may also be found. An abnormal metabolite of fructose is probably responsible for the hepatic and renal damage, and the hypoglycaemia for the convulsions. Fructose intolerance should be suspected in a convulsing child with a normal or high blood sugar (measured as reducing substance) and a low level of true glucose. Treatment consists of excluding fruits and cane and beet sugar from the diet.

GALACTOSAEMIA

Symptoms of galactosaemia may appear in the newborn period, as soon as the infant is given milk. He starts to convulse and often to vomit. The symptoms continue for as long as milk feeding (breast milk or cows' milk formulae) continues. Signs of liver cirrhosis, mental retardation, cataracts, and recurrent infections, particularly otitis media, eventually develop, demonstrating the general toxic effect of galactose. If a reducing substance other than glucose is present in the urine, galactosaemia should be suspected. The reducing substance can be identified through spectrophotometric examination of the urine. The enzyme deficiency can be confirmed through direct analysis of the red blood cells. At least two different enzyme defects seem to exist, one of which produces more serious symptoms than the other. Some galactosaemic infants may therefore have only vague symptoms such as mild feeding difficulties. All infants with galactosaemia must be fed on a diet free of milk sugar. If the diagnosis is established and treatment is started early, the prognosis is good; when the treatment is delayed, the damage caused by the toxic substance derived from galactose is irreversible.

URAEMIA

Kidney insufficiency may cause severe grand mal seizures. As a rule these are due not to the uraemia but to the accompanying increase in blood pressure and electrolyte disturbances, and they respond to procedures that lower blood pressure and correct the abnormal electrolyte levels. It is debated whether uraemia *per se* causes convulsions; if so, the toxic substance is not yet known.

SEVERE ELECTROLYTE DISTURBANCES

Severe electrolyte disturbances may also cause convulsions in non-uraemic patients. Both hypertonic dehydration, with a high osmolarity and high sodium concentration in the serum, and hypotonic dehydration, with a low osmolarity and a low sodium concentration, produce severe grand mal seizures during the acute phase and also when correction of the abnormality is attempted too rapidly. These situations arise particularly in acute gastroenteritis in young children; the risk of convulsions increases if the child is febrile. It is therefore important to try to keep the body temperature down and to prevent the development of hyper- or hypo-osmolarity of the blood by the correct administration of fluids and electrolytes. *Fluids completely free of electrolytes (e.g. pure glucose in water) must never be given intravenously to young children* (newborns, however, constitute a separate problem), *not even for hyperosmolarity, as this must be corrected slowly.*

The reader is referred to textbooks of general paediatrics for details of acute fluid and electrolyte therapy. An acute episode of severe hyper- or hypo-osmolarity may cause permanent brain damage with recurrent fits.

AMINO ACID ABERRATIONS

Many of the amino acid aberrations may cause both convulsions and mental retardation (*see* Chapter 5).

PYRIDOXINE DEFICIENCY OR DEPENDENCY

Pyridoxine (vitamin B_6) is important in cerebral metabolism. If infants are given a diet deficient in pyridoxine, a small proportion of them will develop symptoms of growth retardation, anaemia, and convulsions. These symptoms will respond to the administration of a few milligrams of pyridoxine per day. If this pyridoxine deficiency is not corrected, the cerebral damage becomes permanent, and the infant may have recurrent convulsions that are unresponsive to pyridoxine.

Pyridoxine dependency is probably due to an enzymatic defect inherited as an autosomal recessive trait. Symptoms start with intractable convulsions during the first week of life, often during the first hours, and may occasionally be observed by the mother as convulsions of the fetus. Clinically and electroencephalographically they respond within 10–15 minutes to 100 mg pyridoxine given intramuscularly; they recur after some hours and then disappear again after a further injection. The long-term treatment is pyridoxine orally in a dose of 10–200 mg a day, which is at least 10–100 times the basic daily requirement of pyridoxine. According to present knowledge, this course of therapy must continue indefinitely. If the only therapy given is symptomatic antiepileptic treatment in the acute situation, the infant may survive with permanent severe brain damage, whereas infants treated early with pyridoxine seem to develop normally. The best way to establish a diagnosis is to observe the response to pyridoxine.

A more vaguely defined group consists of children with pyridoxine-responsive seizures. This group contains children of all ages with therapy-resistant convulsions, often with ataxia and mental deterioration, who are empirically found to respond to pyridoxine in an arbitrarily chosen dose of 100–350 mg a day. The need for these high doses of pyridoxine seems to last for a variable period of time, ranging from a few months in some patients to several years in others. This syndrome is probably not a homogeneous disease but may contain several different metabolic disorders.

Cardiovascular factors

Increased blood pressure, regardless of its cause, may produce convulsions, especially prolonged grand mal seizures. This is particularly apparent when the water and electrolyte balance is also disturbed, as is the case in renal disease.

CARDIAC STANDSTILL

Impaired circulation causes brain anoxia and convulsions which may be indistinguishable from ordinary grand mal seizures. Attacks of abolished cardiac activity (Stokes–Adams attacks) may be due to organic cardiac disease, causing recurrent heart block. Cardiac standstill may also be due to a primary brain lesion; animal experiments have shown that stimulation of certain areas of the brain, particularly the temporal lobe, influences the heart rhythm and may cause cardiac standstill. In the absence of obvious organic cardiac disease it is difficult to separate a primary brain lesion causing cardiac standstill from the secondary effect on the brain of repeated attacks of impaired circulation and brain anoxia. Cardiac standstill is probably an unusual cause of convulsions. However, it may easily be overlooked as there may be no opportunity to examine the patient during an attack, and examination between attacks may reveal no abnormalities. Unexplained attacks of cardiac standstill have been described in sibs. These attacks appear to be more common in children with early severe deafness than in otherwise healthy children; the ECG may reveal a prolonged Q–T interval between attacks. If a disturbance of heart rhythm is suspected to be the cause of the convulsions, a cardiologist must be consulted; some of these children may benefit from beta-blocking medication, and others from a pacemaker.

VAGOVAGAL REFLEXES

Vagovagal reflexes may elicit bradycardia, impaired circulation, and brain anoxia. Touching the skin of the auditory canal, pressure on the eyeballs, or coughing may in some sensitive individuals elicit such an effect. Treatment with atropine may be helpful.

CONGENITAL CARDIAC MALFORMATION

In congenital cardiac malformation, with cyanosis and a high haematocrit, brain circulation may be impaired. The incidence of convulsions is therefore increased in children with cyanotic congenital heart disease.

SYNCOPE

Syncope, a simple fainting attack, may occasionally be difficult to distinguish from a convulsion or a vagovagal reflex. A syncope is usually elicited in a predisposed individual with a tendency to orthostatic reactions. Eliciting factors may be fatigue, enforced standing still for a long time, or an unpleasant or frightening experience. In these situations, the patient becomes pale and clammy and faints; he regains consciousness when his head is kept low.

Breath-holding spells

So-called breath-holding spells are seen in children from about 9–10 months to about 3–4 years of age. The attacks are always elicited by an unpleasant experience to which the child responds by 'crying without a sound' against a closed glottis. In this way he produces a Valsalva phenomenon which rapidly impairs cerebral circulation and causes unconsciousness, often with cyanosis and convulsions. As soon as he loses consciousness, the Valsalva phenomenon disappears, the child takes a deep breath and colour and consciousness return. At this point the child is tired and upset and has usually forgotten the event that triggered the attack; he needs the presence of an adult known to him, preferably a parent, for comfort and security, but no discussion of the triggering event.

Breath-holding spells never occur without a preceding unpleasantness. The diagnosis can usually be established from the typical history; rarely, breath-holding spells may be difficult to differentiate from temporal lobe epilepsy, in which case investigations, particularly an EEG, may be indicated. Drug therapy is unnecessary, but it is important to explain to the parents the mechanism of breath-holding and its innocent nature. To parents, breath-holding spells are as frightening as all other types of fits. Parents are not calmed by the general statement, 'this is not dangerous and will disappear'; they must have a full explanation of the mechanism of breath-holding, and must be allowed to talk about their anxiety. The most effective way to reduce the incidence of breath-holding spells is to reduce parents' anxiety; these attacks will always disappear with increasing age of the child.

Programme for the examination of children with convulsions

The suggested programme is a compromise between the likelihood that the result of an investigation will be of significance in the diagnostic procedure and its cost and the difficulties it presents to the patient and the examiner. The higher the value of a negative finding, the lower the cost, and the simpler the procedure is to patient and examiner, the more widely is its use recommended, even when the chance of a positive finding is small.

Basic examinations for convulsions

Besides the history and ordinary physical examination (including the measurement of blood pressure), a complete neurological examination should be performed. As always in children, this should include an estimate of the developmental level on which the child is functioning and an ophthalmoneurological examination. The first EEG should, whenever possible, be recorded without any previous medication, with all provocations including sleep, and at least 1 week after the patient has become afebrile. An EEG recorded in the immediate postictal period is only rarely of great diagnostic value; as a rule, the EEG should preferably be recorded about 1 week after the attack. A lumbar puncture should be performed (for exceptions *see* page 51) immediately in an acute situation to exclude meningitis, encephalitis, and subarachnoidal bleeding. When the investigation is performed in an attack-free interval, the level of protein in the spinal fluid is more important than the cell count.

An ECG should always be performed to exclude arrhythmia and hypocalcaemia (prolonged Q–T interval). The blood sugar should always be determined if the child is convulsing in the hospital; a blood sugar determination performed *during* a fit is of great value, whereas routine blood sugar determinations between fits are meaningless. The urinalysis should include a test for reducing substances in general (Clinitest) and for glucose specifically (Clinistix).

Further metabolic studies

From a clinical point of view further metabolic studies are indicated in the following groups of children:

1. Those in whom convulsions start during the *first year of life*, particularly if they are of the type *infantile spasms* (*see* page 92).

2. Older children with *frequent short fits that are hard to control.*
3. Children with fits, who also show *progressive mental deterioration and/or ataxia.*

The first metabolic studies to perform are amino acid chromatography of urine (possibly also of blood), organic acids in urine, liver function tests, and serum ammonia level. A trial of pyridoxine intake is another metabolic diagnostic procedure (*see* page 103). Blood and urine should always be collected before any treatment, including pyridoxine, is started, as treatment may affect the results of the metabolic studies.

An abnormal result from a screening procedure may provoke further metabolic studies, e.g. if hypoglycaemia or hypocalcaemia is found its cause must be investigated, or if the urine contains a reducing substance it must be identified. Any peculiar *smell* around the child or his urine is also an indication for further metabolic studies.

Neuroradiological examinations

Computerized tomography is indicated in a child with focal fits, except fits diagnosed as benign epilepsy of childhood with Rolandic spikes (*see* page 78); when fits start simultaneously with the appearance of mental and/or other neurological symptoms and signs; and when the fits are remarkably hard to control with the usual therapy, particularly if the child also shows mental signs. Focal EEG findings, i.e. *focal slowing of the background activity* with or without spikes, may be another indication; they are, however, usually connected with some of the clinical symptoms and signs already mentioned. As computerized tomography causes neither risk nor pain, it can be used for a wider range of indications than pneumoencephalography. Occasionally an arteriogram is indicated, particularly if a malformation of blood vessels is suspected.

Ultrasound investigation of the skull is useful, particularly in infants with a fontanelle that is still open. This method, which is less disturbing to the baby than computerized tomography, should be used for a wide range of indications in infancy. In older children it may be used as a screening procedure for revealing a shift of midline structures, when the need for more sophisticated methods is debatable.

Other methods, such as positron emission tomography and nuclear magnetic resonance (*see* pages 69 and 70), are not yet in routine use.

The management of convulsions in the neonatal period

Fits that occur in the neonatal period are often less dramatic than those occurring later in childhood. The infant may have jerks in one or more extremities and/or the face; they may be easier to feel than to see. Occasionally the fits may consist only of a cyanotic spell or an attack of apnoea. The level of consciousness is always hard to evaluate in a sick neonate. Also, it may be difficult to determine by direct personal observation of the infant whether the jerks are normal movements or part of a seizure.

The cause of the fits should be identified and removed whenever possible. Common causes of neonatal fits are listed in *Table 4.3,* the most common being brain hypoxia due to asphyxia or intracranial bleeding or both in combination, none of which can usually be removed.

TABLE 4.3. Causes of neonatal convulsions

1. Intracranial bleeding and/or cerebral hypoxia due to asphyxia

2. Cerebral malformations
   a. Holoprosencephaly
   b. Micropolygyria
   c. Lissencephaly
   d. Other malformations

3. Meningitis or meningoencephalitis (prenatal or perinatal)
   a. Bacterial
   b. Viral
   c. Other, e.g. toxoplasmosis

4. Metabolic disturbances
   a. Hypoglycaemia
   b. Hypocalcaemia
   c. Hypomagnesaemia
   d. Galactosaemia
   e. Pyridoxine dependency
   f. Phenylketonuria
   g. Maple syrup disease
   h. Other amino acid aberrations
   i. Other metabolic disturbances

More than one cause may be present in the same infant. 1 and 2 may be preventable but not treatable. 3 and 4a, b and c may occur alone or be a treatable complication of 1, as asphyxia may impair the infant's resistance to infection or predispose to an abnormality of metabolism of glucose, calcium or magnesium. The metabolic disturbances, even when they are secondary, may cause brain injury or predispose to asphyxia (particularly 4e).

In the investigation of a convulsing newborn infant blood must be drawn for blood sugar determination, an ECG performed for evaluation of the presence of hypocalcaemia, and a lumbar puncture performed for the diagnosis of meningitis or an intracranial haemorrhage extending into the subarachnoid space. If the fits continue, pyridoxine is given intramuscularly or intravenously, preferably under EEG control (*see* page 103). A pyridoxine test should also be performed when the history suggests asphyxia, because the disturbed metabolism may impair the infant's ability to adjust to extrauterine life; asphyxia may thus be added to the metabolic disorder. If an amino acid aberration is suspected, urine should be collected before the pyridoxine test, as pyridoxine may influence the urinary excretion of amino acids.

A low blood glucose must be corrected with the help of food and intravenous glucose infusion, possibly supplemented by an intramuscular injection of 0.3 mg glucagon. If this is not enough to correct the hypoglycaemia, 25–50 mg hydrocortisone per day may be added to the intravenous infusion. If the hypoglycaemic infant has received milk before the onset of convulsions, a diagnosis of galactosaemia must be confirmed or excluded by a blood test; an infant with galactosaemia must be changed to a completely milk-free diet as early as possible.

Hypocalcaemia is corrected by an intramuscular injection of calcium gluconate in a dose equivalent to 45 mg calcium. If this measure fails, hypomagnesaemia must be considered and an intramuscular injection of magnesium given (*see* page 100). Meningitis is, of course, treated according to the susceptibility of the invading organism.

Investigation of a convulsing newborn child should also include ultrasound investigation of the head which will reveal intracranial bleeding, particularly intraventricular haemorrhages. Ultrasound examination does not disturb the infant and can be repeated daily. Only rarely is the intracranial bleeding accessible for neurosurgery. The haemorrhage may lead to expansive hydrocephalus (*see* page 251), which will require an operation. If the intracranial bleeding is found to be a subdural haematoma, neurosurgery is indicated. Computerized tomography is superior to ultrasound examination in the diagnosis of subdural haematoma, but is also more disturbing for the sick infant.

The investigation of neonatal seizures should also include an EEG. Its result is seldom necessary for the acute management of the infant, but is important for the long-term management and prognosis; thus the EEG can be postponed if the infant is in acute distress.

A sick convulsing newborn infant should be handled as little as possible. One may have to refrain from some investigations or postpone them. This applies also to the clinical neurological examinations, some of which should be omitted, e.g. tests involving changes of position and the Moro reflex. Several examinations can be postponed without loss of information of value for the *immediate* management; if carried out they may worsen the infant's condition.

Symptomatic anticonvulsant treatment must be given simultaneously with the diagnostic procedures. Each fit is too short to make its individual treatment meaningful; the aim of treatment must be to prevent the development of new fits, i.e. to *keep the infant seizure-free*. Various drugs can be used. Diazepam and lignocaine have in our experience been effective; phenobarbitone is reported to be effective from many centres. The common factor in any successful treatment is the administration of a high enough dose for a sufficient period of time.

1. Diazepam is given as a continuous intravenous infusion at a rate of at least 0.3 mg/kg per hour. If the infant is not seizure-free, the dose must be increased. The upper dose limit is not known; 0.7 mg/kg per hour can safely be used. The dose that keeps the infant seizure-free is continued for at least 24 hours. The dose is then decreased in steps of 0.03–0.08 mg/kg per hour, preferably in one step, possibly two, per 24 hours, provided the infant remains seizure-free. If not, the dose is increased to the level that keeps the infant free of fits and kept at this level for 24–48 hours, after which a slow decrease is again tried.
2. Lignocaine is given by continuous intravenous infusion. The initial standard dose is 4 mg/kg per hour; if necessary it may be increased, the upper limit being 10–12 mg/kg per hour. If the dose necessary to keep the infant seizure-free is above 4 mg/kg per hour, one should try to decrease it in steps of 1–2 mg/kg per hour every 6–8 hours until 4 mg/kg per hour is reached. From here the dose decrements should not exceed 1 mg/kg per hour and the interval between steps should be 24–48 hours, provided the infant remains seizure-free; if not, the dose is again increased.

   Both diazepam and lignocaine are effective, provided high enough doses are used and dosage is decreased slowly. Diazepam is possibly more effective against generalized convulsions and lignocaine against focal ones; if the fits are clearly focal, the order of preference between these drugs may be reversed.
3. Phenobarbitone is given by slow intravenous injection in a dose of 10–15 mg/kg; it may be repeated after 12–24 hours.
4. Clonazepam can be used in the same way as diazepam; the dose is approximately one-quarter of that used for diazepam. Diazepam and clonazepam have similar effects and side effects; in an individual case one may seem more effective than the other.

It is our policy to give the infant phenobarbitone orally in a dose of 6–8 mg/kg per day (blood level 80–120 μmol/ℓ) for 1 year, provided the infant is seizure-free and shows no side effects. If the infant remains seizure-free and has a normal EEG at 1 year of age, we stop the medication. If these conditions are not fulfilled the situation must be assessed individually and one of three possibilities chosen: continue phenobarbitone, change to phenytoin or carbamazepine, or stop all medication.

For the successful treatment of neonatal convulsions, optimum basic neonatal care is necessary with close attention to the infant's ventilation and circulation, pH, and the balance of water, electrolytes and energy supply. This basic neonatal care is a prerequisite for a good response to anticonvulsant measures. The prognosis most often given for infants with neonatal seizures is 50 per cent surviving healthy children and 50 per cent dead or handicapped children. With optimum basic care and intense anticonvulsant measures as outlined here, it is possible to get 80–90 per cent surviving healthy children.

The acute management of convulsions and status epilepticus outside the neonatal period

Status epilepticus (i.e. a grand mal seizure prolonged for at least half an hour or a series of grand mal seizures between which the patient does not regain consciousness) is a life-threatening condition which, whenever possible, should be prevented and always requires immediate treatment. At the start of a grand mal seizure it is impossible to know whether it will abate spontaneously; treatment should preferably be started long before status epilepticus has had time to develop. To achieve this goal the first line of defence must be available to those closest to the child, in the hands of lay people, i.e. the parents of a child with known grand mal epilepsy must be provided with a rapidly absorbed and effective anticonvulsant drug in a form that can be given rectally. The parents are instructed to use it if a grand mal seizure is not clearly abating within a couple of minutes. The parents are also advised to give the same instruction to the child's teacher and other adults who may take care of the child.

1. There are two drugs available in a form that can be administered rectally and from which the drug is rapidly absorbed: chloral hydrate and diazepam rectal solution. Diazepam is the drug of choice for use by lay people; the dose is 2.5 mg for small infants, 5 mg for older infants and toddlers, 10 mg for older children, and 20 mg for adolescents. These doses are too low to impair respiration, a side effect of high doses. When used by medically trained people who have the knowledge and equipment for assisting respiration, the dose can be doubled. Only diazepam rectal solution can be used in this acute situation. In most countries diazepam is also available as suppositories for rectal administration, but the drug is absorbed too slowly and incompletely from this formulation for it to be used in the acute situation. Chloral hydrate is used in a dose of 0.3 g for small infants, 0.5 g for toddlers, 1 g for older children, and 2 g for adolescents. The side effect of the two drugs are the same: drowsiness and impaired respiration. Both desired effect and side effects last longer after chloral hydrate than after diazepam. In most patients diazepam is more effective than chloral hydrate, but occasionally a patient may show the opposite reaction.

2. It is also wise to initiate treatment in hospital with diazepam rectal solution, as it may take time to establish an intravenous route in a small convulsing child. However, this route must eventually be established, particularly if convulsions continue into status epilepticus. The drug of choice is diazepam intravenously. The usual dose required to stop a convulsion is 5 mg for an infant, 10 mg for a small child, 20 mg for an older child, and 30–40 mg for an adolescent. Half the expected dose is given over 1 minute and administration is continued at a rate of about 1 mg/min, keeping fits and respiration under observation. When the fit has stopped, another 1–2 mg is slowly injected. The doses recommended above may be exceeded if necessary. Measures for assisted ventilation must be available. If convulsions stop after diazepam injection and relapse within a couple of hours, a continuous intravenous infusion is arranged in the same way as described for neonates (*see* page 108); the dose required is usually around 0.1–0.3 mg/kg per hour but must always be individually adjusted. The dose is slowly decreased in principally the same way as described for neonates (*see* page 108). Intramuscular injections of diazepam *must not* be used in the treatment of acute convulsions, as absorption is too slow and too unreliable by this route.

3. Lignocaine is used in the same way and in the same dose as described for neonates (*see* page 108). If the convulsions are clearly focal, the order of choice between diazepam and lignocaine may be reversed. Lignocaine also has the advantage of decreasing wakefulness less than diazepam or chloral hydrate.

4. Clonazepam is given intravenously, in the same way as diazepam, in a dose of approximately one-quarter of that recommended for diazepam. Diazepam and clonazepam have very similar effects and it is hard to say which drug will have the best effect in an individual case.

5. Phenobarbitone is given by slow intravenous injection in a dose of 3–5 mg/kg. It *must not* be given intramuscularly to stop convulsions, as absorption is too slow and too unreliable by this route.

6. Phenytoin is given by slow intravenous injection in a dose of about 5 mg/kg. It *must not* be given intramuscularly, as absorption is too slow and too unreliable by this route.

7. Chlormethiazole is given as a continuous intravenous infusion of a solution containing 8 mg/ml at a rate of 500–1000 ml over 6–12 hours to an older child or adolescent. This drug, which is mainly used for the treatment of delirium tremens in alcoholics, is an effective anticonvulsant. Experience with its use in acute convulsions is limited; to my knowledge it has not been tried in infants and young children. I have found it useful in older children with status epilepticus due to acute encephalitis and recommend its trial in this situation if nothing else helps. Its irritant effect on the venous wall is its most disturbing side effect and precludes its use for any length of time.

8. If nothing else helps, the child is given complete intravenous narcosis with a barbiturate and put in a respirator with slight hyperventilation, which is a good way to counteract brain oedema. Brain oedema will always complicate a prolonged status epilepticus and prolong it further, thus creating a vicious circle.

9. Excellent nursing care is as important as the pharmacological treatment. The unconscious child must be turned regularly, his airways kept free and ventilation adequate. Water and electrolyte balance must be corrected. A child has less resistance to a deficient energy supply than an adult, and an intravenous infusion of a salt solution with added glucose does not supply enough calories. In an infant or a small child, tube-feeding or complete intravenous nutrition must

be considered within 24–48 hours of the attack to supply the energy and protein needed. The body temperature must be kept within normal limits. The hard physical work of grand mal seizures produces heat, and an increased body temperature lowers the threshold for convulsions, thus creating a vicious circle. Woollen blankets are forbidden. If the body temperature rises above 37.5°C, the temperature of the room must be decreased, and the child undressed and sponged with coolish water. Shivering must be avoided. Occasionally these conditions are hard to fulfill if cooling is less active the child's temperature rises, but if cooling is intensified, the child starts to shiver. In this situation salicylate or paracetamol should be tried; both are available in a rectally applicable form. If neither works, chlorpromazine 15–20 mg intramuscularly may be effective, as it removes the child's protection against cooling and stops shivering. However, chlorpromazine also slightly decreases the threshold for convulsions and should therefore be used with caution and only when all other possibilities have been tried.

All children with prolonged seizures are given corticosteroids to counteract the brain oedema. The drug of choice is dexamethasone which is given in a dose of 2–4 mg four times a day for 24–48 hours and then rapidly tapered.

The importance of rapid measures to prevent or to interrupt status epilepticus cannot be overestimated. This condition carries a definite risk to the child's life and may cause a permanent brain injury in surviving children.

The long-term management of children with benign febrile convulsions

The long-term management of children with benign febrile convulsions is discussed on pages 94–95.

Long-term symptomatic antiepileptic therapy outside the newborn period

As a rule the cause of the child's fits can either not be identified or it cannot be removed. Symptomatic antiepileptic treatment is then indicated, beginning as soon as possible after the onset of fits. The basic investigation (see page 105), including an EEG with all provocations, should be performed before long-term treatment is begun, as treatment may influence the findings. A diagnosis of epilepsy is based on the history and not on the findings at investigation. An EEG may be normal in about 5–10 per cent of children with epilepsy, even when all provocative methods are used. Thus, antiepileptic treatment may be indicated even when EEG findings are normal. If the history is convincing, the patient gains nothing by a delay in the start of therapy; the likelihood that the patient will become seizure-free increases as the interval between the onset of fits and the start of therapy decreases. If the history is hard to interpret and the EEG is normal the diagnosis is uncertain and it is usually best to postpone therapy until a definite diagnosis has been established. The aim of antiepileptic therapy is to keep the patient seizure-free with as few side effects as possible. The drugs available will first be reviewed and the practical management then discussed.

Anticonvulsant drugs

PHENYTOIN

Phenytoin has been used for almost 50 years and is usually effective in grand mal seizures, often also in temporal lobe fits, particularly in young children. The initial dose is 6–8 mg/kg per day, divided into two doses approximately 12 hours apart; the higher dose is used for young children and the lower dose for older ones. Blood is drawn for measurement of the serum phenytoin level 2–3 weeks after the start of therapy. The optimal level for children is 60–100 μmol/ℓ, which is slightly higher than that for adults. If the serum level is not within this range, the dose is adjusted and a new serum sample is taken 2–3 weeks later. The programme is continued in this way until the blood level is within the desired range, after which no more adjustments are made. The difference between individuals is so great that treatment with phenytoin can scarcely be recommended unless the facilities for serum measurements are available and are used. After the correct dose has been established, the serum level should be checked in the following situations:

1. At the clinical visits (children may outgrow their dose or the metabolism of the drug may become faster, thus increasing the dose required).
2. Two to three weeks after a dose adjustment
3. If the patient has another fit (is the dose too low or is the drug ineffective?)
4. If the patient shows symptoms that may be due to overdosage

The possibility of drug interaction must also be considered if other drugs are introduced concurrently or withdrawn.

Side effects
A small percentage of children are allergic to phenytoin and react with an exanthema which usually appears 2–3 weeks after the introduction of the drug (*see Figure 4.12*, between pp. 100–101). The exanthema may be associated with fever and swollen lymph glands and thus may easily be misinterpreted as a viral disease, e.g. rubella. In these circumstances the drug must be abruptly withdrawn; this can be done safely in this situation as the child will only have been taking the drug for a short time. Because phenytoin is only slowly eliminated it will take at least a week for the rash to disappear completely. At least one further week must elapse before the next antiepileptic drug is started, otherwise the risk of recurrence of the rash is high.

Ataxia with nystagmus, a staggering gait, and intention tremor are typical signs of overdosage. If possible the overdosage should be confirmed by measurement of the serum level which also helps in the evaluation of the necessary dose reduction.

In children some gingival hyperplasia is an almost inevitable side effect of phenytoin. In otherwise healthy children who can chew and keep good oral hygiene this is seldom a problem and will only rarely be a reason for discontinuing the drug. It will take some months for the hyperplasia to appear after the start of therapy and about the same time for it to disappear after the interruption of therapy. Phenytoin should be avoided in children who, because of severe mental retardation or motor problem in the oral region, cannot chew and have trouble with oral hygiene; in such children the gingival hyperplasia may be severe (*Figure 4.13*) and lead to a gingivitis which causes the patient pain. Rarely there may be hyperplasia of all facial structures, giving the child's face coarser features; if so, the drug should be withdrawn. Hirsutism is another unpleasant side effect, which in adolescent girls may be a reason for stopping the drug.

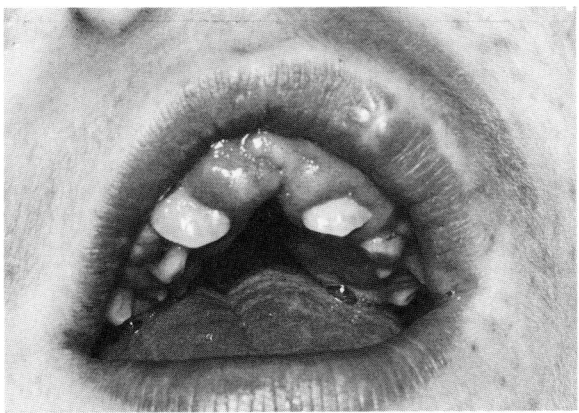

Figure 4.13. Gingival hyperplasia due to the administration of phenytoin in a 12-year-old mentally retarded boy

Very rarely patients have reacted to phenytoin with hypoplastic anaemia, severe megaloblastic anaemia, severe aggressiveness, polyneuropathy, a myasthenia-like syndrome, or collagenosis of any type (disseminated lupus erythematosus, rheumatoid arthritis, dermatomyositis). In such situations the drug must be stopped, and if necessary replaced with another drug.

CARBAMAZEPINE

Carbamazepine is effective against grand mal and temporal lope epilepsy. The dose that is usually tolerable and effective in long-term treatment is 20 mg/kg per day, divided into two doses approximately 12 hours apart. If this dose is introduced immediately, most patients will react with fatigue, dizziness, double vision and unsteadiness, some of them so severely that they may become bedridden. The dose must therefore be introduced slowly. It is recommended that treatment is started with one-quarter of the calculated dose; this is then increased slowly over 2–4 weeks. If side effects appear, the drug can be introduced even more slowly; occasionally the actual final dose may have to be lower than the calculated final dose. A small percentage of patients react with a rash 2–3 weeks after the start of therapy which necessitates its immediate interruption and usually prevents its further use in the same patient. Other reported side effects are hypoplastic anaemia, hepatic insufficiency, various types of collagenosis, and lung infiltrates. Most of these side effects have been reported in adults. To my knowledge, impaired function of liver and bone marrow has been reported in one child only and in this child the damage to both organs was reversible. In my own experience of more than 20 years I have never known a side effect to occur after 1 month of uncomplicated treatment has elapsed (except following an accidental overdosage of short duration).

The serum level of carbamazepine considered desirable is between 20 and 40 mmol/ℓ. It is helpful to measure the serum level, but the correspondence between effect and side effects on one side, and the serum level on the other, is poorer than for phenytoin; a carbamazepine metabolite probably also plays a role but is not routinely measured.

PRIMIDONE

Primidone may be effective aginst both grand mal seizures and various types of short seizures, including temporal lobe epilepsy. The common dose is 15–30 mg/kg per day, divided into two doses approximately 12 hours apart. It may cause an allergic rash, but this is unusual; other serious somatic side effects are rare. However, almost all patients experience some side effects, particularly fatigue, which may be so serious that the child's ability to function at play and in school is impaired. The fatigue is most pronounced at the beginning of therapy, which cannot be started on the calculated long-term dose. The initial dose should be one-quarter to one-fifth of the calculated final dose, which is reached after 4–6 weeks of slowly increasing dosage. Fatigue may be so severe that the higher doses may have to be introduced even more slowly and it may not be possible to reach the calculated final dose. A tired child usually shows short attention span, hyperactivity, and learning difficulties. Primidone may also cause severe aggressiveness, particularly in adolescents. These side effects are not as obvious as the severe somatic ones; they should be familiar to the physician who must specifically ask the patient about their presence. They may seriously impair the child's interaction with his peers, also his education and maturation. Primidone is partly metabolized to phenobarbitone; some of the side effects are therefore common to the two drugs.

PHENOBARBITONE

Phenobarbitone is the oldest drug still in regular use. It is effective against grand mal seizures and particularly useful in febrile convulsions and for grand mal seizures in infants. An allergic rash may occur, but other serious physical side effects are rare. However, phenobarbitone decreases wakefulness and causes hyperactivity (or increases it if already present), short attention span, irritability, and impaired concentration; unlike primidone it seldom produces aggressiveness. The high incidence of mental side effects is the main reason why many physicians are rightly reluctant to use phenobarbitone. The side effects described above occur on a low or adequate dose; they do not improve on dose reduction, and may even deteriorate; if the dose is too high the child may become apathetic and sleepy. The recommended daily dose is 4–7 mg/kg, divided into one or two daily doses. On this dose the serum level will usually be 80–120 μmol/ℓ. The serum level of phenobarbitone is more stable and easier to predict from the dose used than that of phenytoin. Once the dose for a given patient has been established, expressed as mg/kg per day, it can be maintained without frequent measurements, i.e. the total dose must increase with the growth of the child but other adjustments are seldom necessary.

SODIUM VALPROATE

Sodium valproate is considered the drug of choice for petit mal and for most types of minor motor seizures. The dose, when the drug is used alone, is 20–60 mg/kg per day, divided into at least two daily doses. Because of drug interaction a higher dose is often needed when sodium valproate is used in combination with other drugs. The enteric-coated tablets should preferably be used, because they cause less gastric irritation; also, the blood level remains more stable due to their slower absorption. The optimal serum level is probably between 300 and 600 μmol/ℓ. The serum level varies greatly during the day, particularly if only two doses are given; it should therefore be determined on a blood sample drawn at a standard time, preferably in the morning just before the first dose of the day.

The side effects are gastrointestinal irritation, which can be diminished by using the enteric-coated tablets and taking them together with food; weight loss; weight increase; change of hair colour to a more reddish shade; and loss of hair (if the drug is continued in the same dose the hair always grows back again, usually thicker and more curly than before the loss). Tiredness, ataxia, and increased frequency of micturition have also been reported. A transitory thrombocytopenia has been noted in about 10 per cent of patients, but it does not produce clinical symptoms. Serious hepatic failure has been reported in a few patients; in most cases the patients have also been taking other drugs, but a few instances are known in patients on sodium valproate alone. This complication is rare but serious, and it has a high mortality. Most instances have been reported to occur within 3 months after the start of therapy, and to my knowledge all have occurred within 6 months; possibly one is safe after that time. Another rare and serious complication is pancreatitis. At the moment there seems to be no way to predict or prevent these rare but serious complications.

ETHOSUXIMIDE

Ethosuximide is effective against petit mal and a good alternative to sodium valproate. The recommended dose is 15–30 mg/kg per day, in two divided doses approximately 12 hours apart; the optimal serum level is considered to be 300–700 μmol/ℓ. Side effects are common, particularly nausea, fatigue, learning difficulties, and headache. Headache is particularly common in adolescent girls. It is never dangerous and eventually disappears (usually after 3–6 months), but it may, together with the other side effects, impair the child's ability to function in school and together with his peers. Serious somatic side effects are rare, but cases of hypoplastic anaemia are on record.

BENZODIAZEPINES

Diazepam is the drug of choice to stop a convulsion in its acute phase (*see* pages 109–110), but has no place in the long-term treatment of epilepsy.

Nitrazepam is effective against infantile spasms, myoclonic petit mal, and some other types of minor motor seizures. The recommended dose is 0.2–0.5 mg/kg per day, in two divided doses approximately 12 hours apart. If necessary, the dose may exceed this limit, provided the increased dose is introduced slowly. One side effect, particularly on a high dose, is decreased wakefulness with hyperactivity or possibly apathy. Another more dangerous side effect is an increase in the secretion of saliva and mucus, which in an infant or small child may increase the risk of pneumonia.

Clonazepam is effective against short fits and grand mal seizures and may be used alone if the child has both types of fits. The recommended dose is 0.1–0.5 mg/kg per day, divided into two doses approximately 12 hours apart. Its most serious drawback is its tendency to become ineffective after 1–6 months of good seizure control. Side effects are decreased wakefulness with hyperactivity or apathy, and increased secretion of saliva and mucus. Psychotic behaviour and severe aggressiveness have also been reported, particularly in adolescents.

New benzodiazepines are under trial, but none has yet proved safe enough and effective enough to be introduced for routine use.

ACETAZOLAMIDE

Acetazolamide may be used in combination with other drugs, particularly carbamazepine. Several cases are on record in whom neither carbamazepine nor acetazolamide alone controlled the fits but a combination of the two drugs did so. The recommended dose is 20–50 mg/kg per day in two divided doses approximately 12 hours apart. Its most serious drawback is a tendency for the drug to become ineffective after 3–12 months of good effect. Side effects include hyperventilation due to metabolic acidosis, and the formation of kidney stones.

ACTH

ACTH is an unspecific, empirically found treatment for the syndrome of infantile spasms, and occasionally for other types of minor motor seizures. Many schedules have been recommended, but there appears to be little difference in effect between them. Keeping the delay between the onset of spasms and the start of treatment as short as possible seems to be more important to the success of the treatment than the exact schedule used. Our own policy is to start with 60 units twice a day for 2 weeks; this dose is then decreased in steps of 10–20 units, one step being taken every third day, so that the decreasing phase takes about 2 weeks and the whole series 4 weeks. If spasms occur when the dose is decreased, it must again be increased and the course prolonged. Occasionally one must continue for months, but by this time usually only two or three injections per week are necessary.

This treatment has unpleasant side effects. The large number of injections are painful for the child. During treatment the child becomes apathetic, irritable and unhappy, probably not only because of the pain, but also because of an element of depression which also seems to be present. During the phase of decreasing dose, this side effect abates. The child's physical appearance changes: he becomes swollen with a round face and a big abdomen, the facial features become coarser, and the skin develops acne. These side effects disappear slowly over several months after the end of the course. Rare but more serious side effects are an increase in blood pressure and the development of diabetes mellitus. The beneficial effect of a course of ACTH may last for ever, but the incidence of relapse within 6–12 months is substantial; later relapses are rare. A second course of ACTH can be given, but usually has less and shorter effect than the first course. ACTH may be exchanged for corticosteroids, which are given orally and can therefore be used for longer periods than the injections. A common starting dose for prednisolone is 25 mg/day, preferably given as one dose in the morning before 8 a.m. If the infant remains seizure-free on prednisolone given every *second* morning before 8 a.m., he will experience less side effects and will be able to continue with this treatment safely for a longer period. Most examiners find ACTH more effective than corticosteroids, but opinions on this point vary.

Neurosurgery

If the cause of the child's epilepsy is found to be a condition accessible to neurosurgery, such as a tumour, cyst, or arteriovenous malformation, the indication for neurosurgical consultation is obvious. Neurosurgery may also be considered in a child who has partial seizures with elementary or complex symptomatology due to a scar, if the fits occur often enough to handicap him and are hard to control. Before neurosurgery is discussed, drug therapy must first have been tried with all the available drugs in high enough doses and over a long enough period with no success or with unacceptable side effects. The child must be carefully examined with neuroradiological techniques and EEG tracings, preferably also with reduced medication, to prove that he has a localized scar that can be operated on and not a diffuse brain injury. The localization of the scar must also be such that it can be removed without harming the patient; it must not, for example, involve the motor strip or the speech centre, or be bilateral. If an operation is decided upon it is performed with the help of electrocorticography, i.e. electrical potentials are recorded directly from the brain surface to ensure that the whole spike focus is removed. As childhood epilepsy tends to improve spontaneously in adolescence, more operations for epilepsy are performed in young adults than in children. However, in well-selected cases children may also benefit greatly from such an operation.

Neurosurgical splitting of the corpus callosum has been reported as successful in a few cases of epilepsy that were hard to control by other measures.

Treatment of various types of fits

GRAND MAL

In infancy, particularly in the newborn period, the drug of first choice is phenobarbitone, second is phenytoin, and third is carbamazepine. In children above 1 year of age phenytoin is the first choice, with carbamazepine second; however, these two drugs are close with regard to first and second choice; their order may be reversed. If none of these drugs work, carbamazepine may be combined with acetazolamide. The next drug to try would be primidone, and last, for children above 1 year of age, phenobarbitone.

PETIT MAL

It is difficult to state an order of choice between ethosuximide and sodium valproate. Both are usually effective; sodium valproate is often better than ethosuximide. Both have side effects. With ethosuximide they are common and often impair the child's ability to function in school and his interaction with peers; with sodium valproate the side effects are rare, but may be serious or even lethal. Our own present policy is to use sodium valproate as the drug of choice.

TEMPORAL LOBE EPILEPSY

The drug of choice is carbamazepine, with phenytoin second. If both these drugs are ineffective, acetazolamide may be added. The third drug to try would be primidone.

MINOR MOTOR SEIZURES

The drug of choice, particularly in infantile spasms, is nitrazepam. If the child also has grand mal, clonazepam may be considered. In some types of minor motor seizures sodium valproate is effective. For the infantile spasms syndrome a course of ACTH or corticosteroids may be effective.

General considerations

When a diagnosis of epileptic fits has been established and the necessary basic investigation carried out, therapy should be started without delay. The aim is to use one drug only in a dose sufficient to produce an optimal serum level. One drug is introduced at a time. Initial side effects, such as fatigue, dizziness, and double vision, must be accepted for several weeks during the introduction of the drug. These initial side effects usually disappear without a change in either the drug or the dose. Occasionally the side effects may necessitate a decrease in the dose or a slower introduction of it. Each drug must have time to prove its efficiency. If the child has a relapse the serum level must be checked (blood for the test must be drawn as near to the time of the fit as possible), as the relapse may be due to too low a dose. If so, this may be caused either by the physician prescribing too low a dose or by lack of cooperation from the parents. In most cases treatment with a drug in a dose that produces an optimal serum level must continue for at least 1 month before the drug can be judged as ineffective. The effects of sodium valproate take a particularly long time to become apparent. However, drugs must eventually be judged as ineffective and stopped, otherwise there is a risk that new drugs may be added to the regimen and the child may receive an unnecessary and possibly dangerous mixture of drugs. The medication is changed until the best for each patient is established; all changes must be done *slowly* and be *planned*. Liquid preparations are undesirable as they always give an uncertain dosage, varying from the first to the last spoonful from the bottle, depending on how vigorously the bottle is shaken; tablets and capsules are more reliable dosage forms.

Antiepileptic therapy must continue in full dosage (which means that the dose must grow with the growth of the child) until the child has been seizure-free for at least 4–5 years. At this point the EEG is checked with all provocations. If the EEG is normal, the medication can be *slowly* withdrawn. A schedule is arranged, leading to no medication after 3–6 months (possibly longer if the patient has been on several drugs, since only one drug at a time can be withdrawn). It is debated whether puberty is a period of increased risk of relapse, indicating that medication should not be withdrawn during this period. However, no unequivocal evidence for this view has been presented. If the EEG still shows epileptogenic abnormalities, the medication is continued for another 1–2 years and the EEG then checked again; if the EEG is abnormal but free of epileptogenic potentials, the situation must be assessed individually. If the patient is well and has been seizure-free during the treatment, an EEG is seldom of value before the limit (4–5 years of freedom from seizures) has been reached; a normal EEG during medication does not mean that medication can be reduced or stopped at an earlier time. A relapse may occur during the first year after discontinuation of therapy, but after one seizure-free year without medication the risk of relapse is small.

The treatment of epilepsy requires patience and knowledge from physician, patient, and parents and good cooperation between all involved. It is the physician's responsibility to act in such a way that he obtains the parents' cooperation. This work starts in the acute situation. At this point the physician must be aware of and accept the strong emotional reaction the child's first fit always elicits in the parents. They must be allowed to work through their shock and be encouraged to talk about their strong reaction, before they can be reached with factual information about their child's disease, its treatment and prognosis. If this part is neglected, it is difficult to establish confidence, respect and cooperation between the physician and the family.

The parents (and the child, if he is old enough) must be given full *medical* information about the disease. The term epilepsy should be used and explained. Epilepsy is not a mental illness and leads neither to psychosis nor to mental retardation. Admittedly a *severe* brain injury or one of the rare progressive cerebral disorders may lead to both epilepsy and mental retardation, but it is not the epilepsy that causes mental retardation. This point often has to be explained several times and related to the individual patient's problem. The aim of treatment in epilepsy is to keep the patient seizure-free with minimal or no side effects. This requires regular medication (no forgotten doses) and communication between the family and the physician. The parents must not change the medication themselves; lines of communication must be available for them to reach the physician with a report about good effect and side effects. The principle of using serum levels to adjust the dose must also be explained to the parents. Well-informed parents cooperate much better than those who receive only instructions without explanations.

A schedule of two doses a day, morning and evening, should be used. Most youngsters are at home morning and evening, eat, and brush their teeth, and the medication can be 'hung up' on these activities. One dose a day has no advantage over two doses and is unsuitable in children, who metabolize drugs faster than adults. The effect of one forgotten dose is doubled if the total daily supply is given in one dose. A third dose to be taken in the middle of the day, which means at day nursery, in school, or at work, is *a serious social handicap* and is usually forgotten. A schedule of more than two doses a day should never be routinely prescribed. In an *exceptional* case the child may benefit from being on more than two doses a day; in such cases the intervals between doses should be as even as possible.

The use of the 'Dosett' is recommended to facilitate regular medication. The Dosett is a box with compartments for each day of the week and for several doses each day. It can be loaded on a Sunday morning, and it is then easy to check that each dose disappears as expected. The Dosett can be used to train the child to take responsibility for his own medication; such training can begin when the child is 6–8 years of age. Fluid preparations cannot be used in the Dosett and is another argument against this form of medication. Prognosis is also part of the medical information (*see below*) and is better than most parents dare to expect.

The family must also have some *general* information about their child's condition and common reactions from the surroundings. After the frightening experience of a convulsion and the diagnosis of epilepsy in their child, most parents have a tendency to watch their child too much. This is natural and acceptable for a *limited* period, but when it becomes apparent that the medication works and does not produce side effects, the parents must be encouraged to give up this close supervision, which otherwise will harm the relationship between the child and his parents. After, at most, a few months the child must be allowed again to take part in all games, sports, and school activities that are natural and normal for his age.

The parents must be aware of situations that may decrease the threshold for convulsions. All this information must, however, be given in a balanced way, so that the parents can avoid restrictions that are too rigid, which will impair the child's interaction with his peers. Factors that may decrease the threshold for convulsions are as follows:

1. Lack of sleep – a regular but not rigid bedtime is suggested.
2. High temperature – remove blankets and warm clothes if the child is febrile but do not measure his temperature more often than you did before he had a fit.

3. Overheating and *exaggerated* sunbathing – make sure that shade and coolish surroundings are available and let the child move as he wants between sunshine and shade.
4. Flickering light, at least in some patients – when he watches TV, make sure that the child is 3 m away from the screen, and provide him with good sunglasses when he watches sunshine glittering on a water surface.
5. Alcohol – make sure that the teenager is aware of the risk and that parents or other adults never offer any kind of alcoholic beverage.
6. Other medications may decrease the threshold for convulsions and/or interact with the antiepileptic drugs – don't refuse other medication that is necessary for the child (e.g. antibiotics during an infection), but always inform the physician about the child's chronic medication and discuss possible interactions.

The points discussed above mean that a child with epilepsy will take his medication twice a day and go to his doctor once or twice a year, but his life will otherwise be the same as that of his peers. He will have neither more nor less restrictions and requirements than a healthy child of his age. Overprotection and abnormal binding between the child and his parents must be counteracted from the beginning.

The child with epilepsy who reaches adolescence must be considered a new patient and be informed by his doctor in the same way as his parents were informed when his disease started.

Prognosis

The prognosis of fits that start in childhood is generally speaking good; approximately 4 out of 5 patients become seizure-free and remain so, even when medication is stopped after several years' treatment. The prognosis is better than average in benign febrile convulsions, benign epilepsy of childhood with Rolandic spikes, uncomplicated petit mal, and idiopathic grand mal with an onset between 1 and 10 years of age in an otherwise healthy, normally developing child. The prognosis is poorer than average in grand mal seizures with an onset in infancy or around puberty, in temporal lobe epilepsy, and in all kinds of minor motor seizures. However, even in these cases most patients can be kept seizure-free, or almost so, with mild or no side effects, but the medication must continue in adulthood. Some children have fits due to a severe though nonprogressive brain injury, e.g. brain malformation; in these cases the prognosis for complete control of the seizures is poor. In the rare patients in whom the fits are due to a serious disease such as tuberous sclerosis, a degenerative cerebral disorder, or a brain tumour, the prognosis of the fits depends on the prognosis of the underlying disease.

Complete control of the fits during the first year of therapy is a good prognostic sign.

References

AGURELL, S., BERLIN, A., FERNGREN, H. and HELLSTRÖM, B. (1975) Plasma levels of diazepam after parental and rectal administration in children. *Epilepsia*, **16**, 277–283
BAUMER, J. H., DAVID, T. J., VALENTINE, S. J., ROBERTS, J. E. and HUGHES, B. R. (1981) Many parents think their child is dying when having a first febrile convulsion. *Developmental Medicine and Child Neurology*, **23**, 462–464

BEJSOVEC, M., KULENDA, Z. and PONCA, E. (1967) Familial intrauterine convulsions in pyridoxine dependency. *Archives of Diseases of Childhood*, **42**, 201–207

BOHM, E., FLODMARK, S. and PETERSÉN, I. (1959) Effect of lidocaine (xylocaine) on seizure and interseizure electroencephalogram in epileptics. *Archives of Neurology and Psychiatry*, **81**, 550–556

CRAWFORD, J. D. and DODGE, P. R. (1964) Complications of fluid therapy in neurologic disease; water intoxication and hypertonic dehydration. *Pediatric Clinics of North America*, **11**, 1029–1052

DALBY, M. (1969) Epilepsy and 3 per second spike and wave rhythms. *Acta Neurologica Scandinavica*, suppl. 45

GAMSTORP, I. and SEDIN, G. (1982) Neonatal convulsions treated with continuous, intravenous infusion of diazepam. *Uppsala Journal of Medical Sciences*, **87**, 143–149

GRAM, L. and BENTSEN, K. D. (1983) Hepatic toxicity of antiepileptic drugs. *Acta Neurologica Scandinavica*, suppl. 97, pp. 81–90

HEIJBEL, J. (1976) Benign epilepsy of children with centrotemporal EEG foci. Umeå University Medical Dissertations. New Series No 17, Umeå

HELLSTRÖM, B. and OBERGER, E. (1965) ACTH and corticosteroid treatment of infantile spasms with hypsarrythmia. *Acta Paediatrica Scandinavica*, **54**, 180–187

HRACHOVY, R. A., FROST, J. D., KELLAWAY, P. and ZION, T. E. (1983) Double-blind study of ACTH vs prednisone therapy in infantile spasms. *Journal of Pediatrics*, **103**, 641–645

JALLING, B. (1975) Plasma concentrations of phenobarbital in the treatment of seizures in newborns. *Acta Paediatrica Scandinavica*, **64**, 514–524

KONISHI, Y., ITO, M., OKUNO, T., HOJO, H., OKUDA, R., NAKANO, Y. *et al.* (1979) Tuberous sclerosis; early neurologic manifestations and CT features in 18 patients. *Brain & Development*, **1**, 31–37

LOW, N. and PELLOCK, J. M. (1976) Seizure disorders. In *Practice of Pediatrics* Vol. 4, Chapter 18. Hagerstown, Maryland: Harper & Row

METRAKOS, J. D. and METRAKOS, K. (1960) Genetics of convulsive disorders. I. *Neurology* (Minneapolis), **10**, 228–240

METRAKOS, J. D. and METRAKOS, K. (1961) Genetics of convulsive disorders. II. *Neurology* (Minneapolis), **11**, 474–483

NELSON, K. B. and ELLENBERG, J. H. (1976) Predictors of epilepsy in children who have experienced febrile seizures. *New England Journal of Medicine*, **295**, 1029–1033

NELSON, K. B. and ELLENBERG, J. H. (1982) Maternal seizure disorder, outcome of pregnancy, and neurological abnormalities in the children. *Neurology* (NY), **32**, 1247–1254

NORELL, E. and GAMSTORP, I. (1970) Neonatal seizures; effect of lidocain. *Acta Paediatrica Scandinavica*, **59**, suppl. 206, pp. 97–98

NORELL, E., LILIENBERG, G. and GAMSTORP, I. (1975) Systematic determination of the serum phenytoin level as an aid in the management of children with epilepsy. *European Neurology*, **13**, 232–244

NORIO, R. and KOSKINIEMI, M. (1979) Progressive myoclonus epilepsy: genetic and nosological aspects with special reference to 107 Finnish patients. *Clinical Genetics*, **15**, 382–398

O'DONOHUE, N. V. (1979) *Epilepsies of Childhood*. London: Butterworths

RIIKONEN, R. (1984) Infantile spasms: modern practical aspects. *Acta Paediatrica Scandinavica*, **73**, 1–12

SILLANPÄÄ, M. (1983) Social functioning and seizure status of young adults with onset of epilepsy in childhood. *Acta Neurologica Scandinavica*, suppl. 96

THURSTON, J. H., THURSTON, D. L., HIXON, B. B. and KELLER, A. J. (1982) Prognosis in childhood epilepsy. *New England Journal of Medicine*, **306**, 831–836

WALDINGER, C. (1964) Pyridoxine deficiency and pyridoxine dependency in infants and children. *Postgraduate Medicine*, **35**, 415–422

WENNEVOLD, A., MELCHIOR, J. C. and SANDÖE, E. (1965) Adams–Stokes syndrome in children without organic heart disease. *Acta Medica Scandinavica*, **177**, 557–563

WENNEVOLD, A., SANDÖE, E. and MELCHIOR, J. C. (1965) Propranolol (Inderal) in the management of Adams–Stokes syndrome in childhood. *Acta Medica Scandinavica*, **178**, 483–492

5

Mental retardation

Mental retardation, like convulsions, is not a diagnosis but a symptom or sign, and can have many different causes. Mental retardation can be established from the history and/or by repeated examinations in two principally different ways:

1. A child may be found to develop more slowly than expected and pass his milestones later than his peers. When this occurs one must take into account the normal variation and many possible temporary causes for the delay in maturation, particularly if it is found at one examination only. The paediatrician alone may have difficulties in evaluating the child's development, even when it is done in collaboration with the parents; help may be needed from other professionals, such as physiotherapist, speech therapist, psychologist, and teacher.
2. A syndrome may be diagnosed in which mental retardation is an inevitable feature. Such syndromes may be diagnosed in early infancy, occasionally even in the newborn period, when the child's mental development cannot be evaluated. The diagnosis may need support from laboratory studies, X-ray examinations, or other special investigations. In this situation it may be difficult, but still important, to explain to the parents that it is possible to establish such a diagnosis and thus predict that the child is mentally retarded at a time when the mental development cannot be evaluated.

A mentally retarded child is delayed in *all* developmental spheres compared with an average child of the same age. During the first year of life the child's maturation is judged mainly from the speed with which he acquires *motor skill*; the milestones of this development are given in Chapter 2 (page 17). However, diseases of the lower motor neurones and muscles (*see* Chapter 6) may cause severely delayed motor development with virtually no mental retardation. Also, children with cerebral palsy may show a much more severe delay in their motor development than in their general mental development. A delay in motor development *alone* must therefore be judged with caution, as it may not indicate a retardation of general mental development. One must be aware of this source of error when evaluating the maturation of young children. Their general alertness and interest in their surroundings and their ability to pay attention and make social contact tell more about their mental development (provided the child is not deaf or blind) than does motor development alone.

The next stage at which retardation becomes evident is during the *development of language,* both in understanding of the spoken word and in the ability to speak. The main sources of error are defective hearing and an inability to control lip and tongue muscles, e.g. as part of a cerebral palsy syndrome. Apart from these conditions, language development usually follows general mental development, although delayed speech development with only mild or no mental retardation may occur.

In cases of mild mental retardation, early development may not have been delayed enough to cause concern. The first sign may then be a *slow acquirement of practical achievements* such as feeding oneself or toilet training. The child's development in this respect depends not only on his maturation but also on the training he receives, i.e. whether he is encouraged to do these things himself or is regularly helped with them.

During the preschool years the child usually has contact with children of his own age. The mentally retarded child then falls behind his peers in motor skill, swiftness, and ability to learn the rules of games and to follow them. When school begins, the demands on the child increase. Every child who fails to fulfil these demands before starting school or, at the latest, at the start of school is entitled to a thorough examination, which must include tests for mental retardation and other learning disabilities. If mental retardation is proven or suspected, an attempt must be made to establish its cause, regardless of the age of the child. This attempt, which at present is successful in a third or half of the cases, is the responsibility of the paediatrician or the paediatric neurologist. The main part of this chapter is concerned with the diagnostic possibilities and procedures involved.

The physician may occasionally be able to establish a medical diagnosis from the physical appearance of the child; in this situation the cause of the mental retardation is revealed before the retardation is detectable.

The diagnosis must be as exact as possible in order that the physician may give the parents accurate information about the cause of the child's symptoms. An exact diagnosis also forms the basis of the prognosis. Correct genetic counselling can only be based on precise diagnosis. Occasionally, a correct diagnosis in a mentally retarded child may lead to the early detection and early treatment of the same disorder in a younger and still symptom-free sib of the patient. Severe mental retardation may in this way be *prevented*; it can only rarely be *treated* successfully, as the damage is by then usually irreversible.

General causes of mental retardation

In the general population the level of intelligence is scattered mainly according to a normal distribution curve. Thus, some children develop slowly, not because of a lesion or a disease, but because they belong to the *low end of the normal variability curve.* Almost all of these children are mildly retarded and do not differ markedly from their parents and sibs. These children need particularly stimulating surroundings during their preschool years and may lack it in their family environment. It is therefore important to try to identify these children as early as possible through well-baby clinics or day nurseries and to provide them with as much stimulation as possible as support for and supplement to their family.

When infants and young children are *deprived,* for periods of months or years, *of good emotional contact* with parents or with one or two adults acting as substitute parents, their mental development may become seriously and permanently damaged. This has happened in children who grew up in institutions with too few nurses or with nurses unaware of or uninterested in the emotional needs of the infant. Awareness of this danger has led to a decrease in the number of children receiving institutional care and to a higher susceptibility to signals from children who are neglected or deprived within their families. Such signals are delayed mental and physical development with, for example, retardation of growth in spite of an adequate food intake. The risk is particularly high in families where one or both parents have a psychiatric illness or addiction to alcohol or drugs. Good cooperation between social and medical care and between the parents' psychiatrist and the paediatrician is important for the children concerned.

Another general cause of mental retardation is *starvation,* which, when it occurs during the first few years of life, causes permanent impairment of brain development, evident also as microcephaly. The effect of starvation, which can also be produced in animal experiments, can be distinguished from the effect of other social factors, which often occur simultaneously. The damage, once established, cannot be influenced later.

A mild delay in mental development, particularly in gross motor skill, may be seen in children who have *recurrent infections* and are therefore confined to bed more than other children; such children are thus unable to train their motor function in the normal way. The delay is only temporary; they rapidly catch up with their peers when they are free of infections.

Deaf children and *blind* children often show a delay in motor development, particularly in the ability to walk without support. This delay is due to the natural insecurity of an individual without vision or hearing and has no prognostic significance.

Medical causes of mental retardation

Sequelae after prenatal, perinatal, or postnatal brain injury

CAUSES

Rubella
Rubella in the mother during the first trimester may seriously damage the fetus, causing cardiac malformations, cataracts, hearing defects, and brain injury with mental retardation. The viral infection of the fetus may still be active at birth and cause skeletal symptoms and thrombocytopenia; these infants can infect their surroundings. The diagnosis can be confirmed by cultivation of the virus from the saliva, faeces, or urine and/or the finding of IgM antibodies to rubella (antibodies that are produced by the infant and not passively transferred from the mother). The only preventive measure available is mass vaccination which aims to eradicate the virus from the population.

Congenital syphilis
In congenital syphilis the brain may also be involved, and permanent damage may occur. This disease can be entirely prevented in the fetus by giving antibiotic therapy (penicillin being the drug of choice) to all infected women during pregnancy. The treatment for congenital syphilis is also penicillin.

Toxoplasmosis

Toxoplasmosis acquired in childhood or adulthood often produces no symptoms. If a woman is infected during pregnancy, she may transfer the infection to the fetus, in whom it may cause severe brain disease. Occasionally symptoms are mild and appear weeks or months after birth. However, most infants in the acute phase of congenital toxoplasmosis are in poor general condition and have feeding difficulties and cyanotic spells. They often also have hepatosplenomegaly, petechiae due to thrombocytopenia, and jaundice. Chorioretinitis is seen in almost all patients, although some weeks may elapse before it is demonstrable. The spinal fluid shows an increased cell count (mainly mononuclear cells) and an elevated protein content; the parasite can occasionally be found in the spinal fluid. When the active disease subsides after a couple of weeks or months, signs of progressive hydrocephalus due to aqueductal stenosis often develop, and skull X-ray shows intracranial calcifications. Antibodies against toxoplasmosis can be demonstrated in the blood of both the child and the mother. The presence of IgM antibodies in the child's blood means that the child has produced them and has thus been infected, whereas other types of antibodies may be passively transferred from the mother.

The treatment of congenital toxoplasmosis is discouraging. The only available treatment, a combination of pyrimethamine (3–6 mg/day) and sulphonamide (100–200 mg/kg per day), seems of little value. The hydrocephalus can be treated neurosurgically (*see* Chapter 9).

Cytomegalic inclusion body disease

This is a viral disease which usually produces no symptoms in an older child or an adult. The mother may become infected during pregnancy and transfer the infection to the fetus. The clinical picture in the child is indistinguishable from that produced by congenital toxoplasmosis (*see above*); jaundice and hepatomegaly are perhaps more constant findings than in toxoplasmosis. The diagnosis is established by cultivation of the virus from the saliva, urine, or faeces and/or the demonstration of IgM antibodies to cytomegalic inclusion body disease in the infant's blood; such antibodies are produced by the infant and have not been passively transferred from the mother. Surviving children usually become severely retarded. No effective therapy is known. There is no vaccine available for mass vaccination.

Bloch–Sulzberger syndrome

This syndrome, also known as incontinentia pigmenti, affects mainly female infants. It is manifest in the newborn period as a skin disorder characterized by vesicles that are either present at birth or appear within the first few days of life. The vesicles are arranged longitudinally on the limbs and transversally on the trunk. They disappear and recur several times and are finally replaced by dark pigmented streaks, which fade within a couple of years. A substantial proportion of children with incontinentia pigmenti also show eye lesions and involvement of the brain, causing cerebral palsy (mainly spasticity), mental retardation, and microcephaly. Such signs should thus be looked for in an infant with the typical skin lesions. The diagnosis is difficult to establish in an older child with ocular or neurological symptoms, unless the history is typical or fading skin lesions are still present. The condition is usually considered to be inherited; the possibility of a viral infection of the mother has also been discussed. No causal therapy is available.

Influence of chemical agents on the fetus
The most common agent known to be toxic to the fetus is alcohol. The fetal alcohol syndrome was known in Great Britain during the eighteenth century but has been forgotten for 200 years. The larger the amount of alcohol ingested, the greater the risk of damage to the fetus, but no limit has been established below which the mother can be certain that no harm will occur. Women with severe alcohol problems may also have a poor food intake and inadequate prenatal care; although these factors may add to the fetal damage, the main injury is caused by alcohol. Children with the fetal alcohol syndrome are born small for dates, occasionally with severe growth retardation. They have abnormally small heads and facial features characterized by small palpebral fissures (less than 20 mm), short nose with anteverted nostrils, flat nasal bridge and long philtrum, low-set ears, and small chin; the incidence of other malformations, particularly cleft palate and cardiac malformations, is increased. Children with the fetal alcohol syndrome remain small (*Figure 5.1*); both their physical and their mental development are retarded. They are often hyperactive with a short attention span. Understimulation may add to their handicap, but their physical and mental retardation remain, even when they receive optimal nutrition, stimulation, and security; the damage caused by the toxic influence of alcohol is permanent.

* Dr Smith-Lemli optis syndrom

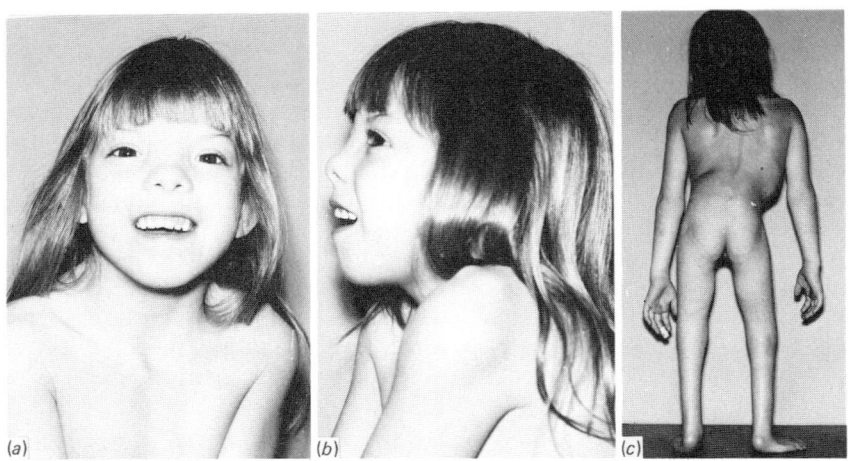

(a)   (b)   (c)

Figure 5.1. A 7-year-old girl, whose mother had ingested alcohol and took phenytoin during the pregnancy. Besides short stature (height 90 cm) and facial features typical of the fetal alcohol syndrome (*a* and *b*), the girl also has a severe malformation of the sacrum (*c*) and cauda equina with neurological symptoms and signs from the legs and impaired control of the bladder

Phenytoin may cause fetal injury similar to the fetal alcohol syndrome. However, women with epilepsy need to continue medication during pregnancy as repeated convulsions may also harm the fetus; close monitoring of the dose is therefore important. If this is done and the pregnancy is otherwise uncomplicated, the risk of fetal injury is small. The possibility that other medical drugs and chemical toxins may cause fetal brain damage is debated.

The possibility of endogenous toxins must also be considered. An example of this situation is the woman with phenylketonuria whose fetus is exposed to the increased phenylalanine level in the mother's blood. Phenylalanine passed to the fetus will harm the fetal brain. A woman with phenylketonuria must therefore start dietary treatment _before_ pregnancy occurs, i.e. at the time when a pregnancy is planned, as the danger is greatest during the early phase of pregnancy. Other amino acid aberrations may conceivably follow the same pattern.

Other prenatal causes
Starvation during pregnancy, particularly during the second trimester, may cause permanent fetal brain injury, regardless of whether the starvation is due to lack of food or to a maternal disease which impairs the mother's ability to eat; the logical measure in the latter situation is complete intravenous nutrition. Lack of specific ingredients in the food, even when the caloric intake is adequate, may damage the fetus.

The possibility that the fetal brain may be damaged by infections other than syphilis, rubella, toxoplasmosis, and cytomegalic inclusion body disease is debated but unproven. Episodes of anoxia in the mother (as may happen during an epileptic fit) may presumably also harm the fetal brain, particularly if they occur frequently.

Perinatal brain injury
Intracranial haemorrhage or cerebral anoxia in the newborn period may lead to permanent brain damage, the localization and extent of which may retard the child's mental development. A complicated delivery or a premature birth will increase the risk of retardation, but neither is regularly followed by a permanent lesion. Brain injury may also occur during an apparently normal delivery. These infants usually have symptoms, such as muscular hypotonia (*see* pages 155–158), convulsions (*see* page 107), increased muscular tone, irritability, cyanotic spells, apathy, and feeding difficulties, during the newborn period. As these symptoms are vague, there is a risk that they may be overlooked and not noted in the record from the newborn period. Jaundice and meningitis occurring during the neonatal period may also cause permanent brain damage and mental retardation.

Postnatal brain injury
Physical brain injury, cerebral anoxia, encephalitis, or meningitis occurring during infancy and childhood may cause permanent brain damage and arrest the child's mental development. Intracranial bleeding, physical brain injury, and meningitis can all cause communicating hydrocephalus, an intracerebral haematoma, cyst, and subdural hygroma (*see* Chapter 9). These conditions, which are surgically treatable, can cause further progressive cerebral damage. It is therefore important to diagnose and treat them as early as possible; computerized tomography of the skull is necessary to demonstrate or exclude these conditions.

Early starvation may interfere with myelination of the immature brain. If the infant cannot eat because of a severe disease, complete parenteral nutrition is essential.

COMPLICATIONS, COURSE, AND PROGNOSIS

Children with mental retardation due to an early brain lesion usually show slow motor development and remain clumsy throughout life, even when they do not show definite neurological signs. Their gait is often broad-based and ungainly and they have trouble learning to hop on one foot and to ride a bicycle. Alternating movements remain slow for age, and the fine finger movements are clumsy and awkward (*see* page 28). Such neurological signs are present in most mild cases. In cases of severe mental retardation due to an early brain lesion, the patient usually also shows definite neurological signs such as abnormal muscle tone, weakness, ataxia, and abnormal reflexes (*see* pages 18–29). If the damage is severe, the growth of the brain may also be arrested, and the child can become microcephalic (*see* page 236).

Many of these children also have other mental symptoms such as restlessness, lack of concentration, and short attention span. These symptoms often deteriorate if the patients are given sedatives, particularly barbiturates.

Many patients have convulsions (*see* page 95); EEG abnormalities are often found. Skull X-ray may reveal skull asymmetry, localized thinning of the skull bones, intracranial calcifications, abnormal sutures, or abnormal growth of the skull (*see* Chapter 9). Computerized tomography of the skull may reveal localized destruction of the brain, porencephalic cyst, hydrocephalus, or subdural hygroma (*see* page 60). Severe cortical atrophy and a considerably enlarged third ventricle (more than 8 mm) are poor prognostic signs for the child's mental development.

A main aim of modern obstetric and neonatal care is to prevent or limit as far as possible a permanent cerebral lesion in the newborn infant. Neurosurgically accessible conditions, such as hydrocephalus, intracerebral haematoma, cyst, and subdural hygroma, must be diagnosed and treated as early as possible. It is worthwhile making an effort to find the best anticonvulsant therapy (*see* page 111), as good seizure control without side effects may increase the child's concentration and attention span and thus his learning ability. Occasionally the mentally retarded child without seizures may also benefit from anticonvulsant therapy, particularly if his EEG is abnormal. Physiotherapy helps to improve the child's motor development. Stimulating surroundings and individually adapted teaching from an early age are also important for the development of the child's potentials.

Prognosis

The prognosis must be given with caution. The attitude must be realistic, but an over-pessimistic prognosis should not be given to the parents of a young infant. An infant, who at an early age appears seriously brain damaged, may make a remarkable recovery. An over-pessimistic prognosis given early may cause the parents unnecessary suffering and may impair their ability to stimulate and train their child. When improvement occurs, it is usually most marked during the first few years of life; the future can therefore be predicted with more certainty in a child 2–3 years of age than in an infant.

Metabolic disorders

During the last few decades the importance of metabolic disorders has been stressed as the cause of mental retardation; many abnormal metabolites may damage the developing brain. Such products can be demonstrated by different laboratory methods; the reader is referred to textbooks on inborn errors of metabolism for details. In several disorders, therapy is now available to prevent the formation of these dangerous metabolites. Therapy is only successful if it is started before the development of symptoms or when only a few symptoms are apparent; it fails if it is started after permanent brain damage has occurred. Screening procedures are therefore designed to diagnose the disorders before they produce symptoms. Although an early diagnosis is extremely important to the individual afflicted, these disorders are all rare, and of all mentally retarded patients only a small proportion are retarded because of any of the known metabolic diseases. New developments are occurring rapidly within this field, and new metabolic disorders are described every year. Most of the metabolic disorders are genetically determined, and their inheritance is usually due to an autosomal recessive gene.

HYPERCALCAEMIA

Hypercalcaemia in infancy may cause vague symptoms, such as failure to thrive, feeding difficulties, and constipation. A finding of hypercalcaemia (serum calcium consistently above 2.3–3.0 mmol/ℓ) establishes the diagnosis. The cause of this disorder is unknown; inheritance due to a recessive autosomal gene appears to be a likely explanation. These children are susceptible to vitamin D, and the usual vitamin D prophylaxis should therefore not be given. Cortisone in the smallest dose that keeps the serum calcium within normal limits (2.1–2.3 mmol/ℓ) is the therapy of choice in severe cases. The metabolic defect seems to disappear within a couple of years, at which time therapy can be stopped. However, some of these children, who have severe symptoms of idiopathic hypercalcaemia early in life, survive with mental retardation, which possibly might have been prevented if the serum calcium had been kept within normal limits. Some of the patients will later show the elfin face syndrome (*see* page 146); the relationship between this syndrome and infantile hypercalcaemia is debated.

ABNORMAL PYRIDOXINE AND LIPID METABOLISM

Three syndromes connected with abnormal pyridoxine metabolism have been described; all three cause seizures and disturbed mental development. They are described in Chapter 4 (*see* pages 103 and 107). The known disorders of lipid metabolism all seem to cause progressive cerebral symptoms and are described in Chapter 13 (*see* pages 295–299).

DISORDERS OF AMINO ACID METABOLISM

The list of disorders of amino acid metabolism is long and increases every year. The metabolic defect is identified by amino acid chromatography of the urine and blood. For a short period after birth (weeks or perhaps months) most of these disorders produce apparently progressive and yet reversible symptoms. Once symptoms of cerebral damage have become established, they are usually permanent and nonprogressive, and most patients will then benefit only slightly from a therapy that corrects the metabolic defect.

Phenylketonuria
Described by Følling in 1934, this is the oldest of the amino acid aberrations known to cause cerebral damage. The metabolic block consists of an inability to convert phenylalanine into tyrosine. This leads to a lack of tyrosine, which accounts for one of the main features of Følling's disease, the relative lack of pigment. These patients thus have fairer hair and complexion than their healthy sibs. Eczematous skin lesions are also often seen. The increased level of phenylalanine is responsible for the cerebral damage. At birth these infants are symptom-free; after a few

months their development is observed to be slow, and mental retardation is obvious at 1 year of age. The mental retardation remains severe; at least 25 per cent of patients have convulsions of the grand mal type. Besides generally slow, clumsy movements, the patients may show rigidity and stereotyped mannerisms.

The increased level of phenylalanine in serum can be demonstrated by a method that is suitable for mass screening and which, in many countries, is performed on all newborn infants. The infants must be at least 3–4 days old and must have received milk for at least 24 hours prior to the test, otherwise the level of phenylalanine remains low, even in phenylketonuric infants. A positive finding on the screening procedure must be checked by more specific methods before a diagnosis of phenylketonuria is established, as other abnormal metabolites may also give a positive reaction. A specific increase in the level of phenylalanine may also be seen in conditions other than phenylketonuria (see below). When the normal metabolic pathway for phenylalanine is blocked, some of it is metabolized abnormally, and the abnormal metabolites appear in the urine, where they can be demonstrated by a positive ferric chloride reaction or a positive Phenistix. These urinary reactions may not become positive until the infant is 2–3 months of age; before the child has reached this age these tests cannot be used as screening procedures. These metabolites are also excreted in sweat and expired air. They have an unpleasant smell, like mouse urine, which is usually noticeable around the child.

Treatment   All infants with a phenylalanine level above 1000 μmol/ℓ must be treated immediately. Those with levels between 250 and 1000 μmol/ℓ should be followed clinically and with laboratory studies; some of them may not need treatment. Treatment consists of feeding the infant a commercially available formula with a low and defined phenylalanine content. This formula is supplemented with extra vitamins and iron and small amounts of other nutrients to keep the phenylalanine level within the range 300–700 μmol/ℓ for children 0–6 years of age and 300–1000 μmol/ℓ for children 7–18 years of age; the plasma amino acid chromatogram must be normal in other respects. It is important to keep the phenylalanine level above the stated lower limit of the range, as the child will otherwise enter a catabolic phase. The child's tolerance for phenylalanine must be tested at intervals, as the time when the strict regulations can be safely mitigated varies from child to child. The need for a strict diet during pregnancy is stressed (*see* page 127).

Prognosis   The prognosis is good for children whose treatment is begun in the newborn period. Dietary restrictions started after 1 year of age may improve the skin condition and the child's behaviour slightly, but appear to have little influence on his mental development. Some individuals have been found to have the metabolic defect of phenylketonuria but with entirely normal development and no dermatological or neurological signs. A diet that is started early is thus not the only factor influencing the prognosis, but other factors are not known.

Increased level of phenylalanine without phenylketonuria
An increased level of serum phenylalanine without phenylketonuria may be seen in prematurely born infants. The increase in the phenylalanine level is slight, and the tyrosine level is also raised. The likely explanation is an inability of the immature liver to metabolize tyrosine at a normal rate; since phenylalanine is converted into tyrosine, this reaction will also be slowed down when tyrosine accumulates. The

administration of vitamin C can correct this metabolic defect, the practical significance of which is debated.

Some patients have been reported in whom an increased blood level of phenylalanine was found together with a normal level of tyrosine and increased urinary excretion of phenylalanine, but no excretion of phenylketones and thus a negative Phenistix. Most patients in this group have had a definitely abnormal level of phenylalanine in the newborn period, but it was still below the level usually found in phenylketonuric infants. Also, without treatment the phenylalanine concentration may drop to a level only two to three times the upper normal level. This condition is termed *hyperphenylalaninaemia*. Its incidence, cause, clinical significance, and treatment are debated. For the full-term young infant with a high blood level of phenylalanine, the safest treatment is probably a diet low in phenylalanine; if hyperphenylalaninaemia is suspected, trials with a normal diet are performed at shorter intervals than in an infant suspected of having true phenylketonuria.

Maple syrup disease
Symptoms usually start with convulsions and impaired general condition during the first few weeks of life. Most of the known untreated patients have died within a few months. The abnormal metabolites are excreted in the urine and give it an odour that resembles maple syrup. Metabolic studies have shown that the metabolism of the branched ketoacids, leucine, isoleucine, and valine, is disturbed. A diet has been constructed to prevent the accumulation of these amino acids. If the diet is started early the prognosis improves, but the treatment is difficult to continue and the ultimate prognosis is uncertain.

The abnormal metabolism of ketoacids can also occur in an intermittent form. Children with this type appear healthy and grow and develop normally. An infection may provoke the metabolic disorder, so that the child becomes seriously ill with vomiting, convulsions, and unconsciousness; the characteristic smell may also be noted. The abnormal metabolite can be identified in blood and urine collected during the episode, whereas investigation performed between attacks gives a normal result. The condition is rare but must be kept in mind if infections provoke disproportionately severe symptoms in a child. These children are not mentally retarded unless they have several serious attacks.

Tyrosinosis
In this disorder the normal metabolism of tyrosine is impaired. This causes generalized and usually severe disease with hepatic and renal impairment, rickets, a tendency to hypopotassaemia and, in many cases, disturbed cerebral function, which may lead to permanent mental retardation. The peripheral nervous system may occasionally be involved. The diagnosis is established by demonstrating an increased amount of tyrosine in the serum and urine. Both hypopotassaemia and rickets need urgent correction. The infant may benefit from an early-instituted diet low in both phenylalanine and tyrosine; this diet is, however, distasteful and it may be difficult to get the child to take it.

Homocystinuria
Patients with this disorder usually have a physical appearance similar to that seen in Marfan's syndrome. They have long thin arms and legs, spindle-like fingers and

toes, and low muscular tone, particularly distally (*Figure 5.2*). Skeletal abnormalities, particularly in the region of the knee and the vertebrae, are often present. The metabolic defect also seems to increase the coagulability of the blood; cortical thrombophlebitis may cause the acute onset of convulsions and neurological signs and is a possible cause of the permanent mental and neurological

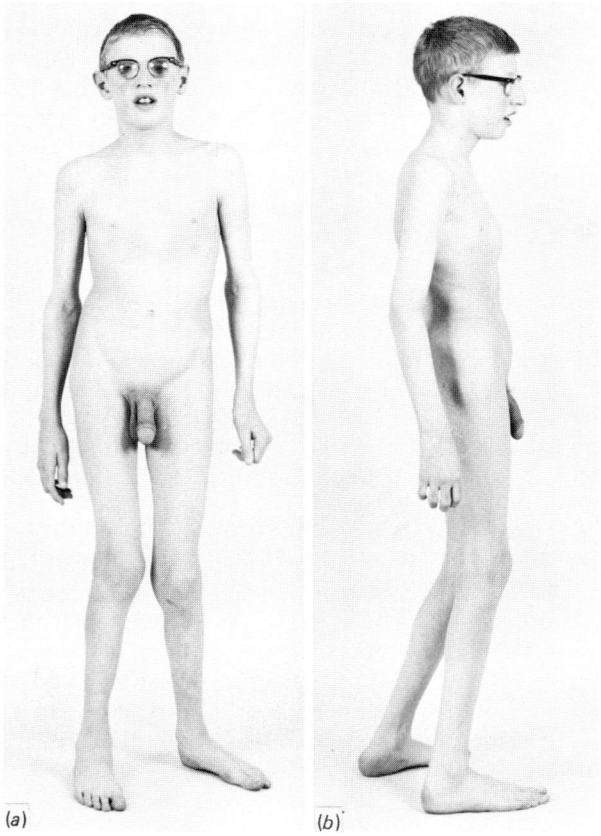

(a)   (b)

Figure 5.2. A 15-year-old boy with homocystinuria. Note the long slender fingers and toes

symptoms. Another common finding, the malar flush (*Figure 5.3*), may also be due to a vascular abnormality. The increased amount of homocystine excreted in the urine can be demonstrated on an amino acid chromatogram. The nitroprusside–cyanide test is a good screening test which is positive when increased amounts of homocystine or cystine are present.

The first described cases of homocystinuria were found through routine screening, with urinary acid chromatograms, of patients in institutions for the mentally retarded. It is therefore not surprising that mental retardation was originally considered a necessary part of the syndrome. However, the number of patients reported with this disorder is rapidly increasing, and several have now been found with normal intelligence; mental retardation may thus not be the result

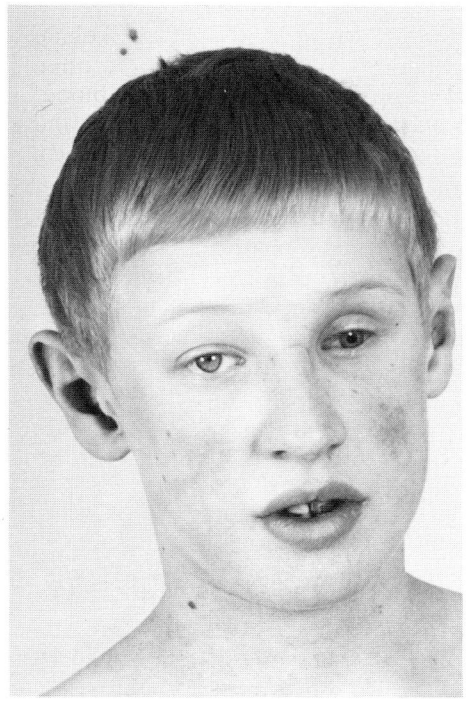

Figure 5.3. The face of a 15-year-old boy with homocystinuria. Note the malar flush

of the metabolic defect but may be due to the vascular complications. A diet that prevents the accumulation of homocystine, and which includes extra amounts of vitamin B$_6$, has been given with encouraging results.

Histidinaemia
In this disorder, speech often appears to be relatively more disturbed than the rest of the mental development, which is normal or at most moderately retarded. The level of histidine is increased in the blood and urine. Abnormal metabolites in the urine produce a positive Phenistix and ferric chloride reaction.

Other disorders
In *prolinaemia*, renal abnormalities have been reported, and in *hydroxyprolinaemia*, haematuria and eye abnormalities have been found. The relationship between the clinical symptoms and the metabolic defect remains uncertain. In *hyperlysinaemia, citrullinaemia*, and *arginosuccinic aciduria* the symptoms are episodes of vomiting, coma, and seizures starting in early infancy. The episodes are connected with a high level of ammonia in the blood. Patients seem to improve on a low-protein diet.

In *hyperglycinaemia* the symptoms are attacks of severe vomiting, associated with ketoacidosis. Thrombocytopenia and neutropenia may develop in patients surviving the first few months. Episodes of ketosis are usually provoked by infections later in the course. These episodes must be treated by intravenous fluids, glucose, and electrolytes to correct the metabolic acidosis. The best long-term treatment seems to be a low-protein diet with or without supplementary amino acids.

Patients have also been reported with increased *cystathionine* and *sarcosine* levels in the blood and urine. The relationship between clinical symptoms and the metabolic defect remains uncertain.

A massive general aminoaciduria is found in the oculocerebrorenal syndrome, *Lowe's syndrome*. This defect is inherited as a recessive sex-linked gene and only affects boys. Symptoms start in the newborn period with severe muscular hypotonia. Psychomotor development is retarded. The eye symptoms are cataracts and congenital glaucoma. The patients also have metabolic acidosis and rickets. There is no available treatment for the cerebral symptoms. The eye lesion responds poorly to most therapies; surgery is, however, often necessary. The metabolic defect can be corrected and the rickets healed by the administration of about 2000 units of vitamin D daily, together with alkali (e.g. calcium gluconate) in a dose of 25–50 mmol/day.

DISTURBED METABOLISM OF URIC ACID

The condition characterized by disturbed metabolism of uric acid, sometimes called infantile gout or Lesch–Nyhan syndrome, is inherited as a sex-linked recessive gene; only boys are affected. They usually show slow development from early infancy. Towards the end of the first year of life movement disorders, particularly choreoathetosis and spasticity, become apparent. These patients seem to have painful paraesthesia, which leads to self-destructive biting around the mouth and on the fingertips; slowly healing sores on the lips are therefore a characteristic feature. Pink urine and rusty spots on the nappy, due to haematuria, repeated urinary tract infections, and the passage of uric acid concrements are common and should alert the physician to the diagnosis of Lesch–Nyhan syndrome. A high urinary excretion of uric acid and a doubled serum level of uric acid are usually present and, if so, establish the diagnosis. However, since both levels may occasionally be normal the safest way to establish the diagnosis is to demonstrate the effect of the lack of the enzyme hypoxanthine-guanine phosphoribosyltransferase. When this enzyme is deficient, excess 5-phosphoribosyl-1-pyrophosphate is produced and can be demonstrated in cultivated fibroblasts, a technique which can also be used for prenatal diagnosis of the disorder. No effective treatment is known, but measures that lower the serum level of uric acid will improve the renal symptoms and may have a beneficial influence on the child's behaviour.

CARBOHYDRATE METABOLISM

In the disorders of carbohydrate metabolism, hypoglycaemia, galactosaemia, and fructose intolerance, convulsions are the dominating neurological symptom (*see* pages 100 and 102). Repeated attacks of hypoglycaemia, particularly together with anoxia, may cause permanent brain damage with mental retardation and often neurological signs. The screening procedure for galactosaemia and fructose intolerance is to test the urine for reducing substances (Clinitest); if this is positive and Clinistix (a test specific for glucose) is negative, urinary chromatography must be performed to identify the reducing substance. It is always imperative to determine blood glucose in convulsing children in order to reveal hypoglycaemia (*see* page 101).

MUCOPOLYSACCHARIDOSIS

Many conditions connected with the abnormal storage of acid mucopolysaccharides have been described; the number is steadily increasing. Hurler's syndrome, inherited as an autosomal recessive trait, and Hunter's syndrome, inherited as a sex-linked recessive trait, are both characterized by dwarfism; broad clumsy hands and feet; coarse features of the face (*Figure 5.4a*), hence the earlier term 'gargoylism'; a large protruding tongue; lumbar lordosis; flexion contractures of the knees and elbows; hepoatosplenomegaly; and hernias (*Figure 5.4b*). The head is

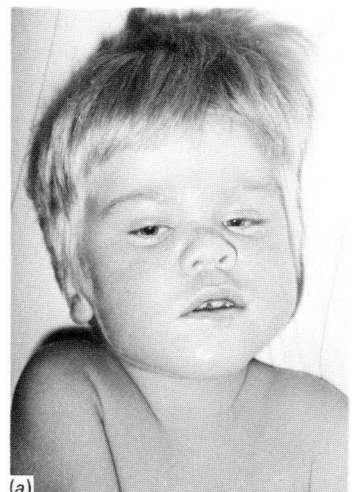 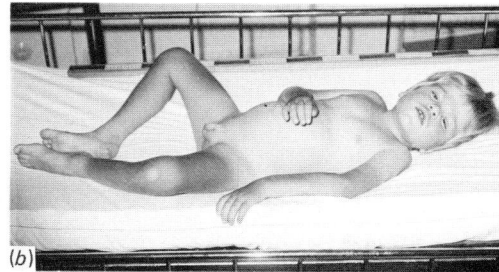

Figure 5.4. A 7-year-old boy with acid mucopolysaccharidosis (probably Hurler's syndrome) showing the typical facial features (*a*). Note contractures of the elbows and knees and the umbilical hernia (*b*)

often moderately enlarged, and a true hydrocephalus with increased intracranial pressure may complicate the clinical picture. On skull X-ray the sella turcica is found to be shallow with the form and appearance of a lying 'J' (*Figure 5.5*). Upper respiratory infections are common and a nasal discharge is an almost constant feature. All features become more pronounced and easier to recognize with increasing age of the patient.

Hurler's syndrome
This condition produces early severe symptoms. Cloudy corneas and cardiac involvement are seen in almost all patients. Death usually occurs within the first two decades from respiratory infection or cardiac failure.

Hunter's syndrome
These patients have normal corneas and only seldom have cardiac involvement. The skin may have an abnormal texture and resemble orange peel. These patients usually survive longer than those with the Hurler type.

   In both conditions, acid mucopolysaccharides are stored in the enlarged liver and spleen. The brain is usually also enlarged and contains a large amount of abnormal lipids. The histopathological picture of the brain is indistinguishable from that seen in lipidosis (*see* pags 295–299).

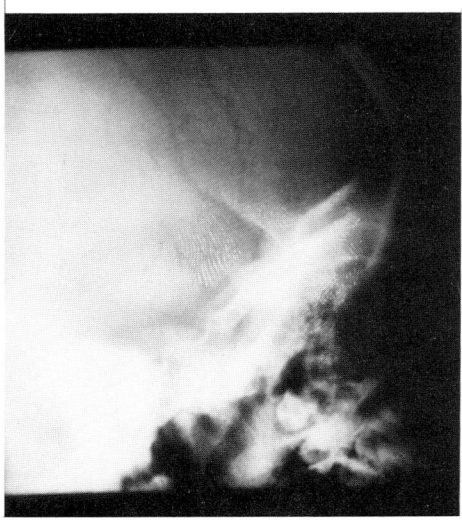

Figure 5.5. Skull X-ray of the boy shown in *Figure 5.4.* Note the shallow sella turcica, shaped like a lying J

Sanfilippo type
In the Sanfilippo condition the physical appearance of affected individuals is normal or almost normal. The mode of inheritance is autosomal recessive. The mental retardation is usually severe, but physical examination reveals no characteristic features. The neurological examination may be normal in early life, but during childhood the patients develop progressive neurological signs such as choreoathetosis and spasticity with severe contractures. Death usually occurs during childhood or adolescence.

Morquio–Ullrich type
This condition is inherited as an autosomal recessive trait. Affected persons are moderately retarded and show the same skeletal abnormalities, though usually milder, as those with the Hunter and Hurler syndromes. The liver and spleen are not enlarged. The disease is milder, and the patients live at least until adult age.

Scheie type
Here, the clinical picture is dominated by cloudiness of the cornea, whereas mental development is normal or almost normal, and other features of gargoylism are absent or mild. The mode of inheritance is probably autosomal recessive.

Other types of mucopolysaccharidosis have also been reported, with and without mental retardation. The feature that is common to all types is an increased urinary excretion of acid mucopolysaccharides, which can be demonstrated by chemical methods. The relative proportions of these abnormal metabolites seem to vary in the different clinical syndromes; they are probably caused by different metabolic disorders. At present no effective therapy is available for any of the mucopolysaccharidoses.

MANNOSIDOSIS

This syndrome is characterized by an appearance similar to that seen in Hunter's syndrome. Growth may be enhanced in infancy, but later becomes retarded. Head

. circumference may become abnormally large. The demonstration of an increased urinary excretion of mannoside establishes the diagnosis.

CRETINISM

Cretinism is the condition caused by congenital hypothyroidism. Children with untreated congenital hypothyroidism become mentally retarded dwarfs with typical facial features and a large protruding tongue (*see* page 388). A screening procedure, applicable to all newborn infants, is now available and used in many countries.

NEPHROGENIC DIABETES INSIPIDUS

This is a genetically determined disturbance of water and salt metabolism, characterized by lack of response of the kidneys to the antidiuretic hormone of the hypophysis. A sex-linked recessive inheritance is assumed, as mainly male infants are affected. It has its onset in early infancy, and the symptoms are attacks of restlessness, vomiting, constipation, and high fever due to dehydration. If the condition is untreated, the patient grows slowly and becomes physically and mentally retarded. With increasing age the child is better able to demonstrate his thirst, and the diagnosis is then easier to suspect than in the young infant, but by this time permanent brain damage has already occurred.

The diagnosis is established by depriving the child of fluid for a few hours under close supervision, with repeated measurements of temperature, body weight, urinary output and osmolarity, and serum electrolytes. In a child with diabetes insipidus signs of dehydration appear within a few hours, body weight decreases, temperature increases, and serum electrolytes rise, whereas urinary osmolarity remains low. As soon as these signs appear, the test must be interrupted to avoid provoking a dangerous state of dehydration. The Pitressin test is used to distinguish diabetes insipidus due to lack of antidiuretic hormone from diabetes insipidus due to lack of *response* to the hormone (nephrogenic diabetes insipidus).

The treatment of nephrogenic diabetes insipidus consists of feeding the infant a diet low in protein (1–2 g protein/kg per day) and in salt and giving him an abundant amount of fluids, both day and night. To ensure normal physical and mental development it is particularly important that this regimen is adhered to during the child's first 3 years. Chlorothiazide 50 mg/kg per day decreases the volume of the urine and increases its osmolarity. An acute attack of severe dehydration is treated with 2.5–3 per cent dextrose in water, intravenously; pure water is given by mouth, as soon as the patient is able to take it.

The prognosis is poor unless the diagnosis is established early and vigorous treatment is started immediately. Death during an attack of acute dehydration has been reported in several patients. The brain damage that occurs in untreated children during their first years is permanent in surviving patients.

'Syndromes'

A constellation of mental retardation and certain physical features characterizes the syndromes to be discussed here. Mucopolysaccharidosis and cretinism could also be described under this heading, but as the general outline of the metabolic defect in these syndromes is known, they have been included in the previous group. In some of the 'syndromes' a chromosomal aberration has been reported; in others the aetiology remains entirely unknown.

CHROMOSOMAL ABERRATIONS

Down's syndrome or mongolism

This is a common cause of mental retardation, occurring in approximately 1 in 600 newborn infants. Common physical features include low birth-weight, short stature, a round face with slanting eyes and epicanthus (*Figure 5.6a and b*), whitish spots in the iris, small flat back of the head, short neck, short broad hands and feet with simian crease on the palms of the hands (*Figure 5.6c*) and a 'sandal gap' between the big toe and the second toe on the foot, other primitive abnormalities of

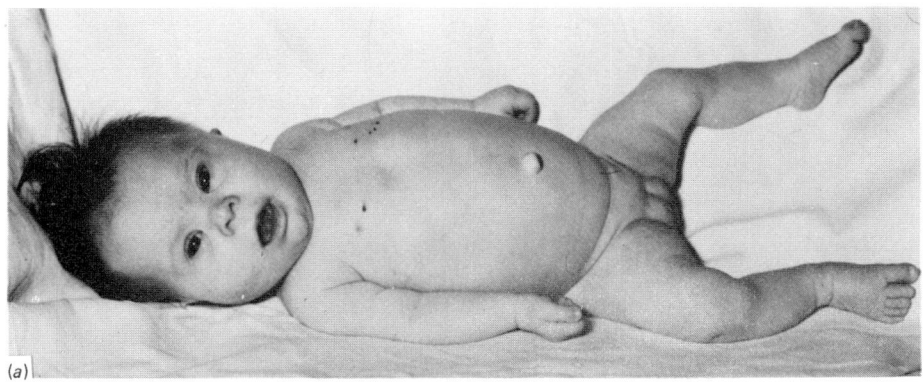

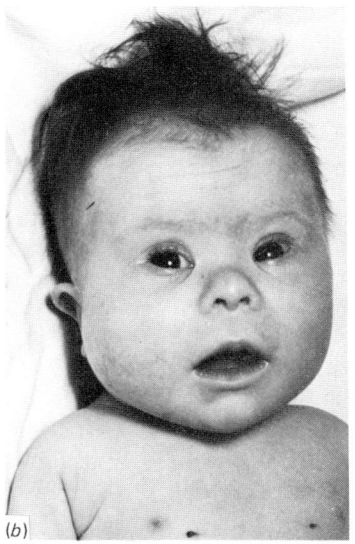
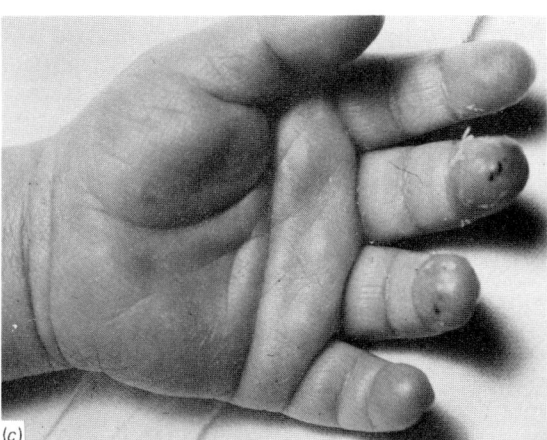

Figure 5.6a, b and c. A 4-month-old girl with Down's syndrome

the pattern of lines on the hands and feet, soft skin, and severe muscular hypotonia. Many more features could be mentioned as characteristic of Down's syndrome; all features are never seen in the same patient. Several of the features may be present in other mentally retarded patients and occasionally also in normal individuals. The newborn mongoloid is often apathetic and has feeding difficulties and sluggish neonatal reflexes. In the diagnosis of Down's syndrome the general impression is even more important than isolated features. Other somatic malformations are common in Down's syndrome. The two most often seen are cardiac malformation and duodenal atresia.

All children with Down's syndrome are mentally retarded. Thus this is a situation in which a diagnosis of mental retardation can be established in a very young infant. There is, however, a great variability in the mental development of children with Down's syndrome from a very low level to a level at which the child can greatly benefit from education in a special school. Almost all mongoloid children learn to walk unassisted (*Figure 5.7*), although they may not pass this milestone until 3–4 years of age. As a rule they learn to speak, although their vocabulary remains small and their articulation poor. Most mongoloid children are pleasant, playful, fondling children, who like to follow and imitate adults; they are therefore often easier to train than other children mentally retarded to the same degree. Individuals with Down's syndrome show a progressive dementia which usually becomes apparent as they approach the age of 40. The morphological abnormalities in the brain, usually already obvious before the age of 20, are identical with those seen in Alzheimer's presenile dementia.

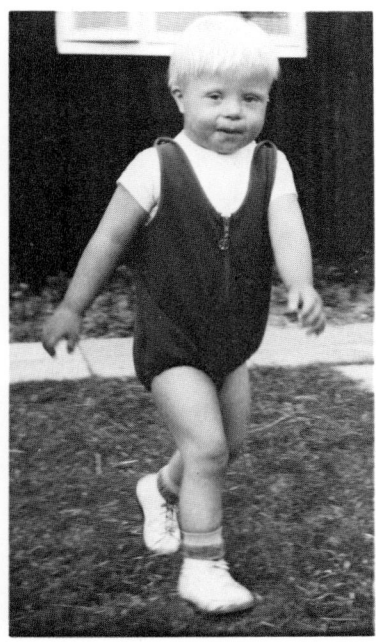

Figure 5.7. A 3-year-old boy with Down's syndrome

In 1959 a chromosomal aberration was described in Down's syndrome: an extra amount of chromosomal material, corresponding to one of the smallest autosomes, was demonstrated. The extra chromosomal material was later identified as chromosome 21, and the common finding is thus trisomy 21. *Figure 5.8a* shows the karyotype of a healthy girl and *Figure 5.8b* the karyotype of a girl with Down's syndrome. Occasionally the extra chromosome is attached to one of the large chromosomes, usually in the group 13–15. These children thus have a normal *number* of chromosomes but the *total chromosome mass* is the same as in trisomic mongoloids, from whom they are clinically indistinguishable. The large *transloca-tion chromosome,* which consists of one chromosome from the 13–15 group and chromosome 21, is often also found in the mother, who then lacks chromosome 21. She thus has only 45 chromosomes but a normal total chromosome mass. The statistical risk of such a mother having another mongoloid child is about 30 per cent, whereas the risk for the mother of a trisomic mongoloid is less than 2 per cent and only insignificantly higher than for any woman of the same age. The likely

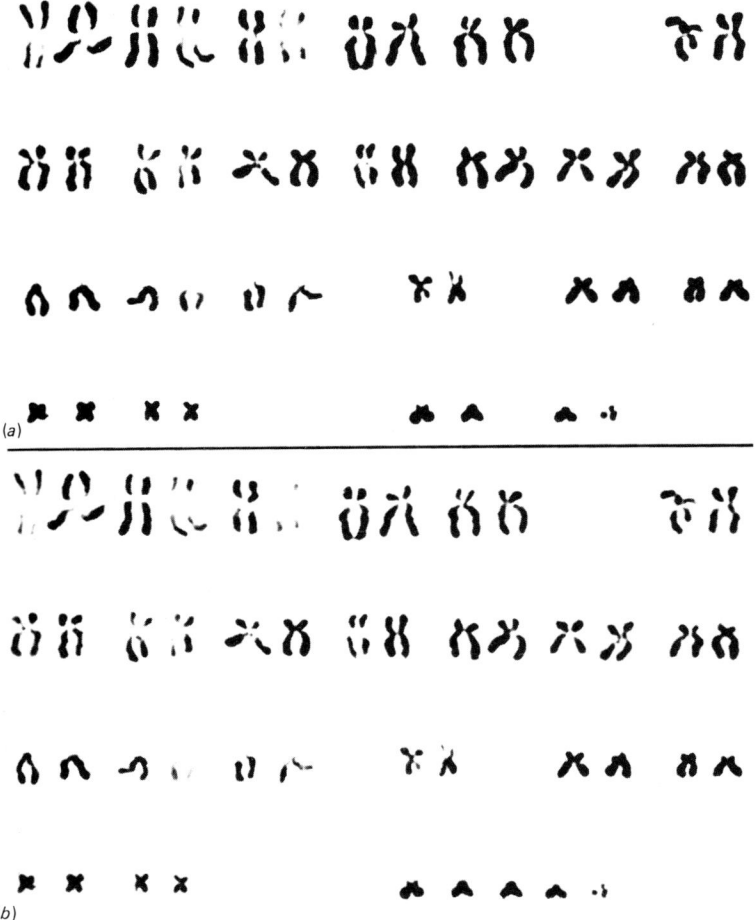

Figure 5.8. The karyotype of an apparently healthy girl (*a*) and of a girl with Down's syndrome (*b*)

translocation between the extra chromosome and a normal chromosome 21 has also been reported. A distinction between Down's syndrome due to trisomy and to translocation has no significance for the diagnosis or prognosis of the child; it is, however, of vital importance for the family who requests genetic counselling as to the risk of more mongoloids being born into the family.

Not all somatic cells of an individual necessarily contain the same number of chromosomes. The term *mosaicism* is used when the number of chromosomes varies in different cells of the same individual. Mosaicism with normal cells and cells with trisomy 21 has been found in a number of individuals with some features of mongolism. The clinical picture varies within this group from practically normal individuals to typical mongoloids. Patients within this group are often difficult to diagnose clinically as mongoloids, and are not all mentally retarded.

Patients have been reported with the chromosomal aberration trisomy 21 but without the physical features of Down's syndrome. Clinically typical mongoloids with an apparently normal number, size, and shape of chromosomes have also been described. The significance of the latter finding can always be debated, as it is impossible to exclude the presence of mosaicism. Down's syndrome is a clinical diagnosis based on the presence of mental retardation and certain physical features; most mongoloids have extra chromosomal material corresponding to chromosome 21.

No treatment is known for Down's syndrome. Prenatal diagnosis, based on analysis of the chromosomes in the amniotic fluid, and legal abortion, if the chromosomal aberration is detected, is at present the only way to prevent the birth of children with Down's syndrome. The risk of the birth of a mongoloid child is increased in two situations:

1. The family who already has a child with Down's syndrome due to a translocation chromosome; in this situation the risk of another mongoloid child being born into the family is high.
2. The incidence of Down's syndrome increases with the age of the mother; however, even for a woman around 45 years of age, it is only 2 per cent.

Trisomy for chromosomes 16–18 and 13–15
Such chromosomal aberrations have also been reported as distinguishable syndromes. These infants are small for dates at birth, develop slowly both physically and mentally, and generally have several somatic defects, e.g. malformation of the eyes, heart, and feet. Most affected individuals die during early infancy, thus the problem of mental retardation does not arise.

'Cri-du-chat' syndrome
In this syndrome one of the short arms of chromosome 5 is absent. Children with this condition are small at birth and grow and develop slowly. They are microcephalic, have a small roundish face with low-set ears, and often have slanting eyes and a squint; their muscles are usually hypotonic. The facial features may, however, be almost normal (*Figure 5.9*). The syndrome gets its name from the patient's typical high-pitched cry, which sounds like the cry of a kitten. Many patients seem to survive infancy and may be found among children with severe mental retardation.

Other autosomal aberrations
Isolated cases of several other autosomal aberrations have been described. Common to them all are severe mental retardation combined with physical signs such as peculiar facial features, low-set ears, and malformation of the brain, eyes, and inner organs of variable severity. Generally speaking, a loss of autosomal material appears more dangerous than an excess. The severity of the clinical syndrome that results from an excess of autosomal material appears to be better related to the quantity of this material than to which chromosome or part of a chromosome is duplicated.

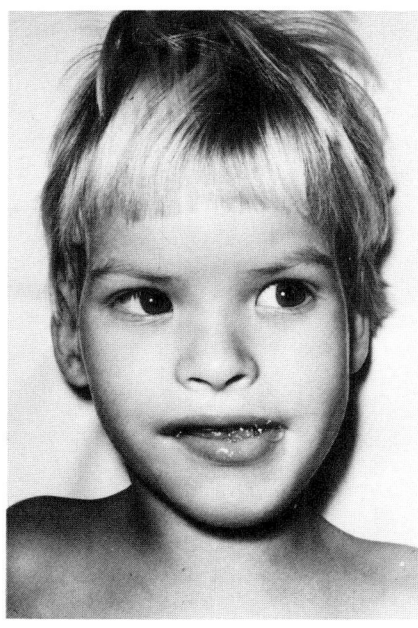

Figure 5.9. The face of a 3-year-old girl with the 'cri-du-chat' syndrome

The *sex chromosomes* may also show abnormalities which, generally speaking, seem to have less serious effects on the individual than autosomal aberrations.

XO syndrome
Individuals with the XO syndrome have a normal female appearance before puberty. As infants they may have a peculiar lymphoedema of the hands and feet and abundant neck skin (the *Bonnevie–Ullrich* syndrome), which, however, is also seen very occasionally in infants with apparently normal X chromosomes. The ovaries are usually absent and replaced by streaks of fibrous tissue. This syndrome of *ovarian agenesis,* which may also occur when both X chromosomes are present and one of them shows structural abnormalities, or, rarely, in individuals with two normal X chromosomes, is called *Turner's syndrome.* Girls with Turner's syndrome are usually already short of stature in childhood (*Figure 5.10a*). As these patients lack the prepubertal growth spurt, their short stature becomes more obvious in adulthood. Secondary sex characters do not develop. The patients often have pterygium colli and a low broad hairline (*Figure 5.10b*); they may have other malformations such as coarctation of the aorta, malformation of the urinary tract, and impaired hearing.

Most girls with Turner's syndrome have an intelligence slightly below normal or within the low normal range. Severe mental retardation is an exception, and high intelligence may be seen. It is difficult to influence the patients' short stature. Endocrine treatment can aid the development of secondary sex characters, which may help their psychological adjustment. No other therapy is available.

XXY syndrome
Most XXY individuals are apparently normal boys at birth and during childhood. At puberty many develop the typical features of the *Klinefelter syndrome,* which is often, though not invariably, connected with the XXY abnormality. The typical

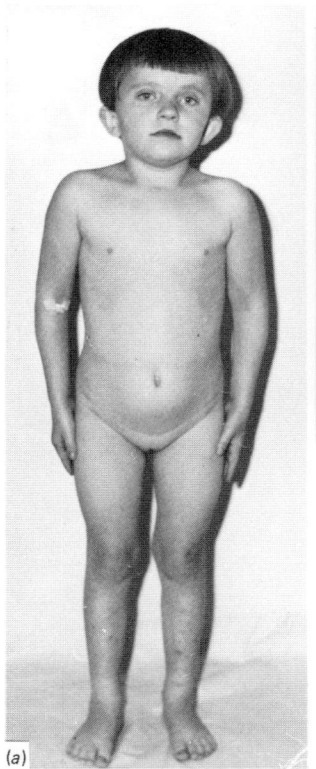
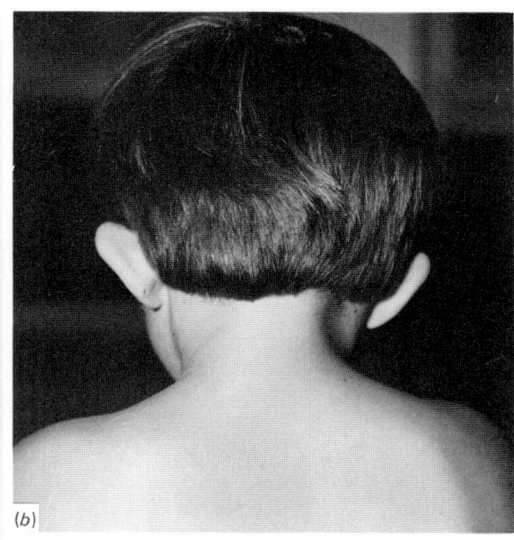

Figure 5.10. A 9-year-old girl with Turner's syndrome (XO), height 110 cm (*a*). Note the low broad hairline (*b*)

features of this syndrome are eunuchoid body proportions with long arms and legs, small underdeveloped testes, and gynaecomastia. Many XXY boys have normal mental development, but there is an over-representation of slightly retarded individuals and perhaps even more of those showing poor adjustment. Endocrine treatment at or shortly before puberty will diminish the physical signs of the Klinefelter syndrome and may also improve the patients' mental adjustment. No other therapy is available.

The XYY karyotype has been reported in a few remarkably tall men with aggressive behaviour. Most known cases of the XYY karyotype, however, have been entirely normal men.

XXX syndrome
Females with the XXX syndrome may be entirely normal, both in physical appearance and mental development. There is, however, an over-representation of mentally retarded individuals and also of patients with convulsions. External features may vary but are seldom grossly abnormal.

Individuals with more than three sex chromosomes
The XXYY karyotype has been reported in some men with the clinical picture of the Klinefelter syndrome. Males with the XXXY syndrome and individuals with more than three X chromosomes are known, both with a Y chromosome and apparently males (*Figure 5.11*), and without a Y chromosome and apparently

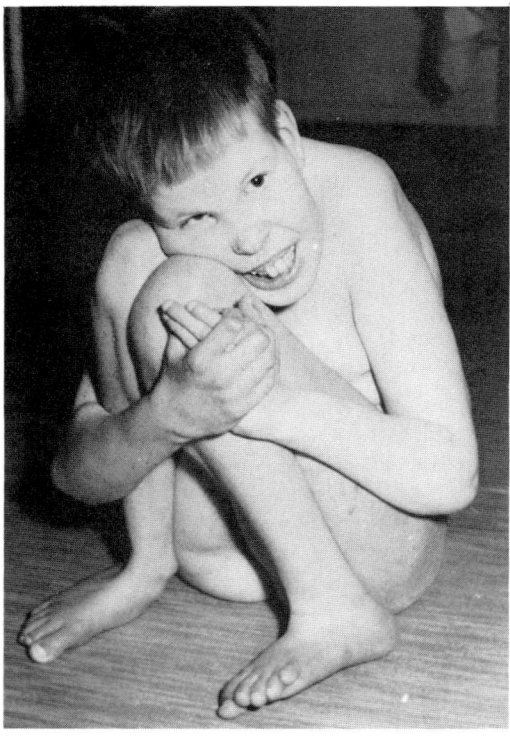

Figure 5.11. A 13-year-old boy with the XXXXY karyotype

females. Most of these patients have severe mental retardation together with various somatic defects; some of them have an external appearance similar to mongolism. Malformations of the genitalia are common (*Figure 5.12*). The severity of both mental and physical symptoms usually increases with increasing number of X chromosomes. Some patients with these severe X-chromosomal aberrations may be found in institutions for mentally retarded individuals. Mosaicism may modify the clinical picture.

Fragile-X-syndrome
A structural abnormality localized to the long arm of the X chromosome (site Xq 28) has been identified in some boys with moderate to severe mental retardation.

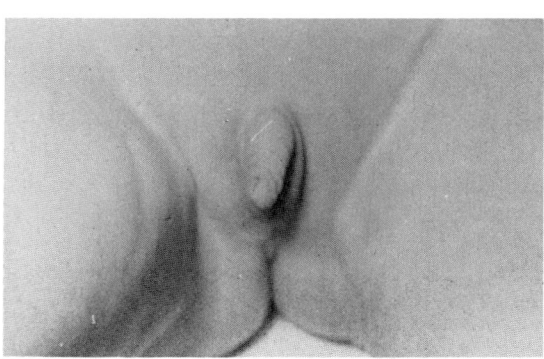

Figure 5.12. Underdeveloped genitalia of the boy shown in *Figure 5.11*

Several of these boys also show abnormally large genitalia (apparent after puberty), and unusually large ears and hands. The female carriers of this marker X may also be identified by chromosomal analysis; most of them have normal mental development, but some show mild mental retardation.

'SYNDROMES' WITH NO DEMONSTRABLE CHROMOSOMAL ABERRATION

Cornelia de Lange syndrome

This syndrome was described in 1933. Its cause is not known; inheritance and chromosomal aberrations have been discussed but none have been proved.

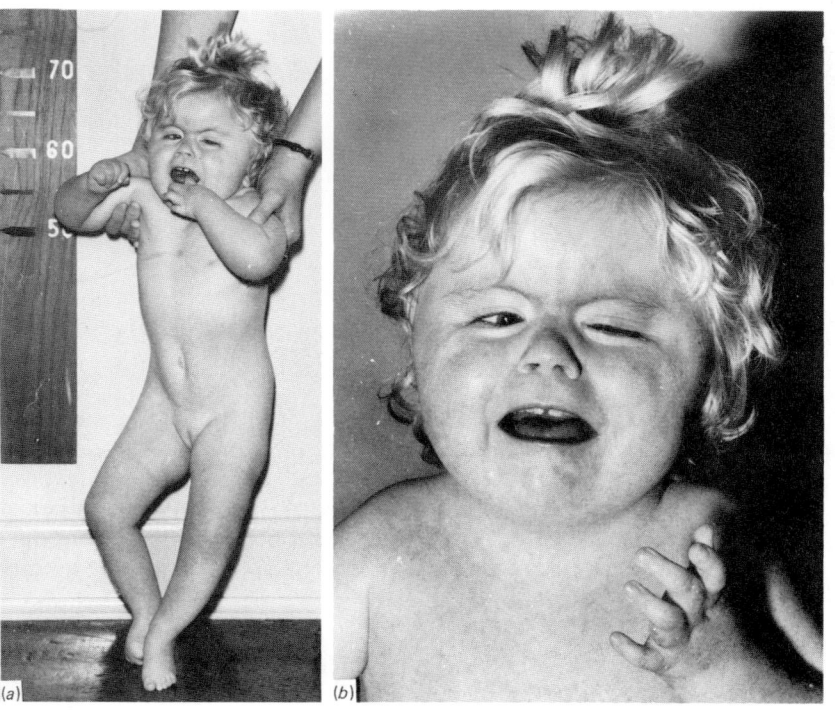

Figure 5.13. A 5-year-old girl with Cornelia de Lange syndrome (Amsterdam dwarf). Note the short stature and the child's inability to stand (*a*) and the characteristic facial features, particularly the eyebrows which meet in the midline and grow down as a tuft of hair on the nose (*b*)

At birth, affected children are small for dates and have a peculiar appearance, which becomes more obvious with increasing growth of the child. The children remain short of stature (*Figure 5.13a*) and usually thin. They have a small head and a peculiar face with marked eyebrows which meet in the midline and often grow down as a tuft of hair on the bridge of the nose (*Figure 5.13b*). The hairline is low on the face. General hirsutism, most marked on the back, is common. The hands and feet are small and thin and have primitive lines. Malformations of the upper extremities are common (*Figure 5.14*). The cry is often hoarse, and mental development is severely retarded. No treatment is known.

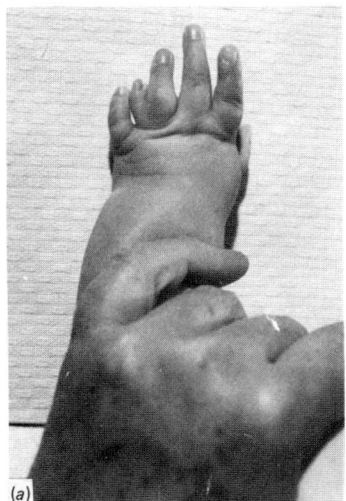 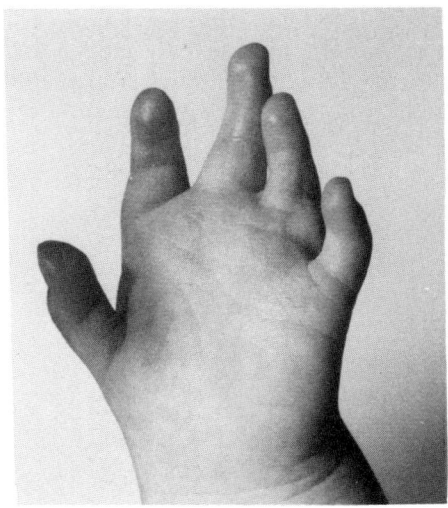

Figure 5.14. The right hand of the girl shown in *Figure 5.13,* before (*a*) and after (*b*) surgical removal of an extra finger

Elfin face syndrome

This is characterized by short stature, a broad forehead, curly hair, heavy cheeks, hypertelorism, and pouting lips (*Figure 5.15*). Squint is a common finding. Another feature of this syndrome is cardiac abnormalities, which consist of a supravalvular aortic stenosis often combined with peripheral pulmonary stenosis. These abnormalities may not be present at birth but develop during the first years of life. In some patients the history suggests the presence of hypercalcaemia during this period (*see* page 129). Autosomal recessive inheritance is a possible aetiology of the disorder. No effective treatment is known, once the mental retardation is established. The cardiac disorder can be corrected surgically.

Laurence–Moon–Biedl syndrome

This is inherited as an autosomal recessive trait. Children with this syndrome may be normal at birth, but most of them have an abnormality of the hands and feet, usually six fingers and toes. During childhood it becomes apparent that their mental development is, as a rule, mildly or moderately retarded. They can usually go to school, although most of them need special education. Their physical development is also retarded; they are short of stature and have a late puberty, during which secondary sex characters develop poorly. The patients are usually obese (*Figure 5.16*). Another cardinal symptom is retinitis pigmentosa which may cause poor vision, particularly in darkness, even in childhood; however, at this age it is usually discovered only on direct examination for this feature. Other eye abnormalities, such as a squint or opacities of the lens or cornea, may be present; some kind of eye abnormality is almost obligatory for the diagnosis. In many cases the extra fingers and toes have already been removed in the newborn period, perhaps even without the mother being aware of it. One should therefore always look for and feel for a scar on the ulnar side of the hand and the fibular side of the foot, as these are common sites for the extra finger and toe respectively.

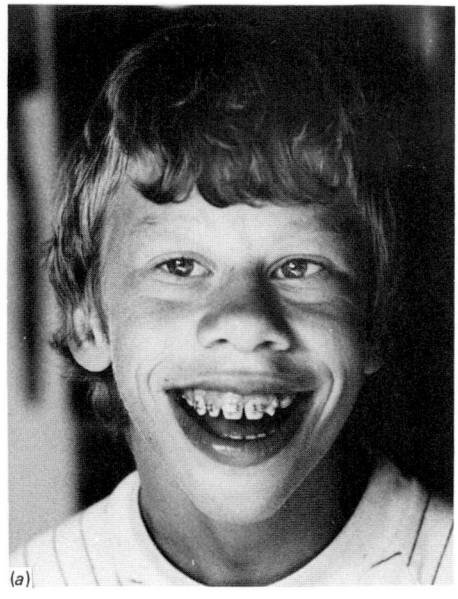

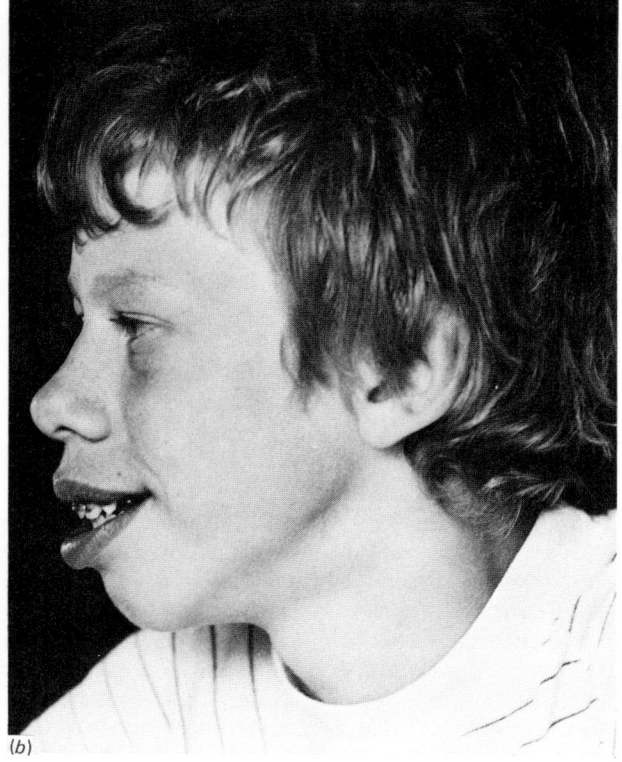

Figure 5.15a and *b*. A 15-year-old boy with the elfin face syndrome

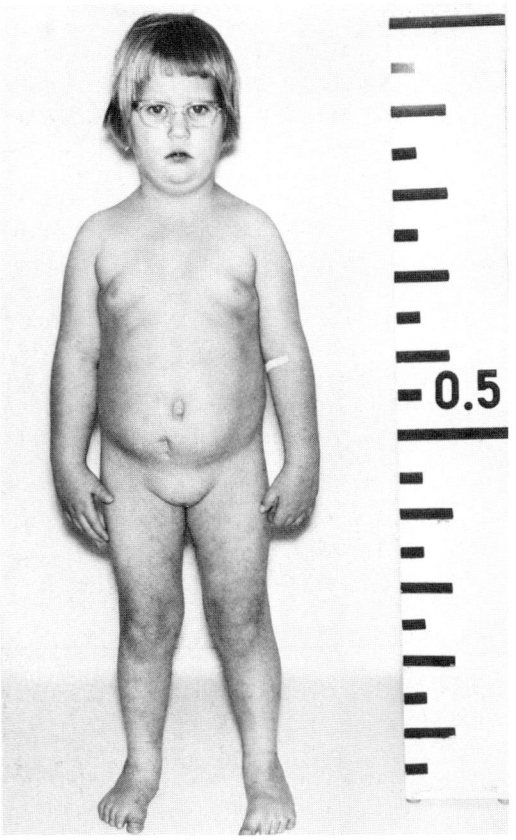

Figure 5.16. A 6-year-old girl with Laurence–Moon–Biedl syndrome. Note particularly the shape and position of the left foot where an extra toe has been removed on the fibular side

The diagnosis is established on the basis of the constellation of mental retardation, short stature, obesity, delayed puberty, six fingers and toes, and eye abnormalities, usually retinitis pigmentosa. There are no characteristic laboratory findings; tests of thyroid function, in particular, are usually normal. At and after puberty the patient may obtain some benefit from treatment with sex hormones; other than this no therapy is known.

Prader–Willi syndrome
The dominating symptom of this disorder is severe muscular hypotonia in early childhood, which is so severe that disease of the lower motor neurones or the muscles is often suspected (*see* page 158).

Myotonic dystrophy
In myotonic dystrophy with onset in infancy, the early dominating symptoms and signs are severe muscular hypotonia, bilateral facial weakness, feeding difficulties, and slow psychomotor development (*see* page 194).

Syndrome described by Sjögren and Larsson
This is inherited as an autosomal recessive trait. It is characterized by mental retardation, ichthyosis, and spastic paraplegia. No characteristic laboratory findings are known; the diagnosis is based on the clinical constellation. No therapy is available.

Rubinstein–Taybi syndrome
This syndrome is characterized by moderate to severe mental retardation, unusually broad thumbs and toes, and characteristic facial features. The thumbs are disproportionately broad in relation to the size of the hands; the distal phalanx, in particular, is short and broad with a flat nail. The big toes are broad and enlarged (*Figure 5.17a*). The characteristic facial features are an antimongoloid slant of the eyes, strabismus, and a prominent beaked nose (*Figures 5.17b* and *5.17c*). The palate is high-arched. Allergic manifestations and recurrent respiratory infections are common. The cause of the syndrome is unknown, and no therapy is available.

Other syndromes
In the phacomatoses *Sturge–Weber syndrome* and *tuberous sclerosis*, mental retardation is a characteristic feature; convulsions are a dominating symptom (*see* page 97). *Gargoylism* and *cretinism* are described on pages 135 and 388. *Microcephaly* as an inherited defect is described on page 236.

Plan of examination in cases of mental retardation

HISTORY

The history must include a family history, events that occurred during the pregnancy, and complications that occurred during delivery or the neonatal period. Whenever possible, the duration of the pregnancy should be estimated (*see* page 2). The developmental history must be taken carefully, always attempting to establish whether or not the patient's neurological and mental symptoms and signs are progressive.

GENERAL PHYSICAL EXAMINATION

The general physical examination must be detailed in order to reveal such features as impaired growth and physical development, a peculiar appearance of the face, low-set ears, abnormal hands and feet, the small scar after removal of an extra finger or toe, cardiac abnormalities, hepatosplenomegaly, or skeletal abnormalities. The smell of sweat and urine should also be noted.

NEUROLOGICAL EXAMINATION

A complete neurological examination, as outlined in Chapter 2, should be performed. It must include careful examination of vision and hearing, as the mental development of a child may be disturbed by defects of the sensory organs, and thus he may be misdiagnosed as mentally retarded. It is also important to detect impaired vision and hearing in a mentally retarded child, as such defects may in some cases provide a clue to the cause of the mental retardation and must in all cases influence the training programme.

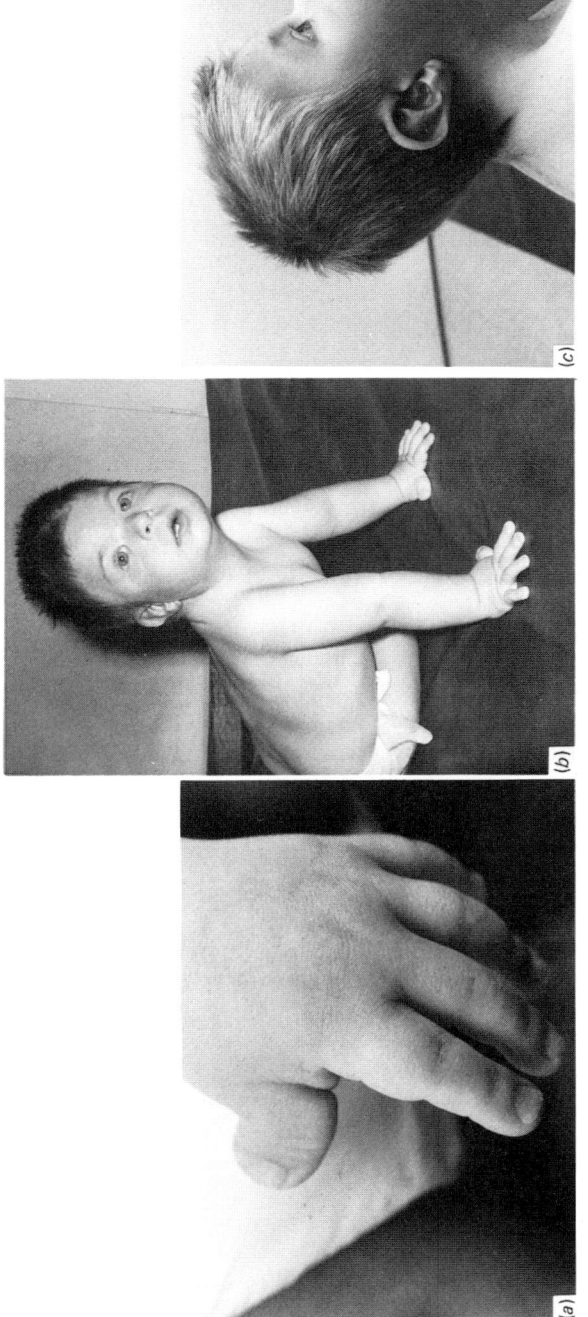

Figure 5.17. A 10-month-old boy with Rubinstein–Taybi syndrome, showing the broad flat nails, particularly on the thumb, and the 'hitch-hiking thumb' (*a*) and the typical facial features (*b* and *c*)

PSYCHOLOGICAL TESTING, NEUROPHYSIOLOGICAL METHODS

Psychological testing should preferably be performed on children with definite or suspected mental retardation. This may reveal that the child has not true retardation but has instead a 'pseudoretardation' due to emotional factors, which requires a different diagnostic and therapeutic approach from a true retardation. It is also important to estimate the patient's level of development and the possible presence of other learning difficulties in order to give advice on the best method of training the child.

An electroencephalographic examination is of value in most children with mental retardation of unknown origin, particularly if the child also has convulsions (*see* Chapter 4). Electroencephalography cannot be used to estimate the child's mental maturation. Occasionally the latency between a visual or auditory stimulus and the evoked response recorded from the brain (visually evoked potential or auditory evoked potential) may be used as a crude estimate of the maturation of these pathways in the brain. Focal spike discharge will usually suggest scarring following an early brain lesion. A severe generalized disorder, on the other hand, suggests a metabolic cause or the acute phase of a brain disease. In simple inherited mental retardation and conditions such as Down's syndrome, the EEG is usually either normal or shows unspecific generalized slowing.

NEURORADIOLOGICAL EXAMINATIONS

These methods will give an estimate of the anatomy of the brain and are particularly useful when a neurosurgically accessible lesion, such as hydrocephalus, subdural hygroma, intracranial bleeding, a cyst, or a brain tumour, is suspected. The use of these methods is justified to demonstrate the presence and extent of a lesion, even when it cannot be treated, since an established cause of the child's handicap is always of great value to the parents. In infants with an open fontanelle, particularly the newborn, ultrasound examination of the skull is the method of choice, as it usually gives good information about the intracranial structures and does not disturb the infant. In slightly older children, and when more detailed information about intracranial structures is needed, e.g. if a tumour is suspected, computerized tomography of the skull is the method of choice. A young child or a mentally retarded child may require sedation for this procedure, but it causes no pain and involves no risk; it may thus be used for a wide range of indications.

METABOLIC EXAMINATIONS

In many countries all newborn babies are screened by means of a blood test drawn during the first week of life, which thus allows the diagnosis of a metabolic disorder before any symptoms are apparent. At present in Sweden, screening is performed for hypothyroidism, phenylketonuria, and galactosaemia. If routine screening has not been carried out, such tests must be performed on all mentally handicapped children. The treatment for these conditions is more effective the earlier it is started (preferably before symptoms are apparent); these conditions must therefore be positively excluded.

Amino acid chromatography of the urine and determination of the urinary excretion of organic acids should be performed for a wide range of indications, particularly if more than one member of a sibship is affected. The mother's urine should also be tested. She may have an undiagnosed metabolic disorder, e.g.

phenylketonuria, and the toxic products may harm her otherwise healthy fetus. In some of the metabolic disorders, e.g. galactosaemia, the enzyme defect can be demonstrated in the blood cells; this is also possible in some of the disorders causing progressive mental and neurological symptoms and signs (*see* Chapter 13). The urinary excretion of acid mucopolysaccharides and oligosaccharides should also be determined. Some of these metabolic disorders produce obvious clinical symptoms and signs, whereas others are impossible to diagnose without chemical investigations. In boys, nephrogenic diabetes insipidus (inability to concentrate the urine in spite of dehydration, i.e. no response to antidiuretic hormone) and Lesch–Nyhan syndrome (increased blood level of urid acid) must also be considered and the appropriate tests performed.

EXAMINATION OF THE SPINAL FLUID

The spinal fluid should be examined, in particular for protein content, and especially in patients in whom slowly progressive symptoms cannot be excluded. Intracranial extracerebral tumours (*see* page 368) may produce an increased spinal fluid protein. This may occasionally also be seen in subdural hygromas. In all types of leucodystrophy (*see* page 301) the spinal fluid protein is high; in this situation electrophoresis of the spinal fluid protein may be helpful.

CHROMOSOMAL STUDIES

Chromosomal studies are particularly indicated in children who are small for dates at birth and have a head size in proportion to the body, peculiar dysplastic facial features, broad hands and feet with a primitive line pattern on the palm of the hand and the sole of the foot, a low broad hairline on the neck, and malformations of inner organs. Another indication for chromosomal studies is abnormalities of the genitalia, such as unusually large or small genitalia; the latter situation is usually combined with late puberty. Fragile X must be asked for specifically. New methods for staining chromosomes are in rapid development, thus the possibility of identifying chromosomal abnormalities is increasing. The diagnosis of a chromosomal aberration does not influence the treatment of the child. Clinically, there is no way of excluding the possibility of a chromosomal aberration, unless another definite cause of the mental retardation has been established. The diagnosis of a chromosomal aberration may give information about the risk of mental retardation occurring in following children in the family and in certain instances will allow prenatal diagnosis during a later pregnancy. A proven cause for the child's handicap is of great value to the parents, even when it does not influence the child's treatment.

Treatment

The disorders that cause mental retardation are only rarely responsive to medical treatment; prophylactic measures are effective in some of them, provided they are diagnosed before they have caused any permanent damage. The possibilities for treatment and prophylaxis have been discussed in the review of the different causes of mental retardation (*see* pages 128–134). Well planned and individually adapted antiepileptic treatment (*see* Chapter 4) may also have a favourable influence on the child's mental development, particularly if the mentally retarded child has convulsions which are brought under control; a beneficial effect may also very occasionally be seen in a child who has no convulsions.

The treatment of the symptom, mental retardation, is mainly a psychological and pedagogic problem; the aim is to find the best way to stimulate and teach the child. As most mentally retarded children also have poor maturation of motor skill, the physiotherapist is of great help in the training. The natural coordinator of all this activity is a paediatrician trained in developmental disorders and their habilitation. The approach must be realistic, based on the individual's ability and limitations, and the goal is to develop this ability as far as possible, particularly in a way that will be useful in the daily life of the child.

Stimulating surroundings are even more important for the development of the mentally retarded child than for the normal child. The child must be talked to, played with, and taught to do things himself as much as possible and not be helped with everything. For the young child, such stimulating surroundings are usually better provided in the home than in an institution. From the age of 3–4 years it is important for most children with mental retardation to be taught by someone outside the family and to have daily contact with children of the same age. This can often be achieved by sending the child to a day nursery for normal children, where he has a special assistant for his training. Daily contact with normal children of the same age is most important for his development, but to get as much as possible out of the day nursery he must also have physiotherapy and special teaching, which may be delivered under guidance by his assistant. Individually adapted teaching must be started as early as possible; it is a great disadvantage to the mentally retarded child to be kept at home without any training during all his preschool years and perhaps even to have the start of school delayed for a year or two. The decisions as to whether and at what age the child should be sent to an institution must be made individually, as it will depend on the child, the family, and the institution. It is just as bad to recommend that all parents send their retarded children to an institution as early as possible as it is to force all parents to keep their children at home, if they there become isolated and untaught, if it is obviously too much for parents, or if it destroys family life for other children in the family. Parents of mentally retarded children are liable to develop guilt feelings; the adviser must be aware of this tendency and try to prevent it.

References

AICARDI, J. and GOUTIÈRES, F. (1981) The syndrome of absence of the septum pellucidum with porencephalies and other developmental defects. *Neuropediatrics*, **12**, 319–329

ANNEREN, G. (1984) Down's syndrome. A metabolic and endocrinological study. Acta Universitatis Upsaliensis, Dissertations from the Faculty of Medicine No 483, Uppsala. Reprocentralen HSC

ANTIA, A. V., WILTSE, H. E., ROWE, R. D., PITT, E. L., LEVIN, S., OTTESEN, O. E. *et al.* (1967) Pathogenesis of the supravalvular aortic stenosis syndrome. *Journal of Pediatrics*, **71**, 431–441

BERATIS, N. G., HSU, L. Y. F. and HIRSHHORN, H. (1971) Familial de Lange syndrome; report of three cases in a sibship. *Clinical Genetics*, **2**, 170–176

BLOMQUIST, H. K., GUSTAVSSON, K.-H. and HOLMGREN, G. (1981) Mild mental retardation in children in a northern Swedish county. *Journal of Mental Deficiency Research*, **25**, 169–186

CHRISTIE, R., BAY, C., KAUFMAN, I. A., BAKAY, B., BORDEN, M. and NYHAN, W. L. (1982) Lesch–Nyhan disease: Clinical experience with nineteen patients. *Developmental Medicine and Child Neurology*, **24**, 293–306

DUNN, H. G., PERRY, T. L. and DOLMAN, C. L. (1966) Homocystinuria. *Neurology* (Minneapolis), **16**, 407–420

DYGGVE, H. V., MELCHIOR, J. C. and CLAUSEN, J. (1981) The Dyggve–Melchior–Clausen syndrome. Follow-up and survey of present literature. In *Frontiers of Knowledge in Mental Retardation*, vol. **2**, pp. 251–259, Ed. Peter Mittler. Baltimore: The University Park Press

GUSTAVSSON, K.-H., HOLMGREN, G., JONSELL, R. and BLOMQUIST, H. K. (1977) Severe mental retardation in children in a northern Swedish county. *Journal of Mental Deficiency Research*, **21**, 161–180

HAGBERG, B. (1978) Severe mental retardation in Swedish children born 1959–1970; epidemiological panorama and causative factors. *Major Mental Handicap: Methods and Costs of Prevention*. Ciba Foundation symposium 59 (new series), pp. 29–51

HAGBERG, B., HAGBERG, G., LEWERTH, A. and LINDBERG, U. (1981) Mild mental retardation in Swedish school-children I and II. *Acta Paediatrica Scandinavica*, **70**, 441–444; **70**, 445–452

HOLMGREN, G. (1974) Inborn errors of amino acid metabolism in children with psycho-neurological diseases. Umeå University Medical Dissertations, No 16

JAGELL, S. (1981) Sjögren–Larsson syndrome in Sweden. Umeå University Dissertations, No 68

KOLODNY, E. H. and CABLE, W. J. L. (1982) Inborn errors of metabolism. *Annals of Neurology*, **11**, 221–232

LEJEUNE, J. (1959) Le mongolisme. Premier exemple d'aberration autosomique humaine. *Annales de Génétique*, **1**, 41–49

NIELSEN, J. and SILLESEN, I. (1975) Incidence of chromosome aberrations among 11,148 newborn children. *Human Genetics*, **30**, 1–12

NIELSEN, J., SÖRENSEN, A. M. and SÖRENSEN, K. (1981) Mental development of unselected children with sex chromosome abnormalities. *Human Genetics*, **59**, 324–332

O'DOHERTY, N. J. and NORMAN, R. M. (1968) Incontinentia pigmenti (Bloch–Sulzberger syndrome) with cerebral malformation. *Developmental Medicine and Child Neurology*, **10**, 168–174

OLEGÅRD, R., SABEL, K.-G., ARONSON, M., SANDIN, B., JOHANSSON, P.-R., CARLSSON, C. *et al.* (1979) Effects on the child of alcohol abuse during pregnancy. *Acta Paediatrica Scandinavica*, suppl. 275, pp. 112–121

RUBINSTEIN, J. H. and TAYBI, H. (1963) Broad thumbs and toes and facial abnormalities. *American Journal of Diseases of Children*, **105**, 588–608

6

Generalized muscular hypotonia and flaccid weakness

Muscular hypotonia, together with wasting of muscles and hypoactive or absent muscle reflexes, is usually considered part of the term 'flaccid weakness', indicating a disease of the motor unit, i.e. the peripheral motor neurone (= anterior horn cell and peripheral nerve) and the muscle fibres innervated by the motor neurone. However, in young infants in particular and occasionally in children, hypotonia is found without evidence of true weakness or muscular atrophy and with normal or even increased muscle reflexes. The strength of muscle reflexes can be assessed in all age-groups. Muscular atrophy is difficult to demonstrate or exclude clinically in infants, as they normally have small muscles covered by a thick layer of fat. Muscle strength may also be hard to evaluate in young infants. Thus, the search for the cause of decreased muscular tone in the paediatric age-group must not be confined to diseases affecting the peripheral motor neurones and the muscles.

In order to evaluate muscle tone it is necessary to know the normal variation with age. The full-term newborn infant normally has high muscular tone, which diminishes and disappears during the second half-year (*see Figure 2.1,* page 6). Characteristic features of some of the conditions described in this chapter are schematically reviewed in *Table 6.1.*

General non-neurological conditions

In these conditions, muscle reflexes are absent, hypoactive, normal, or hyperactive.

Prematurity may be called a physiological cause of muscular hypotonia in the newborn period, as many of these infants are otherwise healthy, although born before term (*see Figure 2.8,* page 11). Their muscle tone will eventually increase but they will never pass through the phase of high flexor tone, characteristic of the term infant.

Any severe disease may cause muscular hypotonia in a newborn infant. The loss of muscle tone in this period of life is an nonspecific finding and usually indicates a serious condition. Thus, a weak, hypotonic, areflexic, sick-looking neonate with a pale, greyish or blue colour may have, for example, a malformation of the heart, renal disease, severe anaemia, adrenal insufficiency, septicaemia, meningitis, intracranial bleeding, a lesion of the spinal cord at the cervical level, or intoxication due to drugs given to the mother.

TABLE 6.1. A schematic review of conditions causing muscular hypotonia and weakness*

When dominating clinical findings are:	The likely or possible cause is:	Special studies of interest:
Muscular hypotonia; no or questionable weakness and atrophy; normal or hyperactive muscle reflexes	Syndromes with mental retardation as part of the syndrome; CNS lesions, cerebral palsy syndromes under development; ALS** (weakness!); early phase of slowly progressive primary muscle disease, e.g. myotonic dystrophy	Various general examinations; EMG and histopathological examination of muscle biopsy (signs of denervation in ALS**, of primary muscle diseases in these, but normal in the rest; i.e. in the majority of patients in this group)
Fluctuating weakness; muscle reflexes varying with the weakness; no atrophy in early cases	Myasthenia gravis Adynamia episodica hereditaria Familial periodic paralysis McArdle's disease Hereditary myopathy with paroxysmal myoglobinuria due to abnormal glycolysis	Tension test; decrement on repeated stimulation; single fibre EMG with jitter Potassium loading Glucose and insulin loading Lactate determination after exercise Oxygen, acid-base, and lactate in arterial and venous blood during exercise
Slow clumsy movements; some weakness (independent ambulation possible) and wasting; areflexia	Peripheral neuropathy	Conduction velocity of peripheral nerves; spinal fluid protein
Weakness and wasting; hypoactive muscle reflexes, with:		
1. Involvement of the facial muscles	Facioscapulohumeral muscular dystrophy Myotonic dystrophy Congenital muscular dystrophy	EMG; histopathological examination of a muscle biopsy specimen; ECG
2. Involvement of the neck muscles	Severe progressive spinal muscular atrophy Facioscapulohumeral muscular dystrophy Myotonic dystrophy Congenital muscular dystrophy Limb-girdle type of muscular dystrophy Myositis	EMG; histopathological examination of a muscle biopsy specimen; ECG
3. Involvement of the tongue and throat muscles	Progressive spinal muscular atrophy Myasthenia gravis Myositis	EMG; histopathological examination of a muscle biopsy specimen; Tensilon test

4. Hypertrophy of calves	Progressive muscular dystrophy of Duchenne type, inherited as a sex-linked or autosomal recessive gene; more benign variants of Duchenne muscular dystrophy (Becker dystrophy), congenital muscular dystrophy, progressive spinal muscular atrophy inherited as a sex-linked recessive (?) symptomatic Duchenne carrier	EMG; histopathological examination of a muscle biopsy specimen; enzyme studies on patients and relatives; ECG
5. Fasciculations	Progressive spinal muscular atrophy	EMG; histopathological examination of a muscle biopsy specimen
6. Involvement of the skin	Dermatomyositis	EMG; histopathological examination of a muscle biopsy specimen; enzyme studies; X-ray study of arm and leg muscles
7. Onset in the newborn period and no apparent progress of symptoms	Central core disease, nemaline myopathy, megaconial myopathy, pleoconial myopathy, myopathy with mitochondrial enzyme hyperactivity, fibre type disproportion, other congenital stationary disorders	Histochemical and electron microscopic examination of a muscle biopsy specimen

* All variations cannot be included in a schematic review; for exceptions and details see text.

** Amyotrophic lateral sclerosis.

In the older infant, the normal muscle tone is lower than in the newborn, and infections and diseases affecting the heart, for example, usually produce more specific symptoms. Thus, these conditions will only cause differential diagnostic problems in young infants.

Muscular hypotonia in infants and children may be caused by other non-neurological diseases, e.g. *malabsorption syndromes,* such as gluten intolerance, and *metabolic diseases,* such as rickets (due to vitamin D deficiency or to a primary metabolic defect) and scurvy. When evidence of such non-neurological conditions is lacking in an infant, the cause of muscular hypotonia should be sought in the nervous or muscular system.

Involvement of the nervous or muscular system, certain or postulated

Conditions with evidence of involvement of intracranial structures or the long tracts of the spinal cord

HYPOTHYROIDISM

Hypothyroid infants may be hypotonic, although rigid hypertrophic muscles with delayed relaxation is a more common neuromuscular disturbance (*see Figure 20.1,* page 388).

PRADER-WILLI SYNDROME

The syndrome described by Prader and Willi (1956) involves several systems (muscular system, brain and endocrine organs), all of which may contribute to the profound hypotonia characteristic of the syndrome. A chromosomal abnormality has been demonstrated in 50–75 per cent of examined patients with Prader–Willi syndrome; the abnormality is localized to one of the chromosomes in pair 15. In most of them the abnormality consists of a complete loss of band q 12 and a partial loss of bands q 11 and q 13. This particular abnormality has been found only in patients with Prader–Willi syndrome. Normal chromosomal findings, with the use of techniques now available, are also compatible with a diagnosis of Prader–Willi syndrome.

The main features of Prader–Willi syndrome are grave muscular hypotonia, obvious in the newborn period and persisting through infancy and childhood, severe proximal muscular weakness, a variable delay in psychomotor development, short stature, disproportionately small hands and feet, hypogonadism (in boys, bilateral cryptorchism), obesity (*Figure 6.1*), and a tendency towards squint and early development of diabetes mellitus. This syndrome has also been termed the HHHO-syndrome, because of the typical findings of hypotonia, hypomentia, hypogonadism, and obesity. Muscle reflexes are usually hypoactive or absent, particularly during infancy. Because of the profound muscular hypotonia, the severe proximal weakness, and the hypoactive muscle reflexes, a disorder of the lower motor neurones or the muscles is often suspected. Electromyography and histological examination of muscle biopsy specimens have, however, been consistently normal in those patients studied.

The difficulties in movement improve with increasing age of the patient. Most patients learn to walk, but because of the proximal weakness they have trouble

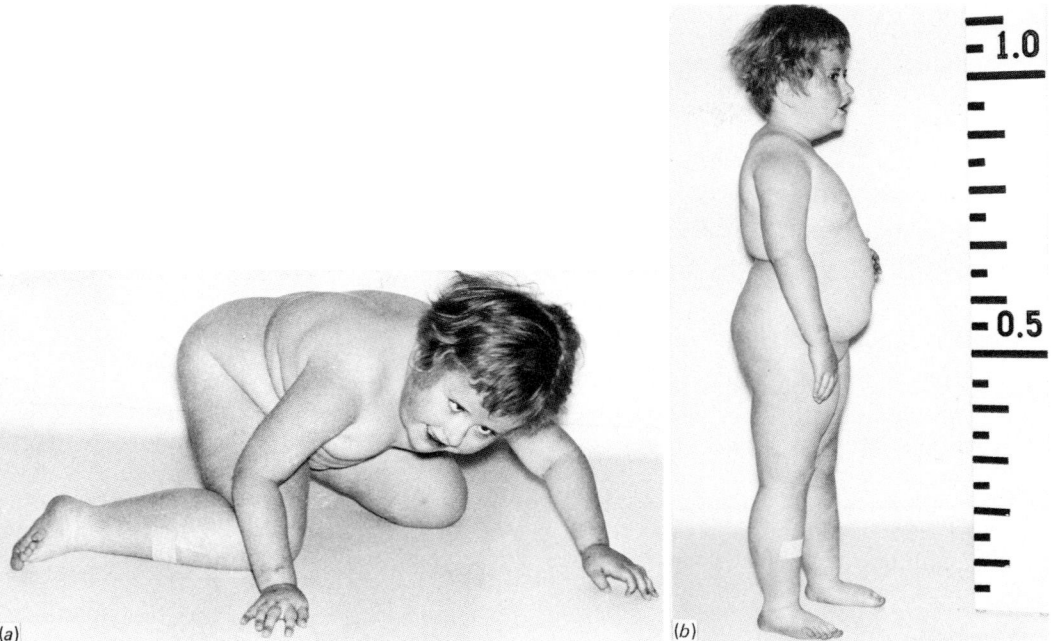

Figure 6.1. A 7-year-old girl with Prader–Willi syndrome, getting up from sitting on the floor to demonstrate proximal muscle weakness (*a*). Note the shortness of stature (*b*), small hands and feet, squint (*a*), and obesity

climbing stairs and cannot run. They must climb on furniture or onto their own knees to get up from sitting on the floor.

A typical physical feature, seen in probably all patients, is disproportionately small hands and feet. Shortness of stature is seen in most patients, but a few otherwise typical cases with normal height are on record. Obesity, which may become grotesque if allowed to develop, usually starts at 2–4 years of age. In infancy, particularly in the newborn period, these infants have severe feeding difficulties and may need tube-feeding. When the feeding difficulties disappear, the child may show an insatiable appetite and from 2–3 years of age this creates great practical problems. Patients with the Prader–Willi syndrome have an increased incidence of diabetes mellitus and of vascular diseases; obesity will increase the risk of complications and also impair the patients' ability to move. Dietary advice to prevent obesity must therefore be given as soon as the diagnosis is established; it might, however, be difficult for parents to accept such advice at a time when severe feeding difficulties have just abated.

Patients with the Prader–Willi syndrome are mentally retarded to a degree which varies from mild to profound. Some patients have been reported to become aggressive in adulthood.

No treatment is available for the disease *per se*. Dietary advice to prevent obesity, physiotherapy to improve muscle strength, and special education are the most important symptomatic measures. The life-span is probably shortened by the vascular complications of diabetes and/or obesity.

LOWE'S SYNDROME

In the oculocerebrorenal syndrome, Lowe's syndrome, severe muscular hypotonia is a cardinal symptom, together with eye lesions and mental retardation (*see* page 134).

CHROMOSOMAL ABERRATIONS

Muscular hypotonia is characteristically found in some chromosomal aberrations, particularly Down's syndrome (*see* page 138).

INTRACRANIAL LESIONS AND DISEASES

Muscular hypotonia is often found during the acute phase of cerebral anoxia, intracranial bleeding, and meningitis in the newborn period and may be seen in infants after the newborn period during the development of movement disorders due to a permanent lesion of the central nervous system, i.e. cerebral palsy syndromes (*see* Chapter 12). In a young infant a lesion of the central nervous system usually produces decreased tone and increased muscle reflexes. This combination, which is rare in older children and adults, strongly suggests a central localization of the lesion.

Different cerebral palsy syndromes develop in different ways during infancy. Muscular hypotonia may gradually be replaced by hypertonia; in some infants this may occur when they are only a few months of age. The increase in tone is first noted in the legs, which are kept crossed, and in the plantar flexors of the foot. The elbows are flexed and the hands are clenched with the thumb tightly across the palm (*Figure 6.2*); this position of the thumb is normal only during the infant's first

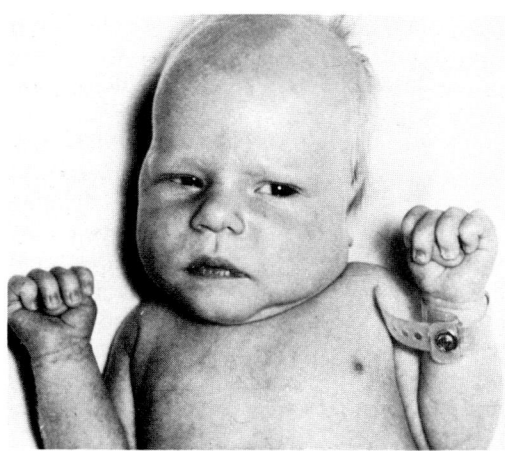

Figure 6.2. Abnormal posture of the hands in a 4-month-old floppy infant with a severe cerebral lesion

few weeks. These originally hypotonic infants thus develop the typical picture of a spastic diparesis during the second and third quarter of their first year (*see* page 284).

Other flaccid newborn infants remain flaccid throughout their first year of life. When they are some months old an abnormal position of the hand is noted. The hand is turned in an unnatural position of extreme pronation, particularly when the

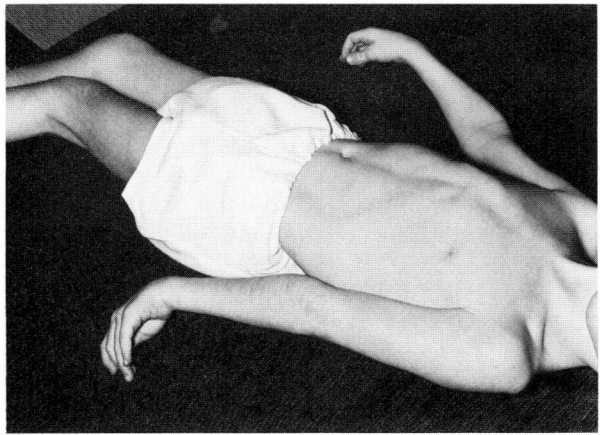

Figure 6.3. Abnormal posture of the left hand in a hypotonic 6-year-old boy with cerebral palsy (brain-stem lesion).

infant tries to grasp an object (*Figure 6.3*). The neonatal reflexes, which should start to disappear at 3–4 months of age (Moro, sucking and rooting, grasp of the hand) persist for months and years after this age. The tonic neck reflex, which should never be strong, becomes abnormally easy to elicit and persists long after its normal time of disappearance (second half-year). From a state of continuous flaccidity the tone starts to alternate between abnormally low when the infant is left alone, and abnormally high when the infant is disturbed by any type of stimulus. Involuntary movements of the choreoathetoid type may also be observed towards the end of the first year of life. These signs point to a lesion of the brain stem including the basal ganglia. They are particularly common in infants who have had signs of serious asphyxia and/or have been deeply jaundiced in the newborn period. These infants are liable to develop a cerebral palsy syndrome characterized by choreoathetosis and alternating muscular tone (*see* pages 277–278).

A small group of flaccid infants remain hypotonic throughout the first year of life with normal muscle reflexes and normal disappearance of neonatal reflexes. Their motor development is delayed, and they can barely sit unsupported at 1 year of age. The clinical picture may be difficult to differentiate, for example, from Prader–Willi syndrome (*see* page 158) or from the primary muscle diseases that produce little reduction of muscle reflexes (e.g. myotonic dystrophy, page 194). However, at the beginning of the second year of life, when the child tries to sit up and to grasp objects, it becomes obvious that his real problem is lack of balance. This is apparent from his staggering way of sitting and the intention tremor that is evident when he reaches out for an object. These infants thus develop a cerebral palsy syndrome dominated by ataxia (*see* page 278). They also remain hypotonic as they grow older, provided the picture is not complicated by involvement of the corticospinal tract; cerebellar lesions also cause both ataxia and muscular hypotonia in older children and adults.

Some of the progressive degenerative brain diseases (*see* Chapter 13) may also, at some stage of their course, produce muscular hypotonia; occasionally this may be due to involvement of the peripheral nerves by the same disease process that affects the brain (*see* page 306).

LESION OF THE CERVICAL CORD DUE TO TRAUMA OR TO IMPAIRED CIRCULATION

Traumatic lesions of the spinal cord at the cervical level may occur during a difficult delivery with breech presentation. However, even infants delivered normally or by caesarean section, may suffer an injury to the cervical cord; this may also occur suddenly after delivery in an apparently normal infant and cause sudden death. In such cases a possible explanation is a vascular malformation, which may suddenly bleed, before or after birth, and be unrelated to the mode of delivery. If the lesion is severe, the surviving infant will have a total flaccid paralysis of all limb and trunk muscles, areflexia, impaired sensation (*see* page 29), and disturbed sphincter

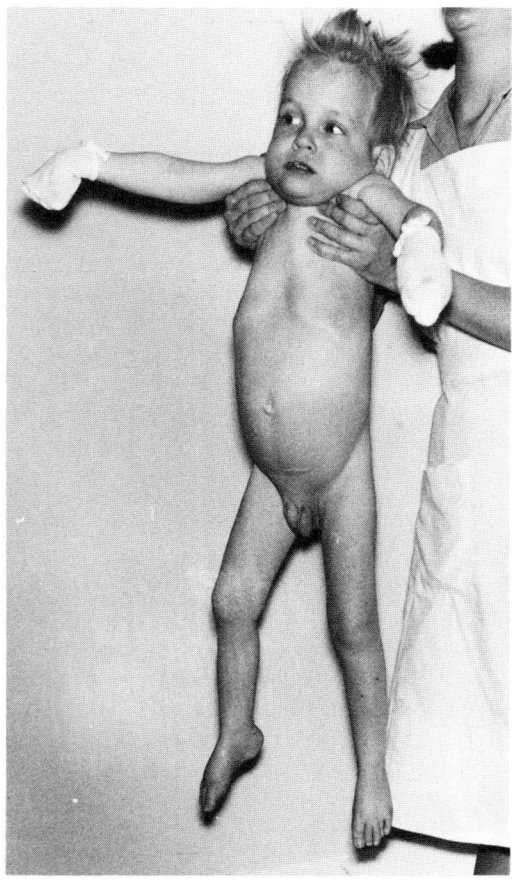

Figure 6.4. A 2-year-old boy with sequelae after perinatal damage to the cervical cord. His hands have been bandaged because of severe sores on the fingers

function. Eye muscles and facial muscles are intact. Episodes of unexplained fever may occur. The mortality is high, mainly due to respiratory paralysis. In surviving infants the tone will return in the legs and eventually become increased. Muscle reflexes appear in the legs and become hyperactive. The older infant and child will therefore have a spastic paraplegia due to damage of the corticospinal tract in the cervical cord. The sensory tract and the anterior horn cells will also be damaged at this level. In the arms there will hence be a mixture of upper and lower motor neurone lesions. The damage to the lower neurone usually dominates, producing a mainly flaccid weakness of the arms with loss of arm reflexes. Atrophy of arm and hand muscles will usually become evident during childhood. Impaired sensation may be suspected from the way the infant bites and maltreats his hands, giving rise to slow-healing ulcers on the fingers (*Figure 6.4*), and may be demonstrable on clinical examination.

If the lesion is serious, surviving children will develop the complications of severe transverse cord lesion, i.e. spastic paraplegia, contractures, bedsores, urinary and faecal incontinence, urinary retention with infection, and subsequent dilatation of the upper urinary tracts (*see also* page 336). Examination of the cervical cord is an important part of the autopsy in all cases of sudden unexplained infant death.

Because of the severely delayed motor development, a cerebral lesion is often suspected in infants with a cervical cord lesion. However, provided no episode of cerebral anoxia complicates the picture, the general mental development is normal, and convulsions and EEG abnormalities do not occur. Spinal fluid examined in the neonatal period is often bloody and may still have a high protein content after a few weeks; when examined at a later stage it is usually normal. Fractures and dislocations of cervical vertebrae may occasionally be seen on X-ray examination; their absence does not exclude the diagnosis. As lower motor neurones are also damaged, electromyography may be of some positive diagnostic help. In a typical case the leg muscles show no electromyographic abnormalities, whereas denervation (*see* pages 45–48) can be demonstrated in the arm muscles.

The late prognosis is poor in infants with severe, perinatal, traumatic damage to the cervical cord. Those who survive the neonatal period will have severe handicaps and many will eventually succumb to respiratory tract and urinary tract infections. Postmortem examination reveals an atrophic spinal cord with destruction of neurones and secondary gliosis. Rests after old haemorrhages in the cord substance may also be found.

OTHER DISORDERS

Encephalomyeloradiculoneuropathy (*see* pages 175–176) and amyotrophic lateral sclerosis (*see* page 173) affect both upper and lower motor neurones. Muscular hypotonia may be present, and the strength of the muscle reflexes varies, depending on whether the upper or the lower motor neurones are the more severely involved; thus muscular hypotonia and normal or increased reflexes may occasionally be found.

Conditions affecting the motor unit, which includes lower motor neurones, neuromuscular junction, and muscle fibres

Most of these patients have a true flaccid weakness. The diagnosis of these conditions requires knowledge of the organization of the lower motor neurone and its connection with the muscle fibres (*see* page 155). The purpose of the diagnostic procedures is to localize the lesion to the anterior horn cells, the peripheral nerves, the neuromuscular junction, or the muscle fibres and, whenever possible, to define the type of lesion. The diagnostic steps will be reviewed before the separate diseases are described in detail.

HISTORY

The history can provide some valuable information.

Inheritance
Knowledge about not only affected individuals but also healthy relatives is necessary to analyse the mode of inheritance. In many situations it is of value to examine both parents clinically and by laboratory methods to reveal healthy gene-carriers of recessive diseases and mild or subclinical cases of dominant diseases.

Age at onset
An exact statement is often difficult to obtain, as most of the diseases under discussion have an insidious onset; fortunately, in most cases, precise information on this point is of secondary importance for the diagnosis.

Symptoms
The first observed symptoms, whether distal or proximal, generalized or localized, and the sequence and speed of development of symptoms are of great diagnostic significance. When distal muscles are the first to be involved a peripheral neuropathy is the likely explanation; early involvement of proximal limb muscles and trunk muscles usually indicates disease of the anterior horn cells or a primary muscle disease.

The symptoms may vary at different times of the day in relation to physical exertion, cooling of the muscles, and food intake. A weakness persisting for weeks or months is probably due to a disease localized either in the peripheral neurones or in the muscle fibres. When the weakness varies considerably over hours or days and perhaps disappears completely for weeks or months, the likely localization of the disease is at the neuromuscular junction. Muscle pains, usually intermittent, are a common complaint in some of the metabolic myopathies. Patients with myositis may complain of aching pains and muscle tenderness, particularly in an acute phase. It is also important to note the appearance, particularly at the onset of the disease, of nonmuscular symptoms such as fever, headache, stiff neck, rash, and sensory disturbances.

PHYSICAL EXAMINATION

Muscle signs
The weakness and atrophy are examined carefully as to symmetry, distribution between proximal and distal muscle groups, and involvement of ocular, facial, neck, throat, and tongue muscles. The presence of muscular hypertrophy, particularly localized to the calves, is found only in primary muscle diseases. Fasciculations, i.e. visible painless twitching of groups of muscle fibres without movement in a joint, are seen only in denervation atrophy and usually suggest a disorder of the anterior horn cells. Suitable muscles are examined for signs of myotonia (*see* pages 213 and 214).

Sensory disturbances
Sensation will be intact in diseases that primarily affect the anterior horn cells, the neuromuscular junction, or the muscle fibres. When the disease is localized to the peripheral nerves not only motor but also sensory nerve fibres are involved, and sensation may be impaired. The presence of sensory disturbances localizes the disease to the peripheral nerves, but their absence does not exclude such a localization. Sensory findings are always difficult to demonstrate and interpret in children.

Muscle reflexes
The strength of the muscle reflexes must always be evaluated in relation to the degree of muscle weakness. A total areflexia combined with only mild weakness usually indicates a disorder localized to the peripheral nerves. As these conditions affect both efferent and afferent fibres, i.e. both legs of the reflex arc, the effect on the reflexes is greater than on the muscle power. In anterior horn cell disease the weakness is more severe before the reflexes disappear. In primary muscle diseases the weakness is usually even more pronounced before the reflexes are lost, and ankle jerks in particular are often preserved to a late stage of the disease.

Non-neurological signs
Non-neurological findings, such as those from endocrine organs, hair, skin, eyes, and heart, usually suggest a primary muscle disease.

SUPPLEMENTARY STUDIES

The history and the physical examination must usually be supplemented by special investigations to establish a definite diagnosis. The four most important special studies are:

1. Electrocardiography
2. Measurement of the serum activities of some enzymes and serum myoglobin level
3. Neurophysiological examination
4. Histological examination of a muscle biopsy specimen.

In special situations other chemical analyses of blood, liver tissue, and muscle tissue may be indicated, as well as ultrasound and X-ray examination and computerized tomography of the soft tissue of the extremities.

Activity of serum enzymes and serum myoglobin level
Of the enzymes that are measurable in serum, two play an important role in the diagnosis of muscle diseases – creatine kinase (CK) and lactic dehydrogenase (LDH).

CK is an enzyme that is specific for muscle tissue (including the heart) and the central nervous system. It can be separated into a muscle component and a brain component, but this is seldom necessary in clinical practice. The blood must be drawn under standardized conditions and compared with the normal value for age. Intense physical exertion, prolonged fasting (more than 24 hours), and blood drawn after the application of stasis and pumping with the hand will all increase the value and thus give a falsely abnormal result. The normal value in the newborn infant is roughly three times that of adults; it decreases slowly and reaches adult level at around 5 years of age. Men have a slightly higher level than women. Women of fertile age have lower normal values than prepubertal girls and postmenopausal women. The normal level is particularly low during pregnancy. The serum level of CK is increased in most primary (myogenic) muscle diseases, particularly during the acute phase of a progressive disorder. In the early phase of Duchenne muscular dystrophy it is always greatly elevated, as a rule to 50–100 times the upper limit of normal. Such a high serum level is a characteristic finding in infant boys with Duchenne muscular dystrophy *before* clinical symptoms or signs of the disease are apparent; it may therefore be used to establish or exclude the diagnosis in a newborn boy. In some countries it is used as a screening procedure to identify affected boys, even in families without a history of previous cases, the main purpose being to give early genetic counselling. Serum levels of CK decrease with age and progression of the disease, but usually remain high until muscular wasting is severe. The determination of CK activity in serum can also be used to diagnose healthy female gene-carriers, as approximately two-thirds of them have an increased level. Standardized conditions for drawing the blood sample and due consideration to the variation in normal values are important factors in evaluating the significance of the level of CK activity found. The serum CK level is also increased in other primary muscle diseases, although usually not to the degree seen in Duchenne dystrophy. It may be normal in stationary or very slowly progressive primary muscle diseases. In cases of muscular atrophy due to denervation it is generally normal, although in about one-quarter of the cases, it is increased to a level about two to three times the normal value.

As LDH is a widely distributed enzyme, an increase in its total activity is a nonspecific finding. The specificity is greatly increased when the enzyme is separated electrophoretically into five isoenzymes, which normally show a decreasing strength from isoenzyme one to five. The same picture, or perhaps a slight increase in isoenzyme one, is seen in muscular atrophy due to denervation. The typical picture seen in all primary muscle diseases and also often in healthy gene-carriers of Duchenne muscular dystrophy is a marked increase in isoenzyme two. This is never found in denervation atrophy and is possibly an even more specific finding than the increased level of serum CK. In patients with traumatic injuries of healthy muscles the typical finding in serum is an increase in isoenzyme five; this is the dominating LDH isoenzyme in healthy muscle tissue.

An increased level of serum myoglobin is seen in the same situations as elevated CK levels. As a rule, serum myoglobin only confirms the findings from the enzyme studies; very occasionally it may make questionable results of enzyme studies easier to interpret.

Neurophysiological examinations
The findings on neurophysiological examinations (conduction velocity of peripheral nerves and needle electromyography) are described in Chapter 3 (*see* pages 45–51).

Muscle biopsy
The muscle biopsy must be performed on a suitable muscle and the specimen correctly handled to make a histopathological diagnosis possible. The muscle must be clinically affected by the disease but not totally destroyed and replaced by connective tissue and fat. Thus, in a mild case, the most involved muscle is preferred; in a severe case the least involved muscle should be used. The arm muscles have certain advantages, as restriction of the patient's activity is unnecessary, and rest is always dangerous for children with weak muscles. The deltoid should be avoided because of the tendency to keloid formation in scar tissue in that region. In smaller children, leg muscles must be used; bed-rest can be avoided if a small biopsy is taken. The gastrocnemius muscle and the anterior tibial muscle are easy to reach. The quadriceps muscle, which is less accessible because it is covered by a thick layer of fat, is only used on special occasions. A biopsy must not be taken from a muscle that has been used for injections or on which a needle

electromyogram (EMG) has been performed during the months before the biopsy, as needles may cause histological changes indistinguishable from myositis. For the same reason local anaesthetics must not be given in the muscle; the biopsy must be taken either under general anaesthesia or after local anaesthesia of the skin only.

For muscle biopsy, several rods of muscle tissue, preferably about 5–10 mm in length and a few millimetres in diameter, are taken out; they must be handled gently without pinching, and put on a moist filter paper with a parallel orientation of the fibres. Two pieces are immediately placed in liquid nitrogen and kept at −70°C, one for histochemical staining and the other for biochemical analysis. Another piece is placed in a Petri dish and covered with a glass lid for 10–20 minutes. At the end of this time the muscle fibres will have ceased twitching and the muscle piece can be put in the fixing solution for routine staining. In many situations it is necessary to take another piece for electronmicroscopy; this piece is put into osmium solution.

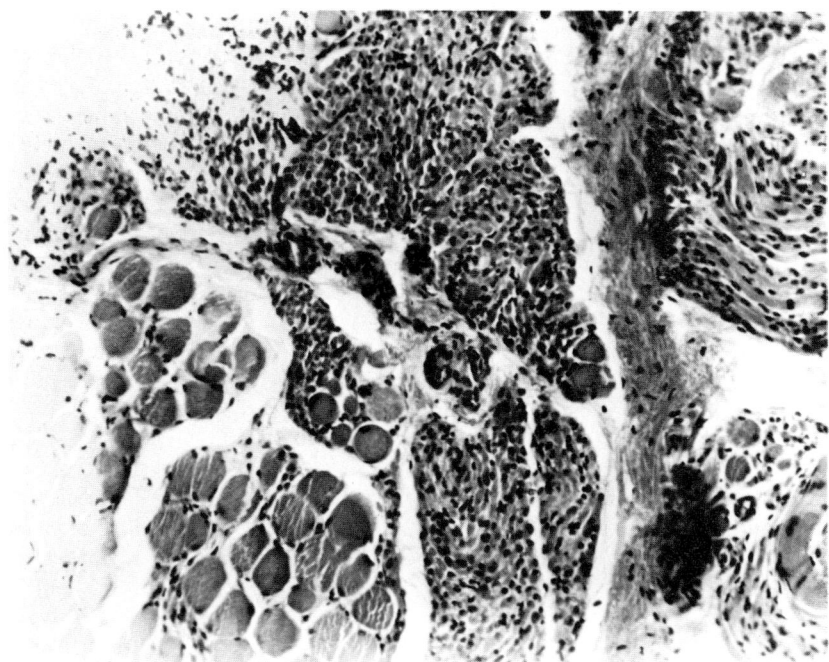

Figure 6.5. The histological picture typical of severe muscular atrophy due to denervation. The biopsy was taken from the quadriceps muscle of a 3-year-old boy with progressive spinal muscular atrophy

In many cases routine and histochemical staining and examination are enough to establish a diagnosis. From these diagnostic procedures the pathologist is able to tell whether there are changes typical of denervation atrophy (i.e. groups of atrophic fibres with only slight or no signs of degeneration intermingled with areas of normal fibres, *Figure 6.5*). or whether the abnormalities are evenly distributed and consist of fibres showing degeneration, hypertrophy, splitting, and rows of central nuclei (such a picture is typical of a primary muscle disease, *Figure 6.6*). Only early cases show isolated clear-cut changes. Any long-standing case of

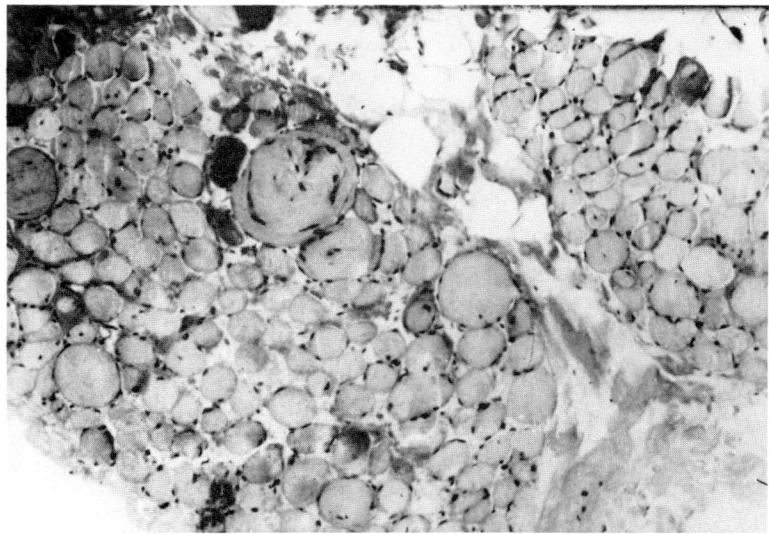

Figure 6.6. The histological picture typical of muscular dystrophy. The biopsy specimen was taken from the anterior tibial muscle of a 7-year-old boy with Duchenne muscular dystrophy

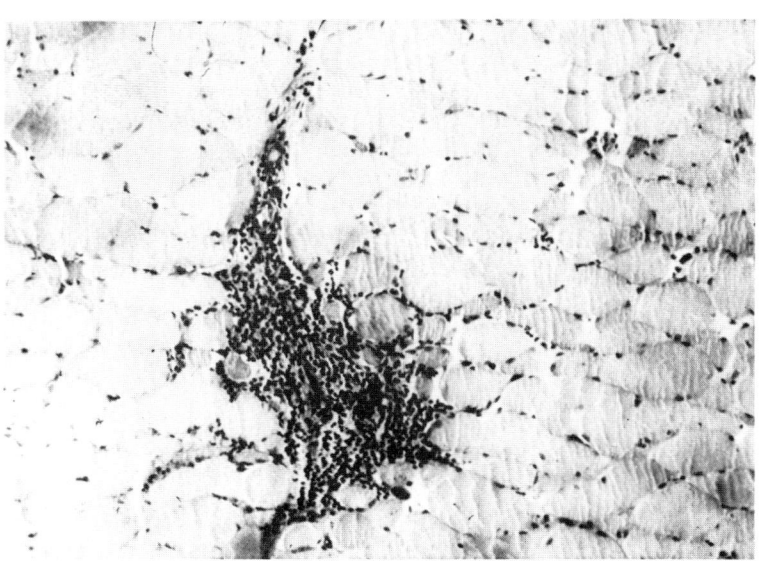

Figure 6.7. An infiltrate of inflammatory cells found on histological examination of a biopsy specimen taken from the quadriceps muscle of a 15-year-old girl with myositis

denervation atrophy will eventually also show signs considered typical of a primary muscle disease. Inflammatory changes, lymphocytic infiltrations seen in myositis (*Figure 6.7*), and abnormal blood vessels, seen also in other collagenoses, can usually be found in the routine preparations. These methods will also reveal the distribution of the different fibre types, the relative size of respective fibres, abnormal glycogen or fat storage and enzyme distribution, and mitochondrial abnormalities. Biochemical analysis of muscle tissue may be needed when abnormal storage appears likely. Good cooperation between clinician, pathologist, and biochemist is necessary to obtain optimal information from the biopsy procedure.

After this general review of the diagnostic procedures, the different diseases will be discussed.

DISEASES PRIMARILY AFFECTING THE ANTERIOR HORN CELLS

Poliomyelitis

The virus attacks primarily the large nerve cells of the lower motor neurones in the spinal cord and the medulla oblongata. As a rule there is an acute phase of the disease with fever and acute meningitis (*see* page 348), but this may be so mild as to be overlooked by the patient, whose chief complaints then will be muscular weakness and wasting. In polio the family history is noncontributory, the onset is rather acute, and the disease is nonprogressive after the acute phase. In a typical case of polio the muscle symptoms are distributed at random and *asymmetrically,* whereas almost all hereditary degenerative diseases cause *symmetrically* distributed weakness and wasting. Polio occurring in infancy, however, often causes symmetrical weakness and wasting. Special studies reveal the typical signs of an anterior horn cell disease. In an unvaccinated individual the demonstration of antibodies to polio may be a useful diagnostic tool.

The main treatment is physiotherapy. In the acute phase its aim is to prevent contractures and overstretching of weak muscles. In later stages active training of the weak muscles is the method of choice. It is always worthwhile to train a polio patient intensely, as the disease is nonprogressive, and surviving nerve cells will reinnervate denervated muscle fibres. Normal muscle fibres can hypertrophy during active training. Orthopaedic measures may also be indicated to give the patient the best opportunity to use his remaining muscle power. No effective treatment exists to prevent or cure the viral attack on the anterior horn cells; mass vaccination effectively protects an otherwise susceptible population. The prognosis depends on the spread of the viral attack.

Progressive spinal muscular atrophy

Various subgroups can be distinguished; those showing different modes of inheritance probably represent different entities. A *sex-linked recessive* inheritance has been reported in a few boys whose symptoms started in late childhood and who also showed calf hypertrophy. Symptoms were slowly progressive and the handicap relatively mild. The first report by Pearn (1978) has so far not been confirmed by other observers.

A type with *dominant autosomal* inheritance is also known. In most reported cases the onset has been in adulthood, but patients with an onset in childhood are on record. The progression of symptoms is slow and the patient may live an almost normal life.

The inheritance in the vast majority of patients with progressive spinal muscular atrophy is due to an *autosomal recessive* gene (or possibly genes). This group contains some variants. The first reported form was described by Werdnig (1894) and Hoffmann (1893). They described infants who appeared to be healthy and developing normally up to their second half-year, when they became weak and floppy and lost their ability to sit up and eventually also to lift their arms, legs and head. The muscles atrophied. Respiratory and tongue muscles were also affected. Mental development was normal. They died from respiratory complications at 4–7 years of age. After the turn of the century several authors reported on the same clinical and morphological picture occurring at an earlier age and with a more rapid progression, causing death usually during the first year of life. A juvenile form with an apparent onset at 2–9 years of age and a slow progression was reported by Wohlfart et al. (1955) and Kugelberg and Welander (1956). The juvenile form was originally described as a separate disease entity, based on its later onset and better prognosis. However, the *stated* age of onset varies with the knowledge and experience of the parents and is always lower in the second than in the first affected child in a sibship. Several transitional forms between the infantile and the juvenile forms are on record. The general rule is that affected members of the same family show the same course, but this rule has enough exceptions to raise some doubt that the various forms are distinct disease entities. Progressive spinal muscular atrophy with autosomal recessive inheritance *may* thus be one disease and its various forms due to modifying genes or environmental influence.

In a case diagnosed as progressive spinal muscular atrophy it is important for the parents to get a reasonable prediction of the expected course. Some early symptoms and signs which may be more useful for predicting the course than the stated age of onset are used to divide the disorder into two types, each with a different prognosis.

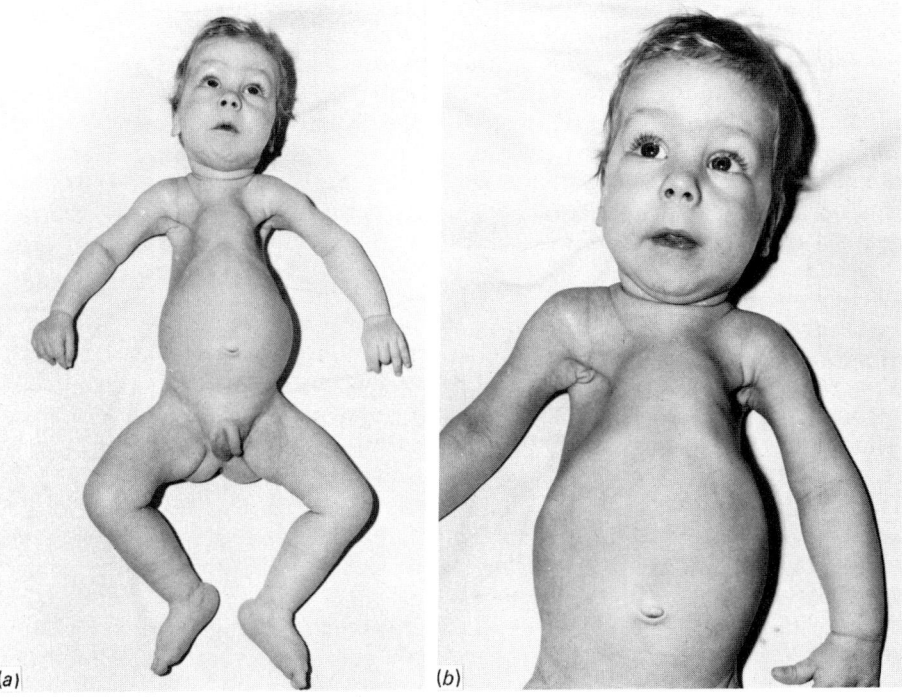

(a)   (b)

Figure 6.8a and *b*. A 7-month-old boy with progressive spinal muscular atrophy of the malignant type I. Note the frog-like position, the deformed chest, the well-preserved facial muscles, and the obvious alertness of the child

In patients with *type I,* muscle symptoms are observed before birth or during the first year of life, usually during the first few months. The mother may have noted unusually weak fetal movements. The weakness is *generalized* from the beginning and involves the trunk, neck, and proximal limb muscles severely, so that the infant cannot lift his head, elbows, or knees from the bed. The distal limb muscles are less involved, and facial and extraocular muscles are entirely spared (*Figure 6.8*). The intercostal muscles are usually severely involved, and the infant breathes with the abdominal muscles. The shoulder muscles are weak and give way if one tries to lift the child as shown in *Figure 6.9a.* Kyphoscoliosis and thoracic deformities develop early. Involvement of the bulbar muscles is common, causing atrophy and fasciculations of the tongue and swallowing difficulties. These are bad prognostic signs. A fine finger tremor is often also observed.

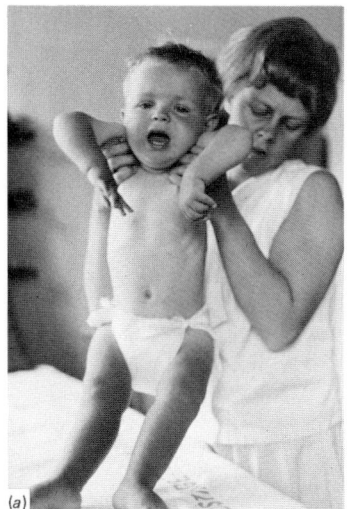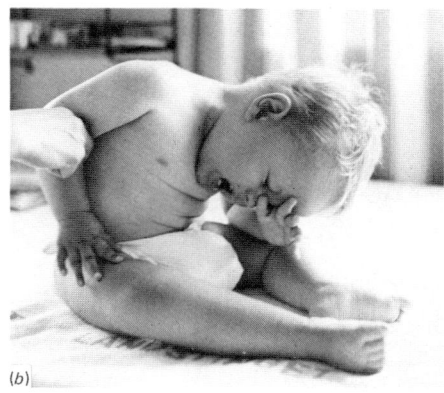

(a)   (b)

Figure 6.9. A 1½-year-old boy with progressive spinal muscular atrophy of the malignant type I. Note his inability to support himself on his feet and weak shoulder muscles giving way when he is lifted up (*a*), also his inability to sit unassisted (*b*)

The disease is progressive, and most of these patients do not learn to sit up unassisted (*Figure 6.9b*). Death occurs from respiratory complications during infancy in the most severely affected patients; few survive their fourth birthday. The progression is slower in some patients; they may learn to sit but not to walk. A few survive to late childhood and adolescence with very little muscle strength and severe deformities (*Figure 6.10*); their mental development is normal.

In patients with progressive spinal muscular atrophy of *type II,* the weakness may be noted as early as in patients with type I or a little later, i.e. during the first 3 years. At the onset it is *localized* to the hip and thigh muscles. The first noticeable symptoms are therefore weak kicking movements and abnormally thin thighs. The muscles of the neck and the upper part of the back are not involved; these children learn to lift their head and to sit up at a normal age. Most of them also learn to walk. They are then observed to have an abnormal waddling gait with protruding abdomen, and abnormal lumbar lordosis (*Figure 6.11a*), and they cannot climb stairs or squat. The proximal limb muscles and trunk muscles are the most severely involved, but within this group of muscles there is no selective weakness or wasting,

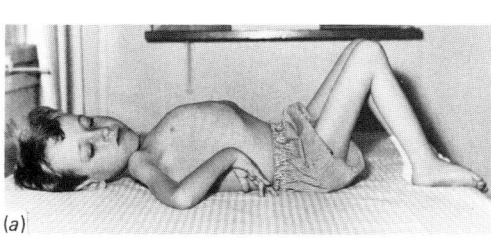
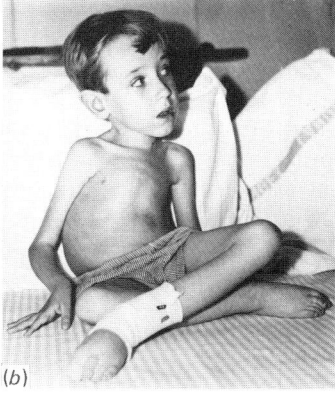

Figure 6.10a and *b*. An 8-year-old boy with progressive spinal muscular atrophy of the malignant type I. Note the severe muscular atrophy, kyphoscoliosis, and other deformities

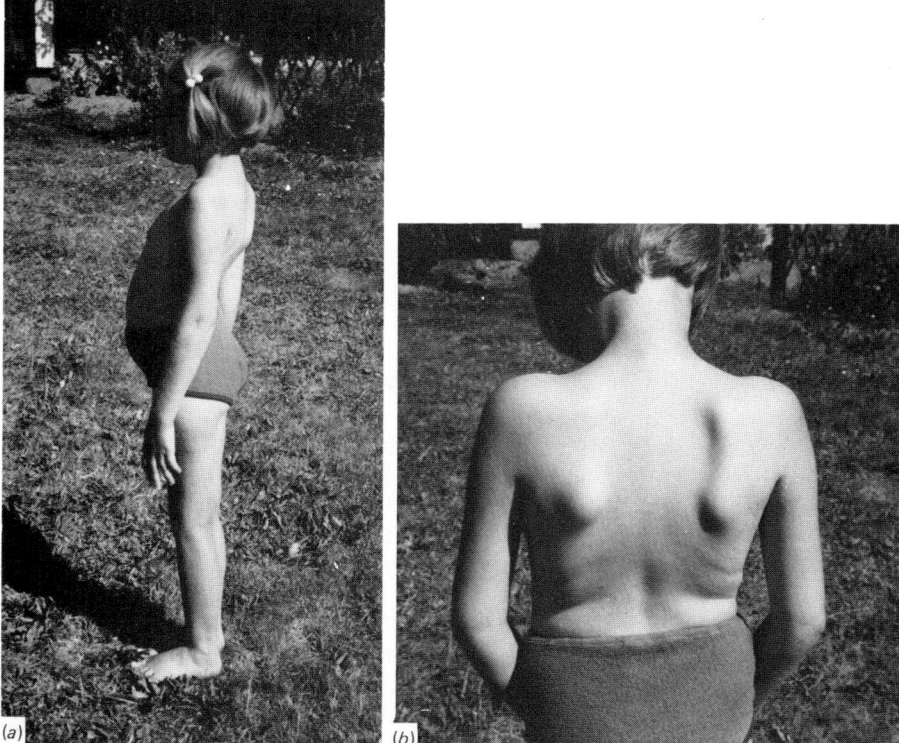

Figure 6.11. A 9-year-old girl with progressive spinal muscular atrophy of type II. Note her thin thighs and her posture with protruding abdomen and marked lumbar lordosis (*a*) and her atrophic shoulder muscles (*b*)

as is typical in Duchenne muscular dystrophy (*see* page 185). The disease is progressive, although at a slower rate than type I. The low back muscles are involved early, in some patients so severely that they have to climb with their hands on their knees and thighs when getting up from sitting on the ground (*Figure 6.12*). This sign, which has been erroneously described as pathognomonic for muscular dystrophy, thus indicates weakness of back muscles but not the *cause* of this weakness. In some children the weakness is mild or moderate (*Figure 6.13*) and appears to be nonprogressive, at least for several years. A rapid progression of

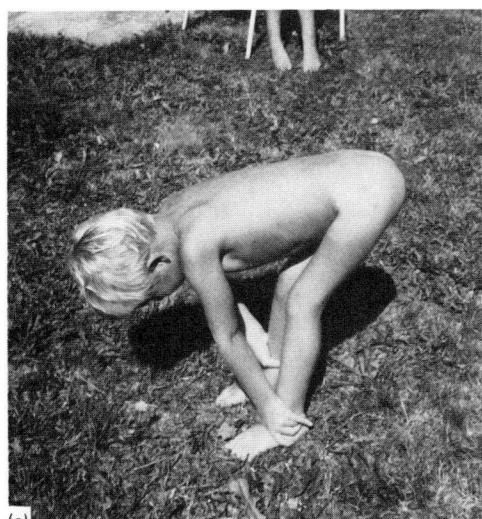 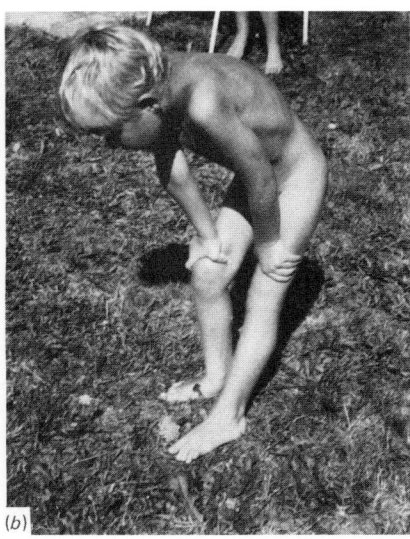

(a)   (b)

Figure 6.12a and *b*. A 5-year-old boy with progressive spinal muscular atrophy of type II, climbing with his hands on his legs in order to attain an upright position

symptoms is common at puberty, when many patients develop contractures (*Figure 6.14*) and some become confined to a wheelchair. This apparent deterioration is probably caused by the prepubertal growth spurt, which in these patients increases the length of the levers without the normal increase in strength of their proximal attachment; it is not therefore a true progression of the disease. After puberty, symptoms seem to remain stationary or progress very slowly in most patients. Atrophy of the tongue and tongue fasciculations (*Figure 6.15*) may appear without being a bad prognostic sign; the patients do not develop swallowing difficulties or a tendency to aspiration. Most patients with progressive spinal muscular atrophy of type II reach adulthood; they may be severely handicapped. The ultimate prognosis is not known in detail.

Juvenile amyotrophic lateral sclerosis may be considered a subgroup of type II. Involvement also of the upper motor neurones is characteristic of this variant. These patients thus have extensor plantar responses and a tendency to increased muscle reflexes. The combined effect of an upper and lower motor neurone lesion may be hyper- or hypoactive or even normal muscle reflexes. The course of this variant bears more resemblance to that of the childhood progressive spinal muscular atrophy of type II than to that of amyotrophic lateral sclerosis seen in adulthood.

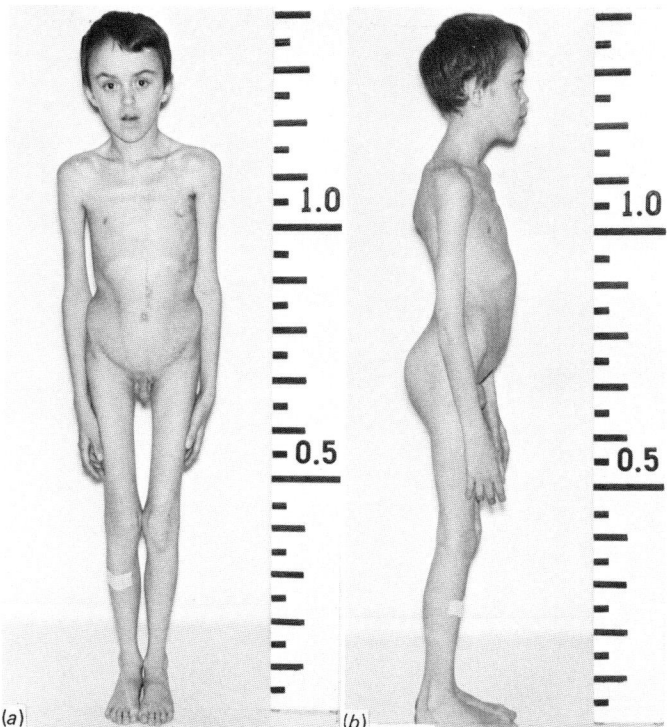

Figure 6.13a and *b*. An 11-year-old boy with progressive spinal muscular atrophy of type II and a remarkably benign course for this type of the disease

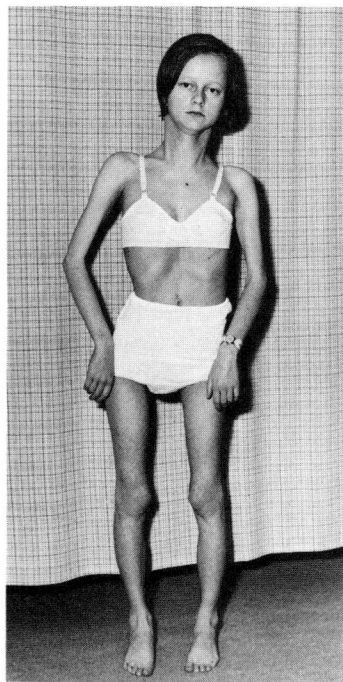

Figure 6.14. A 15-year-old girl with progressive spinal muscular atrophy of type II. Note the scoliosis and contractures of the hips and elbows

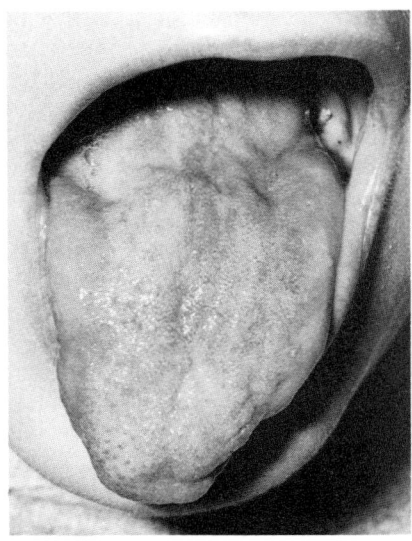

Figure 6.15. Atrophy of the tongue in a 12-year-old boy with progressive spinal muscular atrophy of type II

The diagnosis in all forms of progressive spinal muscular atrophy is based on evidence, from the history, physical examination, and special studies, that the disease is progressive and localized to the anterior horn cells. Only the history and follow-up can distinguish between the two types of the recessively inherited form.

There is no specific treatment for progressive spinal muscular atrophy. Physiotherapy helps to postpone severe atrophy and contractures as long as possible; bed-rest is always dangerous. Obesity will increase the patient's difficulties and must be avoided. Because the mental development of these children is normal, technical aids and the best possible school education are very important. All general measures described under Duchenne muscular dystrophy (*see* pages 188 and 189) are also applicable in progressive spinal muscular atrophy.

On postmortem examination a reduced number of anterior horn cells is found. Occasionally other parts of the central nervous system are also involved in the degeneration.

DISEASES PRIMARILY AFFECTING THE PERIPHERAL NERVES

From a clinical standpoint the peripheral neuropathies can be divided into three groups: an extrinsic cause proven or likely, inheritance proven or likely, and no apparent cause. Involvement of the peripheral nerves may also occur in diseases that produce symptoms primarily from the central nervous system (*see* pages 301–303 and 305–308). The degree of severity may vary in all groups from an involvement so mild that it can only be demonstrated electrophysiologically, to an affection so serious that it confines the patient to bed.

Extrinsic cause

The Guillain–Barré syndrome   This syndrome is considered to be an autoimmune disorder which requires both an altered immunological response and an extrinsic triggering factor. The latter is usually, at least in childhood, a viral infection, e.g. influenza, infectious mononucleosis, or mycoplasma; the triggering factor may vary from case to case. The syndrome has a higher incidence in adulthood than in childhood, but it exists in children and has even been reported in the newborn period. The first symptom is weakness which has an acute onset and progresses for a few days. It usually involves both the distal and proximal muscles and may affect the respiratory muscles. Mild bilateral facial weakness is a common finding; the extraocular muscles are not involved and the bulbar muscles only in rare severe cases. Sensory disturbances, such as paraesthesia and impaired vibration and position sense, may occur but are often absent and always hard to evaluate in children. Muscle reflexes are usually lost, but are occasionally hypoactive.

Involvement of the central nervous system may also occur and may precede the peripheral symptoms. Ataxia and abnormal eye movements have been reported in cases with features of Guillain–Barré syndrome by Miller Fisher; the exact border between Fisher's syndrome and Guillain–Barré syndrome is unclear. Brain-stem involvement is seen, causing abnormal eye movements, decreased wakefulness, and involvement of corticospinal tracts, which changes the muscle reflexes from absent or weak to normal or hyperactive; rarely this evidence of central involvement may precede that of peripheral involvement. Bilateral papilloedema is also common in cases without other evidence of involvement of the central nervous system. Reversible EEG abnormalities are common. Abnormal fatigue persists for 6–12 months after the acute phase and causes fretfulness and irritability. It is debatable how far involvement of the central nervous system should be accepted under the term Guillain–Barré syndrome. As such involvement seems to occur often enough to cause semantic difficulties, it might be better to use the broad descriptive term *encephalomyeloradiculoneuropathy*.

The typical finding in the spinal fluid is a normal or slightly elevated cell count (usually less than 10–20 cells/mm^3) and an increased concentration of protein. Electrophoretic separation shows an unspecific relative increase in the globulins, suggesting damage to the blood-brain barrier with leakage of serum proteins. The spinal fluid may occasionally be normal during the first stage of the disease, and typical abnormalities may be delayed until 1–2 weeks after the onset of neurological symptoms.

The conduction velocity of peripheral nerves often remains normal for a few weeks after the onset of neurological symptoms. It then decreases and remains low long after clinical recovery has occurred, occasionally for several years.

The usual course in children is progress of symptoms for a few days, stationary symptoms for a few weeks, and then recovery over several months. In the acute stage it is important to prevent the stagnation of mucus in the bronchi, atelectasis, and pneumonia. Antibiotics are given when indicated because of infectious complications, but they do not influence the disease *per se*. Assisted respiration and tracheotomy may be necessary. The value of treatment with steroids has been debated. They may possibly shorten the acute phase of the disease but do not influence its outcome; they are not needed in children. Immunosuppressive drugs have also been used but have no proven value. Plasmaphaeresis has been used with a beneficial influence on the acute phase in a few severely ill children; its value is hard to assess due to the variable natural course of the disease and the small number of serious cases in childhood. Physiotherapy is important in the acute phase to keep the airways clear and to prevent contractures, and in later stages to build up muscle strength.

On the whole, the prognosis is good. Most children recover with only mild or no sequelae. Death may occur from respiratory complications during the acute phase;

very occasionally patients survive with severe permanent weakness. Parents must be informed that the fatigue and irritability that is so often seen for 6–12 months after the acute phase is a common and reversible symptom for which nothing can be done. Rarely the course becomes protracted for months or even years, perhaps undulating with exacerbations and periods of spontaneous improvement. In this situation the need for treatment is great but its effect is very difficult to evaluate.

Toxic substances   Almost any drug can cause polyneuropathy in a susceptible person; nitrofurantoin, sulphonamides, and isoniazid are among the drugs most often incriminated. Polyneuropathy due to toxic drugs is unusual in childhood. The effect of isoniazid is not considered toxic but due to competition between isoniazid and pyridoxine; the simultaneous administration of pyridoxine will prevent this complication. Heavy metals (e.g. lead) may cause a peripheral neuropathy characterized by bilateral symmetrical weakness of the wrist extensors. Although lead intoxication in children usually produces symptoms of increased intracranial pressure (*see* pages 396–397), typical lead neuropathy has also been described. Adults may be exposed in their work to neurotoxic substances, such as acrylamide and organic solutions. In children the possibility of exposure to organic solutions and glue in hobby activities must be considered. Diphtheria toxin (*see* page 360) is a well-known cause of polyneuropathy in children. Toxic substances, accumulating because of an intrinsic metabolic defect, are probably the cause of the polyneuropathy in porphyrinuria (*see* page 396) and Refsum's disease (*see* page 263). Another metabolic disorder that may cause polyneuropathy is inherited amyloidosis; it does not seem to produce symptoms before adolescence.

Beriberi, thiamine deficiency   The dominating symptoms in children are progressive polyneuropathy with motor and sensory symptoms and general fatigability and irritability; in infants cardiac failure and convulsions appear to be more common. The disease occurs in the Orient; although it is rare in Western countries it may occur as part of a severe malnutrition syndrome or when the child is on a special diet that is mistakenly too low in thiamine. The administration of thiamine will prevent and cure the disease.

Diabetes mellitus   Involvement of the peripheral nerves is found in at least one-third of adult diabetics. In diabetic children, clinical signs of neuropathy are rare and, when they occur, consist of impaired sensation and absent ankle jerks. Decreased conduction velocity is found in about 10 per cent of diabetic children.

Inheritance

Chronic hereditary polyneuropathy   On histological grounds two kinds of chronic hereditary polyneuropathy may be distinguished, one due to *axonal* degeneration and the other to *demyelination* and remyelination, leading to hypertrophy of the nerve. The latter is the most common type. The two types may be impossible to separate on genetic or clinical grounds alone. Inheritance in both may be due to an autosomal dominant, an autosomal recessive, or a sex-linked recessive gene, although autosomal recessive inheritance is the rule in the axonal type and autosomal dominant in the demyelinating type, whereas sex-linked recessive inheritance is rare in both. Both may show any degree of severity, although the axonal type is usually more severe and shows more involvement of the proximal muscles than does the demyelinating type.

In chronic hereditary polyneuropathy the symptoms may be mild enough to be overlooked by the patient. A family history can therefore never be accepted as negative without examination of both parents. Clinical symptoms may appear at any age or be absent throughout life; such a person may still transfer the disorder to his children, thus dominant inheritance with decreased penetrance is a possibility.

The first vague symptoms are usually observed when the children are a few years old. As a rule they start to walk at a normal age, but continue to fall often and to walk unsteadily, and they do not learn to run. All their movements remain slow and clumsy. Muscular tone is low. In most cases true muscular weakness is insignificant, and the disturbance of movements must, to a large extent, be due to diminished muscle sense. Impaired sensation to pinprick and touch can seldom be demonstrated; occasionally impaired position and vibration sense is found. Muscle reflexes are usually absent or hypoactive. Adiadochokinesis is a common finding. The gait is unsteady. There is a tendency to develop contractures. High-arched feet are the most common deformity and may even be seen at birth. Tight heel-cords are found; kyphoscoliosis may be seen (*Figure 6.16*). In some cases weakness and muscular atrophy may be so severe that a diagnosis of spinal muscular atrophy or muscular dystrophy may be discussed. However, even in very weak patients the distal muscles are more severely involved than the proximal ones.

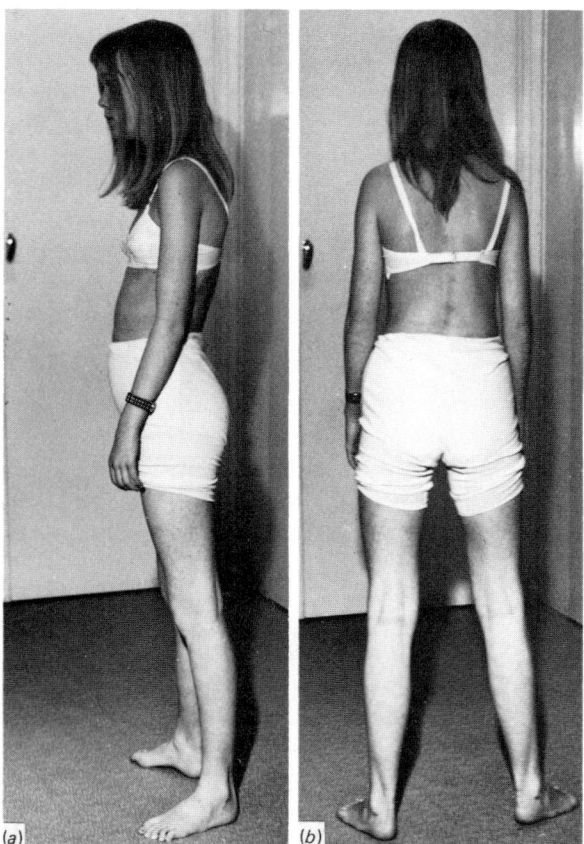

Figure 6.16a and *b*. A 15-year-old girl with chronic hereditary polyneuropathy. Note the scoliosis, high-arched feet, tight heel-cords, and inability to stand with the feet together

Progression of symptoms is the rule but it may be so slow that for years or even decades the disease may appear stationary. Distal weakness and wasting usually start in the feet and may slowly progress to the lower legs and then affect the hands. A period of apparent rapid progression, particularly of the scoliosis, is often noted at around puberty, mainly for the same reason as mentioned for progressive spinal muscular atrophy of type II (*see* page 173). Some of these patients may then show a clinical picture similar to that described by Charcot, Marie and Tooth and carrying their names, i.e. severe weakness and wasting of the hands, feet, lower legs, and the distal third of the thigh. Most patients with chronic hereditary polyneuropathy, though definitely limited in their choice of a profession and leisure-time activities, can expect a normal life-span and a fairly normal life. Exceptionally, however, a patient may be severely handicapped.

The important diagnostic procedure is measurement of the conduction velocity of peripheral nerves. In the demyelinating type, values are very low, often down to a quarter of the value normal for age. If the disease is inherited as a dominant, the affected parent will have a value of the same magnitude, even if he has no subjective symptoms. In the axonal type the value is usually also decreased but often only to a borderline or mildly abnormal value; it may then be difficult to differentiate it from progressive spinal muscular atrophy of type II. A low conduction velocity is seen in all types of chronic demyelinating polyneuropathy; its hereditary character must be proved by a positive family history or by positive findings on examination of family members. Electromyography and histological examination of a muscle biopsy specimen will show long-standing denervation, particularly in the distal muscles. Histological examination of a nerve biopsy specimen, preferably taken from the sural nerve, will show either demyelination and remyelination or axonal abnormalities. The spinal fluid protein is normal or slightly elevated. In most cases the diagnosis is established without the three last-mentioned examinations; thus muscle biopsy, nerve biopsy, and lumbar puncture are seldom necessary for the diagnosis.

There is no treatment for the disease *per se*. These patients often benefit greatly from orthopaedic measures and physiotherapy.

Disorders of the peripheral nerves which are probably inherited and which give symptoms other than generalized weakness and hypotonia are discussed in Chapters 10 and 21 (*see also* pages 227–228).

No apparent cause
The chronic cases in this group resemble clinically those described under the heading chronic hereditary polyneuropathy. The Guillain–Barré syndrome could have been included here, as its cause is unknown. Subacute cases of polyneuropathy also occur in children for no apparent reason; they have a fluctuating course over several years and eventually tend to show definite improvement. This spontaneous course makes it difficult to evaluate the effect of treatment. Corticosteroids and immunosuppressive drugs have been suggested, but their value remains debatable.

DISEASES PRIMARILY AFFECTING THE NEUROMUSCULAR JUNCTION

Myasthenia gravis
Myasthenia gravis, once considered a homogeneous disease, can now be separated into several entities. Two symptoms are common to all types of myasthenia gravis:

1. *Muscles innervated by cranial nerves* are particularly early and seriously involved.
2. The typical finding in involved muscles is an abnormal *fatigability,* occasionally described by children as a kind of painful sensation.

The classic common type of myasthenia gravis is an acquired autoimmune disease in which antibodies to the acetylcholine receptors of the muscle end-plates can be detected in about 90 per cent of the cases. It usually has its onset in young adulthood, but it may start at any age, including infancy.

Juvenile myasthenia gravis is the same disease as adult myasthenia gravis. The first symptoms usually involve the extraocular muscles and consist of ptosis, various forms of strabismus, and restricted eye movements. In some patients the symptoms are confined to the eye muscles; this form of the disease is termed *ocular myasthenia.* In the early phase it is impossible to tell whether the myasthenia will remain confined to the eye muscles or become generalized; the duration of the period of purely ocular symptoms after which one can be sure that generalization will not occur is also unknown. In most cases, clinical and/or electrophysiological signs of generalization are present from the onset. Facial and chewing muscles, tongue and throat muscles, and neck muscles are involved early, and often also the muscles of the trunk and of the extremities. Symptoms are mild or absent in the morning and progress during the day. The first few movements are performed with good muscle strength but the following movements become increasingly weaker. At the beginning of a meal the patient can chew and swallow normally but after a few morsels chewing becomes weaker and the patient may choke when trying to swallow. Exercise of other muscles may also increase the weakness; thus ptosis may increase if the patient squats and gets up again several times.

The clinical diagnosis is confirmed by pharmacological and electrophysiological tests and by the demonstration of receptor antibodies in the blood. Receptor antibodies are abnormally high in 80–90 per cent of children with generalized myasthenia gravis, but are usually absent in pure ocular myasthenia. It is debatable whether a borderline titre in ocular myasthenia may signify the beginning of generalization.

The electrophysiological tests consist of single fibre electromyography and repeated supramaximal stimulation of a peripheral nerve with recording of the amplitude of the muscle response; in a rested myasthenic muscle the amplitude of the first response is normal and in the following responses decreased by at least 25 per cent; the decrement disappears if the test is done immediately after a short exercise of the muscle. The single fibre EMG may reveal an instability of neuromuscular transmission, evident as increased jitter and blocking of end-plates (*see Figure 3.12,* page 49). This method requires good cooperation from the patient and can seldom be used in children below 10 years of age.

The pharmacological test consists of the intravenous injection of an anticholinesterase drug, preferably edrophonium bromide, and observation of its effect on the muscles involved. A small dose is given first, followed after 1 minute by a full dose, provided neither disappearance of weakness nor side effects (abdominal pains, cramps, visible muscle fasciculations) have occurred. In adults and older children (above 35–40 kg) the small dose is 2 mg and the full dose 10 mg; these doses are halved in younger children; in neonates the small dose is 0.5 mg and the full dose 2 mg. The effect is seen within 1 minute after the injection and lasts for 5–10 minutes. Neostigmine given by mouth may also be used (*Figure 6.17*).

Pharmacological and electrophysiological tests may be combined; the normalization of an abnormal muscle response to repeated nerve stimulation after edrophonium bromide proves the diagnosis of myasthenia gravis.

The symptomatic treatment consists of the administration of drugs with anticholinesterase activity, pyridostigmine being the most commonly used drug. The size of the dose and the interval between doses must be individually adjusted. A reasonable dose is 20–80 mg every 4 hours during the day and every 8–10 hours during the night. The best way to establish the optimal dose is to adjust the dose until the patient has the maximal desired effect with minimal side effects. These consist of increased salivation, increased mucus secretion, abdominal pains, nausea, and diarrhoea. The side effects are unpleasant but never dangerous and can always be reversed by decreasing the dose; they may also improve if a small dose of atropine is added to the regimen.

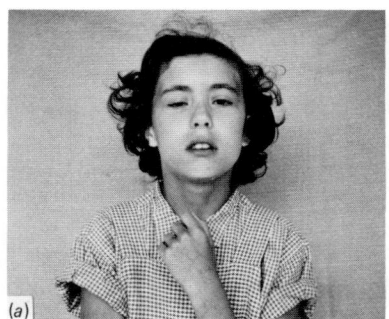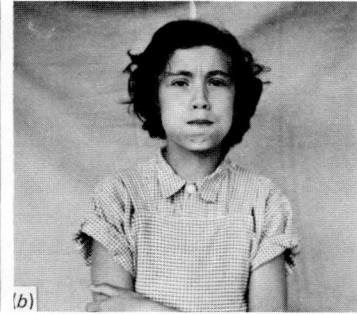

Figure 6.17. An 11-year-old girl with myasthenia gravis, trying to blow out her cheeks: before neostigmine (*a*) and after neostigmine (*b*)

Thymectomy is considered a more causal treatment, as it may intervene in the autoimmune process. If the patient's condition is good, the operation carries only a small risk. No sequela, such as impaired immune defence, has been noted after thymectomy, even in infants. The effect on generalized myasthenia gravis is usually good and the operation is also recommended for infants and children. There is no need to perform the operation urgently but there is no advantage in delaying it.

Corticosteroids are widely used in the treatment of adults with myasthenia gravis. Their place in the treatment of children is still questionable. The most important side effect in children is growth retardation, which can be minimized by giving the drug every second morning before 8 a.m. If corticosteroids are used at all, they must be used in this way and in the lowest effective dose. Immunosuppressive therapy has also been used in adults, but experience in children is scanty. Plasmaphaeresis is used for the acute crisis in adults, but as myasthenic crisis is rare in childhood the effect of this expensive method is hard to evaluate.

The prognosis of juvenile myasthenia gravis is similar to that of the adult form. Spontaneous remissions occur and treatment is usually effective enough to enable the patient to live a fairly normal life. Mortality has decreased considerably during the last two decades; myasthenia gravis probably has only a small influence on the child's expected life-span.

Neonatal transitory myasthenia gravis also belongs to the classic form of the disease; it affects approximately 15 per cent of infants born to mothers who have the disease. Within the first day of life the infant is found to be weak and floppy with a weak cry and has difficulty in breathing, sucking, and swallowing. It may be noted that the infant can suck and swallow normally a few times and then gets tired and chokes. Muscle reflexes may be normal but are usually weak. If the mother's disease is undiagnosed, there is a risk that these weak floppy babies with respiratory and swallowing difficulties will be diagnosed as cases of perinatal brain injury. The diagnosis of neonatal transient myasthenia gravis is established by electrophysiological and pharmacological tests (*see* page 180).

The treatment is pyridostigmine bromide 5–10 mg four to six times per 24 hours; the dose must be adjusted individually. The infant usually needs tube-feeding and may also need assisted ventilation, particularly before the optimal dose is found. The prognosis is poor in untreated infants, thus treatment may be life-saving. Treatment can usually be tapered and stopped after 6–8 weeks without recurrence of symptoms. Most of these children probably remain healthy; a few, however, may show signs of a stationary permanent myopathy. The cause of neonatal transient myasthenia gravis is thought to be the transfer from the mother to the child of antibodies to acetylcholine receptors which damage the end-plates; such antibodies have been demonstrated in both the mother's blood and the child's blood. Symptoms usually disappear within 6–8 weeks, i.e. the time it takes for the child to break down passively transferred antibodies. Some infants seem also to produce their own antibodies to the receptor; this production may conceivably have something to do with the more permanent symptoms in the child.

The *myasthenic syndrome* described by Eaton and Lambert occurs almost exclusively in adults, although a few cases have been reported in children aged 9–16 years. It is an autoimmune disorder, which in adulthood is usually connected with carcinoma, mainly of the lung. The defect in neuromuscular transmission differs from that in classic myasthenia gravis. The amplitude of the first muscle response is abnormally low and decreases further on repetitive stimulation at a rate of less than 10/s; if the rate is greater than 10/s, a marked increase in amplitude occurs instead. Patients may improve with corticosteroid treatment.

In patients with congenital onset of permanent myasthenic symptoms at least four different *congenital myasthenic syndromes* have been identified, based on different defects in neuromuscular transmission. In one of these syndromes there is good evidence for a dominant inheritance; in the others, autosomal recessive inheritance appears likely. Autoimmune reactions have not been found. Besides the fatigability, some permanent weakness may also be present, particularly of muscles innervated by cranial nerves and of proximal limb muscles. The myasthenic syndromes may therefore be impossible to distinguish on clinical grounds from congenital disorders of the muscle fibres. The necessary diagnostic procedure is an analysis of the defect in neuromuscular transmission. In all but one of the myasthenic syndromes there is a decrement in the amplitude of the muscle response to repetitive supramaximal nerve stimulation. In the syndrome lacking this sign the characteristic finding is a double response to a single stimulus. A recording of the muscle response to nerve stimulation will thus reveal some abnormality in all the congenital myasthenic syndromes. No receptor antibodies are demonstrable in the blood. A slight improvement may be seen on treatment with anticholinesterase drugs, but the effect is usually insignificant and outweighed by the side effects. No effective treatment is known. The symptoms usually appear stationary or may show some improvement with increasing age; the ultimate prognosis is not known.

Botulism

Botulism is an infection with the toxin-producing bacteria *Clostridium botulinum*. This infection is rare but may occur in children, even in infants. The toxin produces a defect in neuromuscular transmission similar to that seen in Eaton–Lambert myasthenic syndrome (*see* page 182). The symptoms are paralysis of both extrinsic and intrinsic eye muscles and of bulbar muscles and weakness and floppiness of the limb and trunk muscles. Paralysis of bulbar and respiratory muscles may be fatal.

Botulism is treated by supportive measures, particularly assisted ventilation and tube-feeding or feeding through a gastrostomy, until the symptoms have subsided, which may take weeks or months.

Familial periodic paralysis and adynamia episodica hereditaria

Both of these disorders are characterized by attacks of muscle weakness and attack-free intervals, during which there are usually no symptoms. They are hereditary, and the inheritance is autosomal dominant. Potassium metabolism is involved in both disorders. The localization of the abnormality, although unconfirmed, is probably the neuromuscular junction.

Familial periodic paralysis   This disease seldom has its onset before puberty. Attacks usually start during the night, last for several hours, and are severe, often with involvement of respiratory muscles but seldom of muscles innervated by cranial nerves. The attack-free interval may last for weeks, months, or years. The attacks are accompanied by a decrease in serum potassium and electrocardiographic signs of hypopotassaemia. For diagnostic purposes an attack can best be provoked by giving the patient 50 g glucose in pure water by mouth every hour until an attack occurs, which may take many hours. The patient may drink water freely but must not eat or drink anything else. The attack can be terminated by the oral administration of potassium, preferably as an organic salt, equivalent to 60–250 mmol potassium. Coated tablets of a potassium salt are ineffective in this situation because they are absorbed too slowly.

Organic potassium salts can also be used prophylactically in a dose equivalent to 60 mmol potassium, administered several times daily or when the patient knows that an attack is imminent, i.e. after intense exercise or a high-carbohydrate meal. Some patients may benefit from the intake of 250–500 mg acetazolamide two or three times a day.

Death may occur from respiratory paralysis. Slowly progressive, permanent, proximal weakness is rare, but may eventually develop.

Adynamia episodica hereditaria   This disease usually has its onset in childhood. Attacks often occur during the daytime. They are frequent, short and moderately severe. In childhood the average patient has many attacks per week, each lasting for less than an hour, which prevent him from standing and walking but not from sitting or moving his arms. Some patients complain of muscle pains (soreness and aching) occurring after the attack, which last for days or even weeks and cause the patient more discomfort than the attack itself. The involvement of respiratory muscles is rare; muscles innervated by cranial nerves may be weak. The clinical picture varies considerably, however. Myotonia (*see* page 213) is demonstrable in some but not all patients. The attacks are accompanied by an increasing serum potassium and electrocardiographic signs of hyperpotassaemia. Attacks occur during rest after exercise and can be provoked experimentally by the oral administration of potassium salts in an amount equivalent to 25 mmol (for a small child) to 60 mmol (for an adult) of potassium; this test is performed in the morning before breakfast. If no weakness is provoked the test can be repeated another day with a larger dose, but the first test dose must be kept small as some patients are very sensitive to potassium.

As the attacks are usually short and mild, treatment during an attack is unnecessary. Acetazolamide 250–500 mg two to three times a day is usually effective in mitigating or preventing attacks; occasionally another diuretic (with no added potassium) may be more effective. Mexiletine hydrochloride 50–100 mg three to four times a day may be effective in some patients. The patient is instructed to adjust the dose until he finds the smallest dose that keeps him reasonably free of symptoms. The disease usually has a spontaneous seasonal variation; if possible, treatment should be interrupted during the summer, when most patients are better. As the disease is lifelong and benign and the treatment is purely symptomatic and not entirely free of side effects, there need be no hurry to start therapy; it is advantageous to postpone it until adulthood. No patient is known to have died from adynamia episodica hereditaria. The disease limits the patient's free choice of a profession and of leisure-time activities but does not prevent him living a fairly normal life.

DISEASES PRIMARILY AFFECTING THE MUSCLE FIBRES

Muscular dystrophy

The term muscular dystrophy includes those primary muscle diseases that are genetically determined and characterized by a progressive degeneration of muscle fibres. Common to them all are a progressive course, lack of effective treatment, and a deleterious effect of prolonged rest, particularly bed-rest. The classification given here follows mainly that of Munsat (1980). A classification is important in every case of muscular dystrophy because, although it does not lead to specific treatment, it enables the physician to give the parents correct information about genetic risks, course, and prognosis.

Duchenne type muscular dystrophy   This is the most common type of muscular dystrophy in childhood. It was first described in 1868 by Duchenne de Boulogne. Its inheritance is due to a sex-linked recessive gene, which often also produces some abnormal laboratory findings in female heterozygotes (*see* page 166), and exceptionally causes mild clinical symptoms and signs in them. For genetic counselling to the family it is important to diagnose the female gene-carriers. Serum enzyme levels and myoglobin levels (if available) are determined on as many female relatives as possible, connected with the affected boy through the X-chromosome line. Unfortunately no way exists to *prove* that a woman is *not* a gene-carrier, as approximately one-third of known carriers has normal enzyme activity. Through a careful family history, including information about both sick and healthy individuals, and enzyme determinations on all available female relatives, it may be possible to calculate the statistical risk of a woman being a carrier.

Early motor development is normal, and the patients learn to walk, at most a few months later than the majority of healthy children. The parents usually become concerned when the children are 2–3 years of age, because they continue to walk unsteadily and have frequent falls, from which they have difficulty getting up again;

they do not learn to run or to climb stairs. Physical examination at this age reveals weakness of the pelvic girdle, hip, and thigh muscles, in which some atrophy is usually noted. At this age, also, the child may already have a tendency to walk on his toes, with protuberant abdomen and marked lumbar lordosis. When asked to run the child increases his pace and walks with swinging shoulders like a walker in a walking race (*Figure 6.18*). Weakness can usually also be found in the shoulder girdle, and the pectoral muscles are atrophic. A disproportionately severe atrophy of the pectoral muscles is a typical finding in Duchenne muscular dystrophy. Bulging hypertrophic calves are usually noted at this age. Special studies to establish the diagnosis, even before clinical symptoms and signs are apparent, are discussed on page 166.

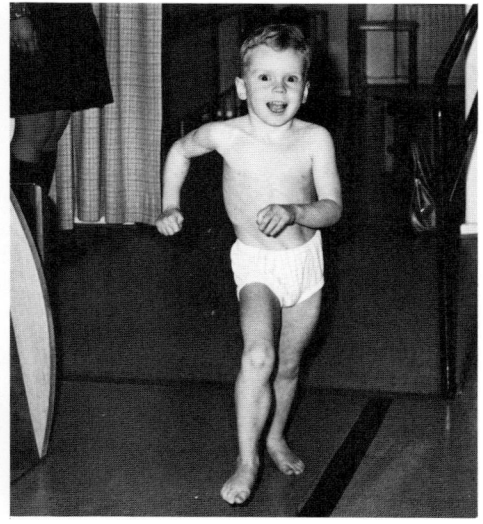

Figure 6.18. A 5-year-old boy with Duchenne muscular dystrophy, trying to run. Note the swing of his shoulders, reminiscent of the style of a walker in a walking race. Note also the selective atrophy of his pectoral muscle and the hypertrophy, particularly of his calves and to a slight degree also of his proximal antebrachial muscles

All symptoms show a slow and steady progression. At 4–5 years of age the difficulties in walking are obvious. At this age the patient must climb with his hands on furniture or on his knees to get up from sitting on the floor (*Figure 6.19*). The heel cords start to become tight. At 8–10 years of age the patient is barely able to stand or walk (*Figure 6.20*). He then becomes confined to a wheelchair, which he soon becomes unable to wheel himself because of increasing weakness of his arms. At this stage contractures in flexion quickly develop in the knees and hips. Kyphoscoliosis usually starts to develop when the patient is confined to a wheelchair. Pronounced lumbar lordosis seems to offer some protection, at least partially, against scoliosis. The small hand muscles also start to lose their strength, but the coordination of hand and finger movements is not lost (*Figure 6.21*).

In his late teens the patient finds it increasingly difficult to sit and may contract complications such as pneumonia or urinary tract infection. Myocardial involvement can usually be demonstrated by an abnormal ECG, often also by increasing dyspnoea. At this late stage the neck muscles may also become involved. Extraocular, facial, throat, and tongue muscles are usually spared. Death usually occurs in the patient's early twenties. Complicating infections can be treated, though not always successfully; they are, together with cardiac failure, the main causes of death.

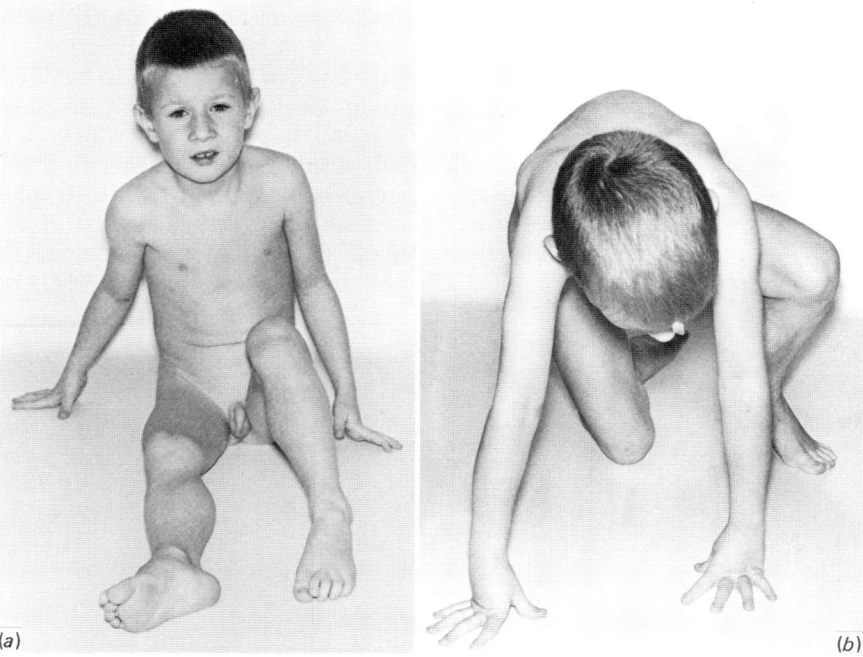

(a)

(b)

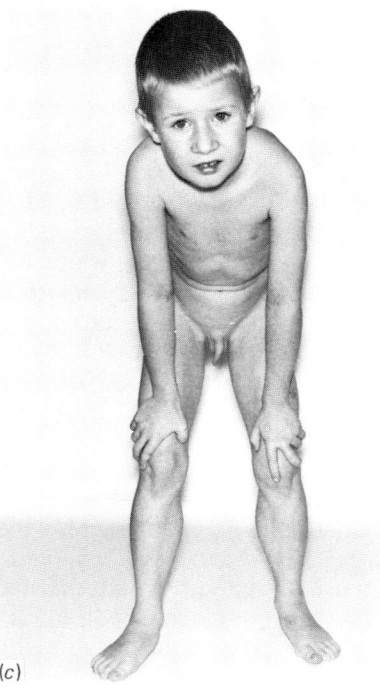

(c)

Figure 6.19a, b and *c.* A 6-year-old boy with Duchenne muscular dystrophy, climbing up from the floor in a typical way. Note also his hypertrophic calves and atrophic pectoral muscles

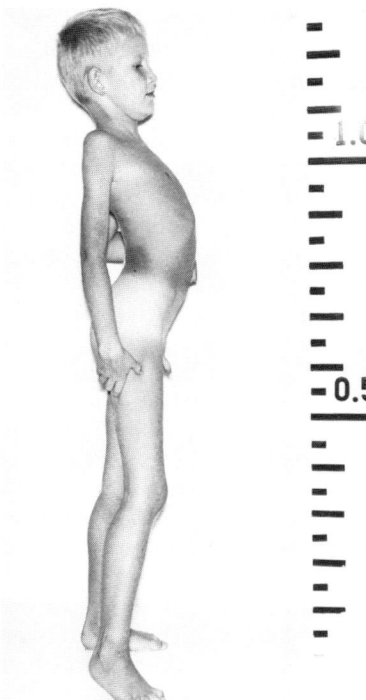

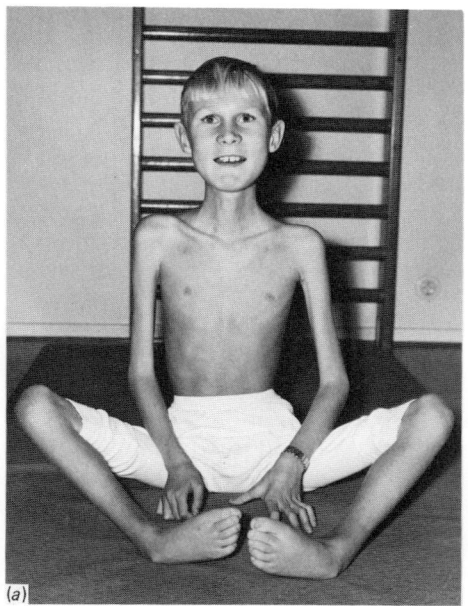

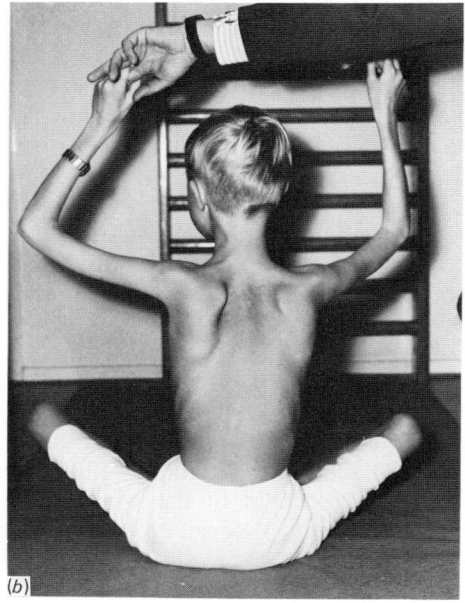

Figure 6.20. A 10-year-old boy with Duchenne muscular dystrophy, barely able to stand without support

Figure 6.21a and *b*. A 13-year-old boy with Duchenne muscular dystrophy. Note the severe muscular atrophy, involving also the small hand muscles, winging of the scapulae, inability to lift the arms, and normal face

A possible involvement of the central nervous system is likely in some patients with Duchenne muscular dystrophy. An increased proportion of patients with an abnormal EEG has been reported. Several examiners have found that the incidence of mild to moderate mental retardation, learning difficulties, and short attention span is higher in patients with Duchenne muscular dystrophy (even when the effect of their physical handicap is accounted for and eliminated as far as possible) than in the general population. Computerized tomography of the skull has in some examined boys shown widened lateral ventricles and mild cortical atrophy. The boys who have shown no evidence of involvement of the central nervous system by 6–7 years of age will not develop them later, nor will other Duchenne patients in their family. The gene for Duchenne muscular dystrophy and involvement of the central nervous system may be a different one from that causing the muscle symptoms alone, or two genes may be working in close connection.

No causal treatment is available; many remedies have been tried and were initially claimed to be effective, but none has yet proved to be so on long-term follow-up. However, much can be done to diminish the influence of the disease on the child. Physiotherapy is started as soon as the diagnosis has been established. At this stage the patient is usually ambulant and can move around actively on his own. He has, however, a tendency to develop contractures and this tendency must be counteracted. At this stage physiotherapy consists of instructions to the parents to stretch the tendons daily, preferably twice a day. Postponement of flexion contractures of the hip and of tight heel-cords is the main aim at this stage. Night braces may be of some help and may be tolerated if used *before* contractures have developed. It may be malposition of the joints rather than muscle weakness that confines the patient to a wheelchair. At the stage when he is about to lose his walking ability, he usually has contractures. Surgical lengthening of the iliotibial band and the heel-cords may then be helpful, provided it is done with a technique that enables the child to get up on his feet 1–2 days after surgery and provided he is immediately trained to stand and walk in braces. This programme may keep the patient ambulant 2 years longer than he would otherwise be. When he is unable to walk independently it is important to get him to stand on a tipping-board as much as possible. Standing diminishes the risk of kyphoscoliosis and the speed of decalcification of the bones and thus the risk of fractures and kidney stones. Eventually flexion contractures develop at the hips and knees, and a point is reached when it is no longer worthwhile to fight them. The risk of kyphoscoliosis is now imminent; a well-fitting corset may be better accepted if prescribed early (but not until the patient is confined to a wheelchair) rather than when the scoliosis is severe.

During the whole course training of the respiratory muscles is important, as are instructions to the parents on how they can help the child to get rid of mucus during a respiratory tract infection. Obesity is a common complication which should be prevented, as far as possible, through early information and instruction.

The diagnosis of Duchenne muscular dystrophy affects not only the life of the child but also that of the whole family. As with all serious diseases, the first information must be given to the parents in a relaxed and unhurried fashion, allowing the parents to show their emotional reactions openly. The facts about the disease must be given honestly. The physician must be aware that parents can only partly take in this information because of the emotional block provoked by the bad news. The information must therefore be repeated on several occasions, preferably by the same physician or team. Attention must be paid not only to the sick child but also to the whole family, including healthy sibs. Parents need help, also, with the many practical problems; the help of a social worker is necessary. The family must be stimulated to live as normal a life as possible and the patient should have ample contact with his peers. School education must be planned according to the patient's mental ability and interests; his physical handicap must never be allowed to prevent him receiving normal school education in a normal class; transportation can always be arranged and electrically operated technical aids to enable the patient to move himself around are available.

Other sex-linked recessive types of muscular dystrophy   Other forms of muscular dystrophy with sex-linked recessive inheritance exist. They are probably separate diseases, as different types do not seem to occur in the same family. The most benign type is that described by Becker and Kiener (1955). Its onset is in late childhood and its progression is so slow that most patients can walk and are even able to do some work in middle age.

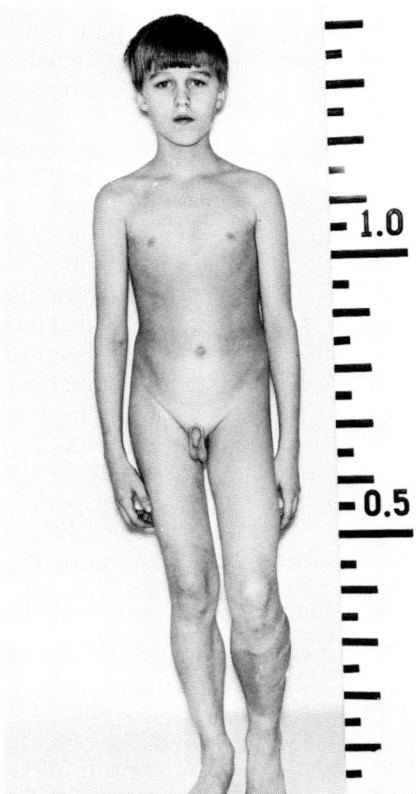

Figure 6.22. A 13-year-old boy with many features of Duchenne muscular dystrophy, but with a more benign course. Note the atrophy of pectoral muscles and the hypertrophy of calf muscles

At least two more distinct types have been suggested with a course between the classic Duchenne type and the Becker type (*Figure 6.22*). The mode of inheritance, the distribution of the muscle weakness, and the presence of hypertrophy are the same in all types.

Duchenne-like type muscular dystrophy with autosomal recessive inheritance   This type thus occurs also in girls. It is similar to the sex-linked type, with severe atrophy of the pectoral muscles, hypertrophy of the calves, and a tendency to tight heel-cords (*Figure 6.23*). However, it appears to be slightly more benign, as the age of onset is usually higher, the progression is slower, and the myocardial involvement is less prominent.

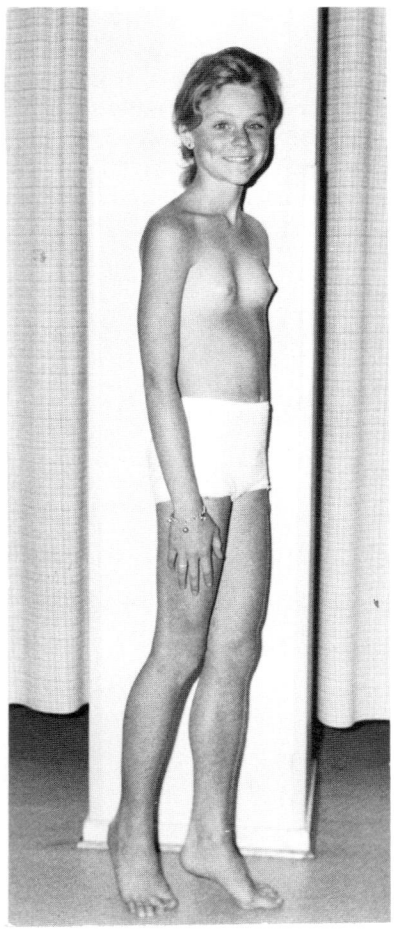

Figure 6.23. A 13-year-old girl with the Duchenne-like variant of muscular dystrophy with autosomal recessive inheritance. Note the atrophy of pectoral muscles, hypertrophy of calf muscles, and tight heel-cords

Limb-girdle type muscular dystrophy   The existence of this type in childhood is questionable; most childhood cases, presented under this diagnosis, have proved to be cases of polymyositis, progressive spinal muscular atrophy of type II, or a congenital stationary muscle disorder. Limb-girdle muscular dystrophy is not a homogeneous disease; if it exists at all it is better labelled limb-girdle syndrome. Childhood cases of this syndrome have usually been sporadic; autosomal recessive inheritance is a possibility. Symptoms are first noted in the proximal limb muscles, usually in the shoulder girdle; hypertrophy is not seen and the facial muscles are not involved (*Figure 6.24*). The disorder is slowly progressive and usually leads to severe disability in adulthood; its prognosis varies.

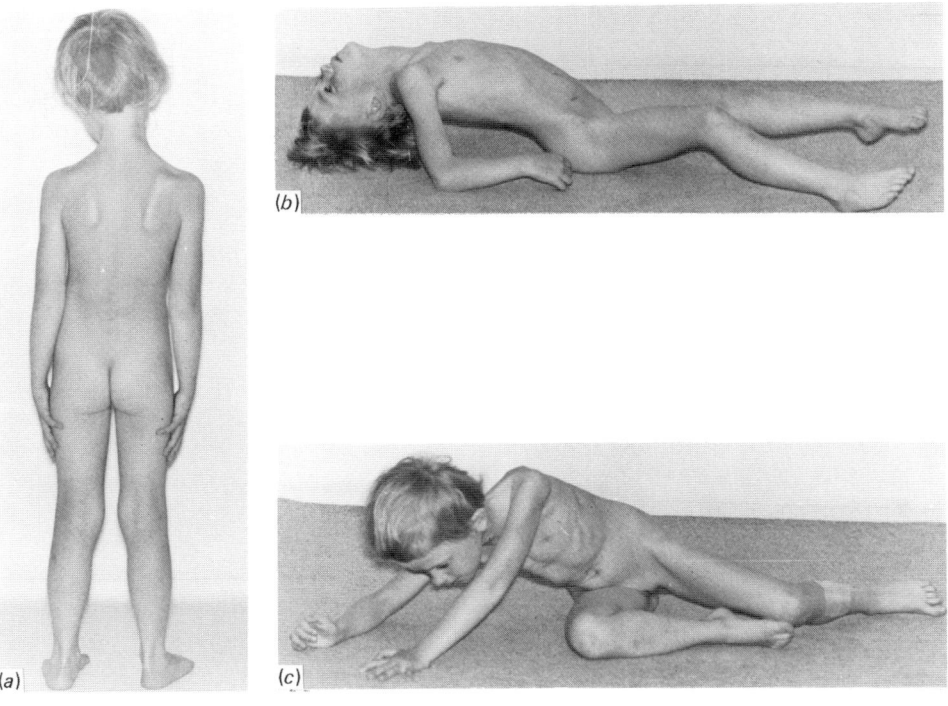

(a)   (b)   (c)

Figure 6.24a, b and *c.* A 6-year-old girl, diagnosed as a case of limb-girdle type of muscular dystrophy. Note the weak neck and shoulder muscles, winging of the scapulae, slight atrophy of the thigh muscles, absence of hypertrophy of calf muscles, and normal face

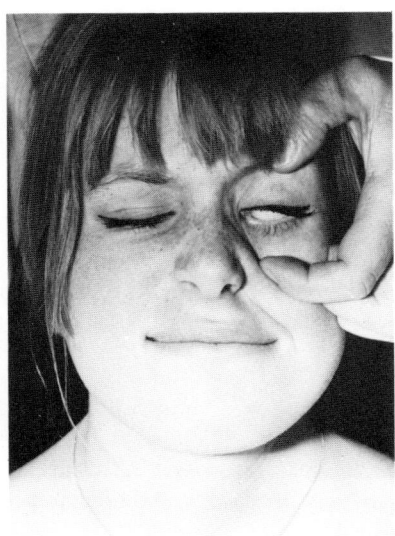

Figure 6.25. A 15-year-old girl with facioscapulohumeral muscular dystrophy. Note her inability to close her eyes tightly

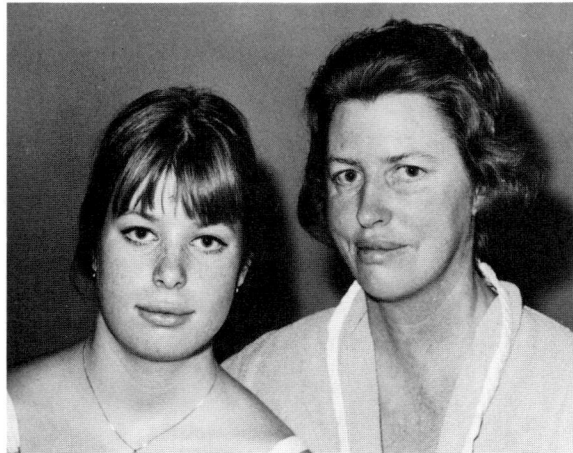

Figure 6.26. Facioscapulohumeral muscular dystrophy in mother and daughter. Note the muscular atrophy obvious in the face of the mother

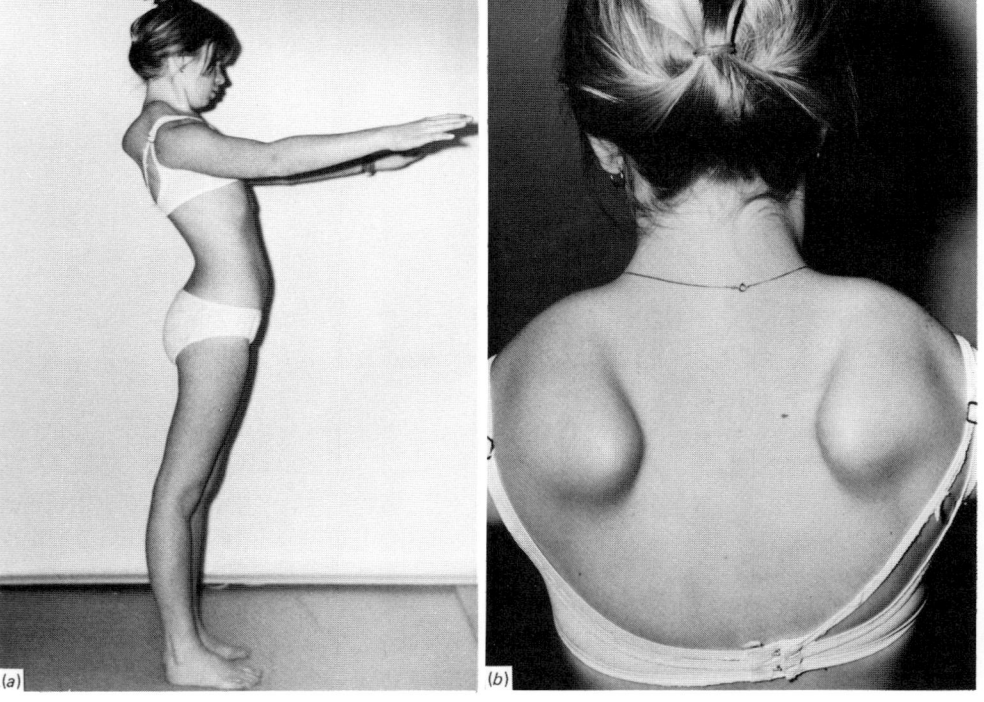

Figure 6.27. A 15-year-old girl with facioscapulohumeral muscular dystrophy. Note her inability to lift her arms to shoulder level (*a*) and severe winging of the scapulae (*b*)

Facioscapulohumeral muscular dystrophy   This type is inherited as an autosomal dominant trait. The disease may be mild, and it may be necessary to examine both parents to establish a dominant inheritance. The onset is usually in childhood, but it is difficult to date it exactly because of the insidious course. The first symptoms are noted in the face. The patients have difficulty closing their eyes tightly (*Figure 6.25*), whistling, and sucking through a straw. The facial muscles become atrophic, and the face remains free of wrinkles (*Figure 6.26*). The weakness and atrophy slowly spread to the muscles of the shoulders and the upper arms, causing the patients difficulty in lifting their arms and in carrying heavy things (*Figure 6.27*). The course is slowly progressive, and hip and low back muscles become involved after a variable time, making it difficult for the patient to climb stairs or to get up from sitting on the floor (*Figure 6.28*). The life-span is little if at all shortened, and working capacity is retained although the choice of profession is limited.

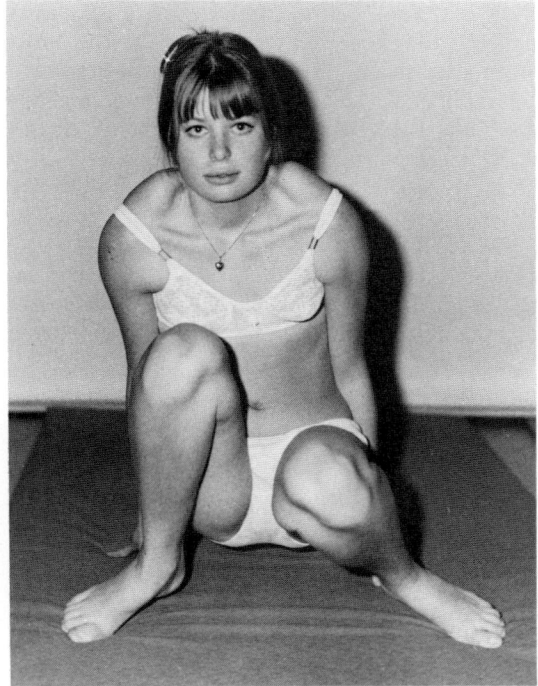

Figure 6.28. A 15-year-old girl with facioscapulohumeral muscular dystrophy demonstrating some weakness of the hip muscles, evident when she tries to get up from sitting on the floor

Ocular muscular dystrophy   This type is usually inherited as an autosomal dominant trait. Its onset may occur at any age. The first symptom is bilateral ptosis, followed by limitation of eye movements in all directions. These symptoms progress slowly over several years. In some patients the weakness may also spread to the facial muscles and possibly to the shoulder muscles. The influence on life expectancy and working capacity is slight.

Oculopharyngeal muscular dystrophy   This type is inherited as an autosomal dominant, and also involves the pharyngeal muscles; it has its onset in adulthood.

Distal myopathy   This disease was described under the name myopathia distalis tarda hereditaria (Welander, 1951) and is inherited as an autosomal dominant. The first symptoms are seen in the hand muscles; its onset is in adulthood. A distal myopathy with an onset in infancy and first symptoms involving the feet has also been described.

Myotonic dystrophy   This disease is inherited as an autosomal dominant with incomplete penetrance. The disease may be mild and a negative family history must not be accepted without examination of both parents. Its manifestations are widespread, even outside the muscular system, and it is debatable whether it should be described together with the muscular dystrophies or as a separate group.

Myotonic dystrophy may give symptoms in the newborn period. If so, inheritance is almost exclusively from the mother. The infant may be extremely weak and floppy and have severe breathing difficulties. Most infants with this malignant clinical picture die during their first days of life, often before a diagnosis has been established. Even at autopsy the diagnosis may be difficult, the most characteristic finding being a paper-thin diaphragm. Various malformations are often present (*see* page 196).

In the milder neonatal cases the clinical picture is dominated by severe generalized muscular hypotonia, inactivity, atrophy of the temporal muscles, an expressionless face with a triangular-shaped mouth and drawn-up upper lip (*Figure 6.29*), and sucking difficulties due to weak lips. Attacks of cyanosis may occur. Muscle reflexes are usually normal. Myotonia, even when carefully sought (*see* pages 213–214), may be impossible to detect on clinical examination. It can, however, be demonstrated electromyographically (*see* page 47). It is thus not surprising that these cases are usually misdiagnosed as cases of perinatal brain injury (*see* page 160).

Myotonic dystrophy is a slowly progressive disease; it is so slow that the child's normal development predominates for several years. These infants therefore seem to improve, they learn to sit up and to walk, although they pass their milestones late. The muscular hypotonia improves, but weakness and eventually wasting become more evident. Both the distal and proximal muscles are involved, the proximal muscles severely enough to cause difficulties in getting up from sitting on the floor (*Figure 6.29c*) and a waddling gait with protuberant abdomen and increased lumbar lordosis. This is unlike the usual picture in adulthood in which the dominating symptoms are from the distal limb muscles. The neck muscles usually become involved in late childhood.

The feeding difficulties improve, mainly because with increasing age the patient learns to eat without sucking. The facial weakness remains severe, and facies myopathica is a typical finding in patients of any age with myotonic dystrophy. The face has no expression, the mouth is half-open and the patient drools (*Figure 6.29a* and *b*). The eyes cannot be closed tightly. The temporal muscles are atrophic.

As the children grow older it becomes apparent that not only their motor development but also their general mental development is delayed. Practically all children with an early onset of the disease are mentally retarded to a variable degree, possibly with a slowly progressive dementia. Weakness of the lip muscles causes articulation difficulties with a disproportionately severe delay in speech development.

Myotonic dystrophy may also have an insidious onset later in childhood, particularly if the child has inherited the disease from the father. Delayed motor

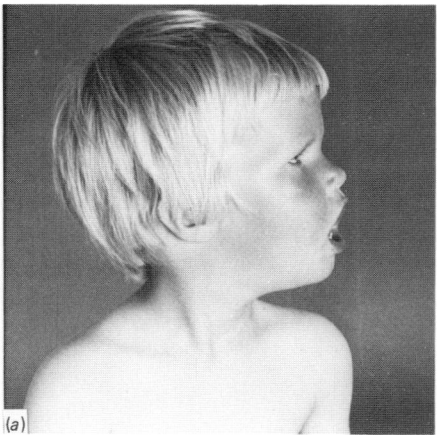
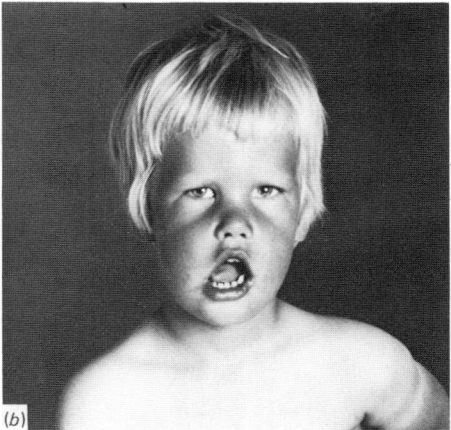
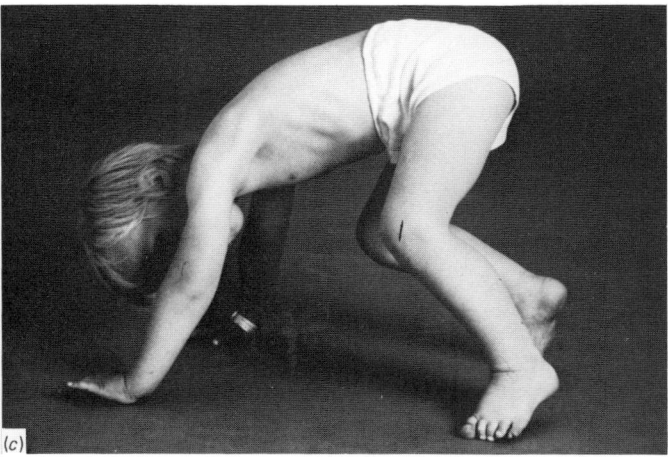

Figure 6.29. A 4-year-old boy with myotonic dystrophy inherited from his mother. Note the facial weakness with hanging chin and triangular mouth (*a*) and atrophy of temporal muscles (*b*). Note also the proximal weakness, making it difficult for him to get up from sitting on the floor (*c*)

development with slow clumsy movements is usually the first symptom. Facial weakness is usually present but not severe enough to attract the parent's attention. The upper lip and the mouth are shaped normally (*Figure 6.30*); the triangular-shaped mouth seems to require prenatal onset of the facial weakness. Myotonia can usually be demonstrated clinically, but is seldom a complaint of the patient. All patients with myotonic dystrophy show a tendency to slowness, tiredness, and lack of initiative.

Myocardial involvement is common, causing electrocardiographic abnormalities, even in childhood, although children seldom have cardiac symptoms. Lens opacities may be found in children with myotonic dystrophy; this manifestation of the disease is more common in adulthood. The endocrine abnormalities and frontal baldness, which are characteristic findings in adults with myotonic dystrophy, are rarely seen in childhood.

Myotonia, for which symptomatic therapy is available (*see* page 216), is practically never disturbing enough in children to require treatment. For the other aspects of the syndrome no therapy is known. The course is slowly progressive; mental retardation and muscle weakness are the most handicapping symptoms. Life-span is probably shortened by the disease, and working capacity is severely impaired.

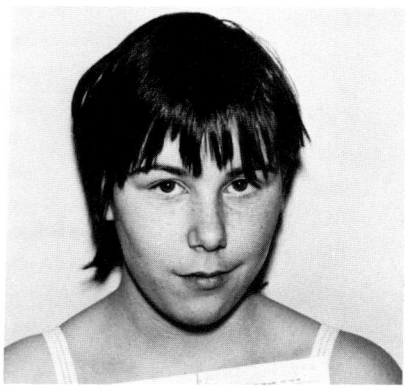

Figure 6.30. A 15-year-old girl with myotonic dystrophy inherited from the father. Note slight atrophy of the temporal muscles and a normally shaped, closed mouth

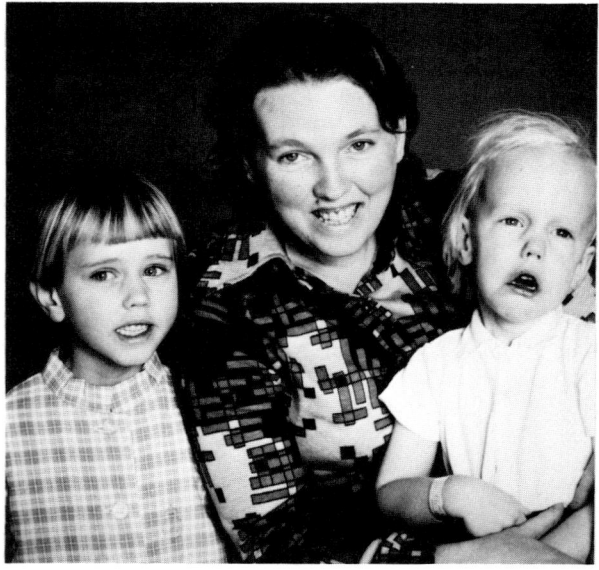

Figure 6.31. A mother and her two children, all afflicted with myotonic dystrophy. All three have atrophy of the temporal muscles. The children, particularly the boy, have a triangularly shaped mouth which the mother lacks (she inherited the disease from her father). The boy also has hydrocephalus, for which a shunt has been inserted

Women with myotonic dystrophy show an increased incidence of obstetric complications, particularly hydramnios. Their children have an increased incidence of malformations (*Figure 6.31*), especially club feet (*Figure 6.32*). Half of their children have myotonic dystrophy. The diagnosis in the mother and correct information to her about her risk of developing obstetric complications and of

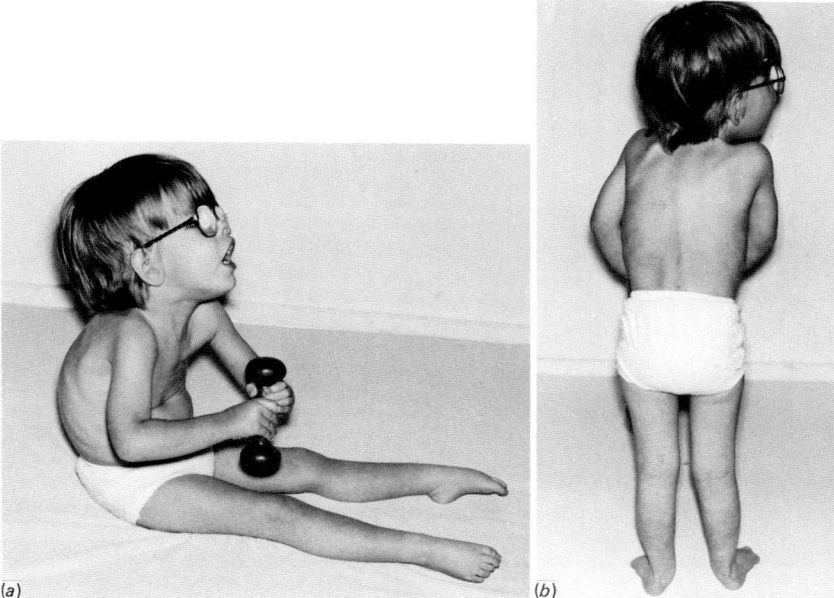

(a)   (b)

Figure 6.32a and *b.* A 3½-year-old boy with myotonic dystrophy inherited from his mother. Note his triangularly shaped mouth, the malposition of his feet (congenital), and the severe hypotonia and weakness of his neck, trunk and limb muscles, which make it difficult for him to balance his head and to sit with a straight back, and which delay his motor development generally

having a sick infant and/or an infant with malformations is the most important practical effect of the diagnosis of myotonic dystrophy in a newborn infant; this diagnosis is thus also important when the infant dies soon after birth.

Other congenital muscle disorders

A group of congenital myopathies, distinguishable mainly on the histological findings in the muscles, have been reported. *Central core disease* and *nemaline myopathy* were originally described as stationary disorders due to autosomal dominant inheritance. In the originally described family with central core disease the condition was found in five members in three generations; they were floppy as infants and remained moderately weak but had little wasting and were able to live a reasonably normal life. Proximal weakness is usually present (*Figure 6.33*). The histological picture consists of central cores appearing in most of the muscle fibres (*Figure 6.34*). These patients have a tendency to develop malignant hyperthermia (*see* page 397). Nemaline myopathy appears to be poorer delineated, inheritance may be dominant or recessive, and progression may occur. The facial and neck muscles are often seriously involved (*Figure 6.35a*); the patient often has a long face and high-arched palate. Both the proximal and distal muscles are involved (*Figure 6.35b* and *c*), and wasting is common as well as a great tendency to contractures, particularly kyphoscoliosis, and foot deformities. Milder cases also exist, with an apparent onset during late childhood or adolescence, usually with weakness of the limb muscles only. Respiratory failure is a common and serious threat to the patient with nemaline myopathy and may even occur in a mild case after physical exertion or in connection with a respiratory tract infection. The

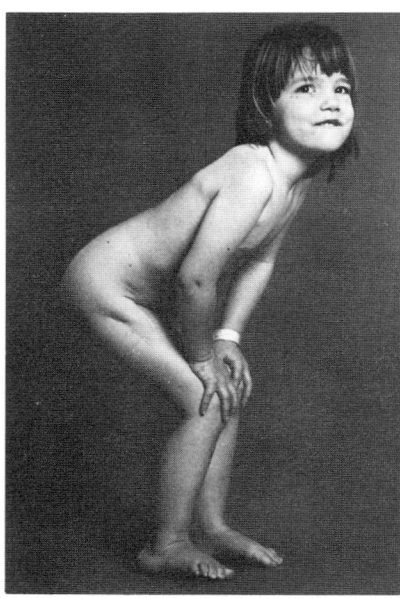

Figure 6.33. A 4-year-old girl with central core disease. Note the weakness of her proximal muscles. (Published with the permission of *Acta Paediatrica Scandinavica*)

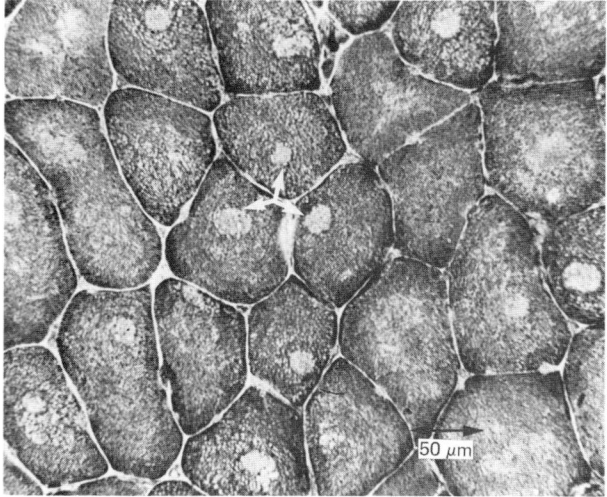

Figure 6.34. The histological picture typical of central core disease. The biopsy was taken from the father of the girl shown in *Figure 6.33*. The father was found to have some proximal weakness which was so mild that he himself was unaware of it

histological picture consists of characteristic threads in most of the muscle fibres (*Figure 6.36*).

Myotubular myopathy or *centronuclear myopathy* are terms apparently used at random for the same although heterogeneous condition. The onset is usually in the newborn period, when the affected infant is found to be floppy. The weakness is usually worst in the proximal limb muscles (*Figure 6.37a*), but the facial and extraocular muscles are as a rule also involved (*Figure 6.37b*). The characteristic

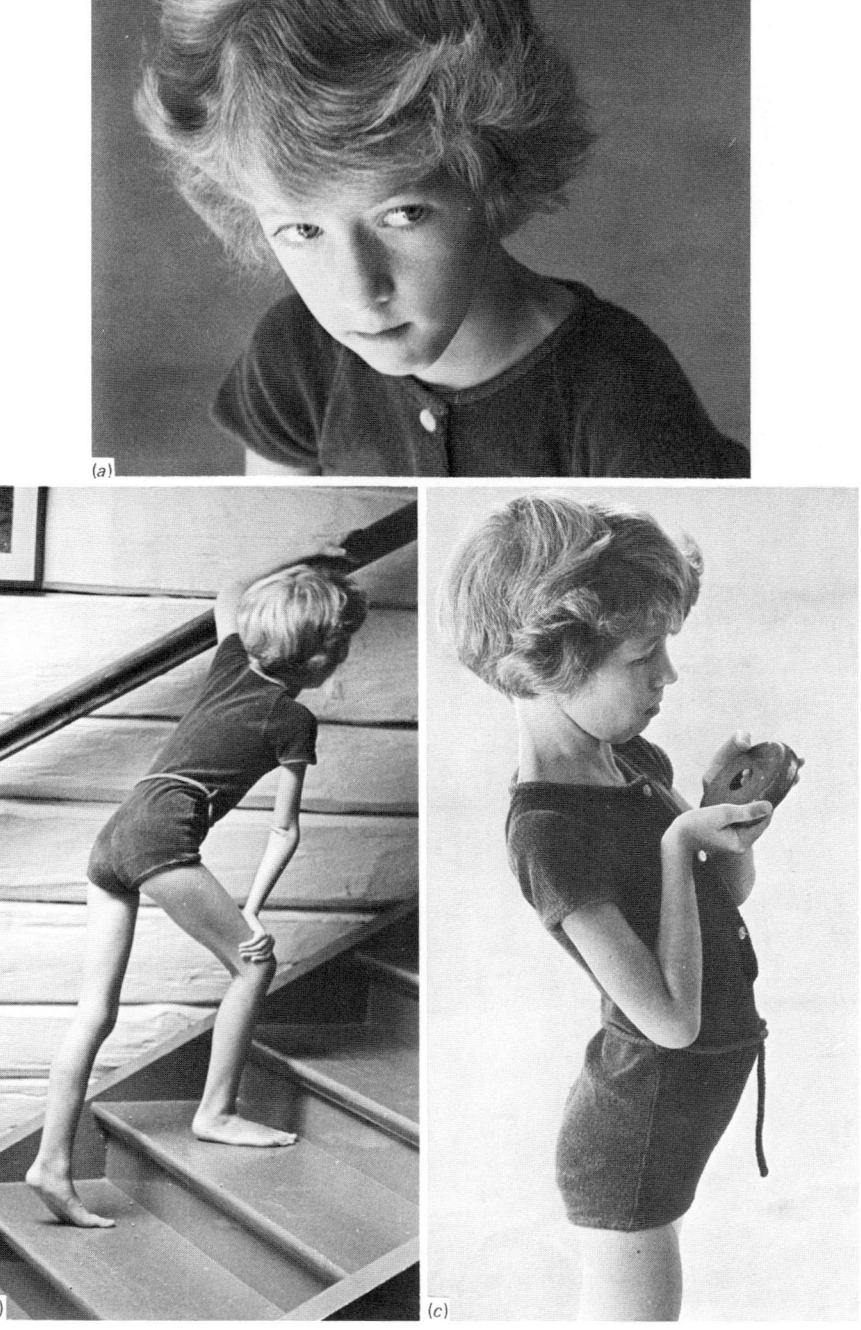

Figure 6.35a, b and *c*. A 7-year-old girl with nemaline myopathy. Note the mixture of proximal and distal weakness, involving also the facial muscles (*Figure 6.35a* is published with the permission of *Acta Paediatrica Scandinavica*)

histological picture consists of rows of central nuclei with no myofibrils but aggregates of mitochondria close to the nuclei. Families showing dominant, recessive, and sex-linked inheritance are on record.

Other congenital muscle disorders are *megaconial myopathy, pleoconial myopathy, fibre type disproportion (Figure 6.38), minicore myopathy, fingerprint*

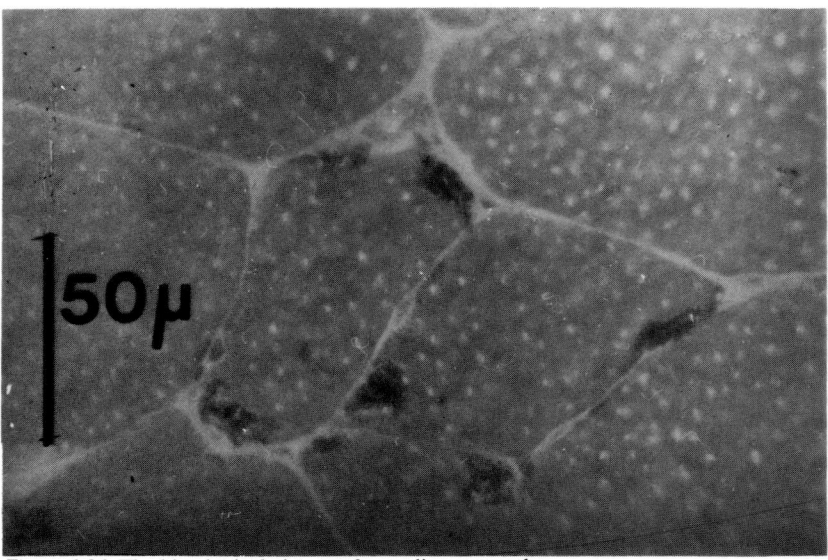

Figure 6.36. The histological picture of nemaline myopathy

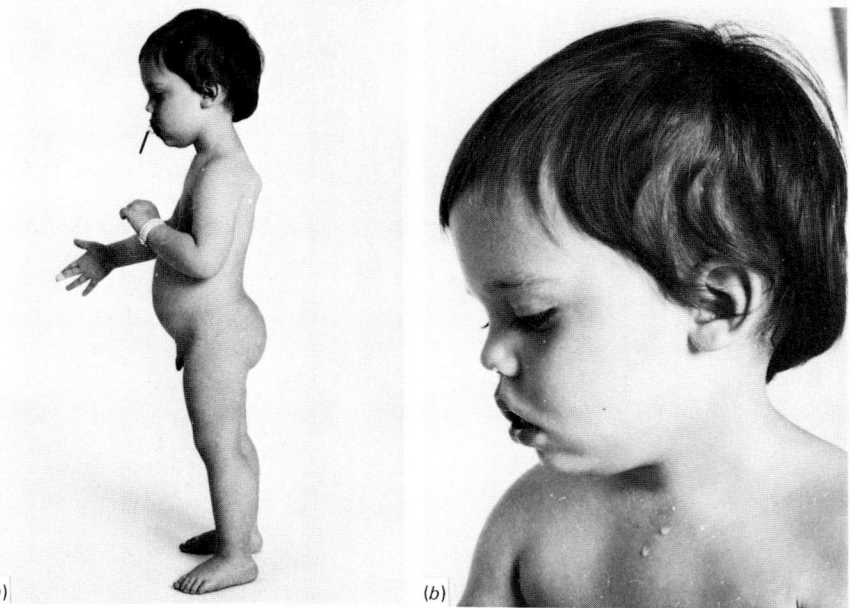

(a)   (b)

Figure 6.37. A 2-year-old boy with myotubular myopathy. Note the posture with protuberant abdomen and increased lordosis due to proximal weakness (*a*) and the facial weakness (*b*); the triangularly shaped mouth is produced by prenatal facial weakness, regardless of its cause, and is thus not confined to myotonic dystrophy (*see Figures 6.29, 6.31* and *6.32*)

body myopathy, and *sacrotubular myopathy.* Symptoms that are common to them all include the onset of muscular weakness and hypotonia in the newborn period, usually involvement of the facial muscles, and no apparent progression of symptoms, at least in early life. Special staining techniques and the investigation of a muscle biopsy specimen are required to separate these disorders. It is questionable whether each of these disorders represents a separate disease entity.

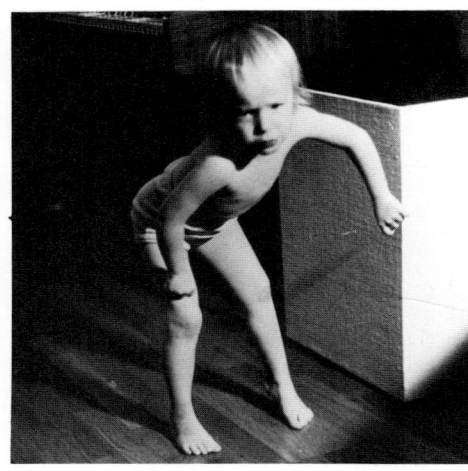

Figure 6.38. A 3½-year-old girl with fibre type disproportion. Note her proximal weakness. (Published with the permission of *Acta Paediatrica Scandinavica*)

For another group of congenital myopathies, the term *congenital muscular dystrophy* seems appropriate, as symptoms in these children are progressive and the histological examination of muscle tissue reveals changes that are typical of muscular dystrophy. Also, this group is heterogeneous. A type of congenital muscular dystrophy with autosomal recessive inheritance, mental retardation with progressive dementia, convulsions, abnormal findings on computerized tomography of the skull, and death during childhood has been described from Japan. A few patients of non-Japanese origin are also on record.

In another type of congenital muscular dystrophy the weakness and wasting may have the same distribution as in Duchenne muscular dystrophy, i.e. wasting particularly of the pectoral muscles, and hypertrophy of the calf muscles (*Figure 6.39*). In most cases of congenital muscular dystrophy the weakness and wasting are mainly proximal but the facial and neck muscles are also involved (*Figure 6.40*); otherwise it is nonspecific in its distribution. Contractures are common. In most cases symptoms progress and the patient is severely handicapped (*Figure 6.41*); death may occur in childhood or adolescence. The serum enzymes are generally normal or mildly elevated. The EMG shows myogenic abnormalities. A muscle biopsy must be performed to confirm the diagnosis of muscular dystrophy and to exclude other diagnoses, particularly myositis.

Mitochondrial and *metabolic myopathies.* A heterogeneous group of disorders can be distinguished, based on the finding of 'ragged-red fibres' in the muscle tissue taken at biopsy. With the use of modified Gomorri-trichrome stain, accumulation of red-staining material can be demonstrated in the subsarcolemmal and intermyofibrillar regions of irregularly shaped fibres (*Figure 6.42*). With the aid of oxidative enzyme stains and electronmicroscopical examination it can be shown

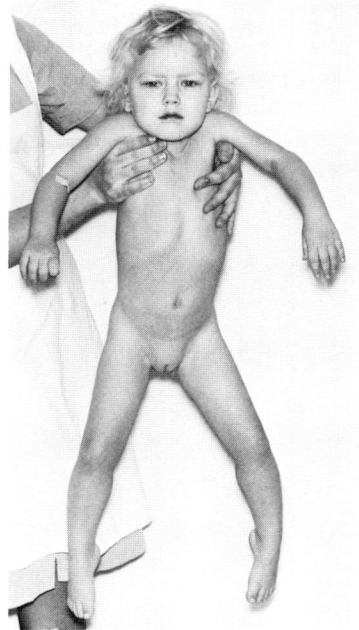

Figure 6.39. A 4-year-old girl with congenital muscular dystrophy of a Duchenne-like type with hypertrophy of the calf muscles, weak shoulder muscles, contractures, and a normal face

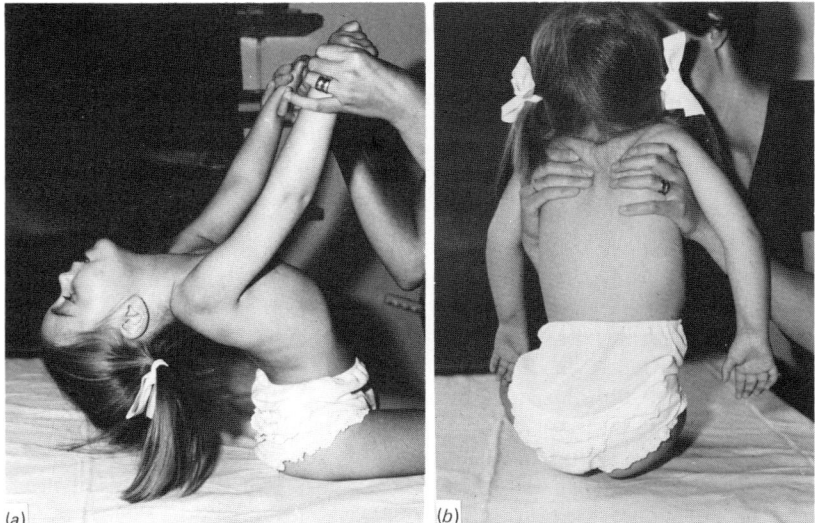

(a)   (b)

Figure 6.40a and *b.* A 4-year-old girl with congenital muscular dystrophy. Note the contractures, the normal face, and weak neck, trunk and proximal limb muscles

that such areas consist of aggregated abnormal mitochondria. Different mitochondrial abnormalities may be identified on electronmicroscopy, which is an important examination in these cases. To this group belong also the myotubular myopathies described on page 198. Some of the patients in this group show only muscle symptoms and signs, such as weakness, hypotonia and wasting, almost always also involving the extraocular muscles. Many patients with 'ragged-red fibres' in the muscles have a more extensive disorder, involving the heart and

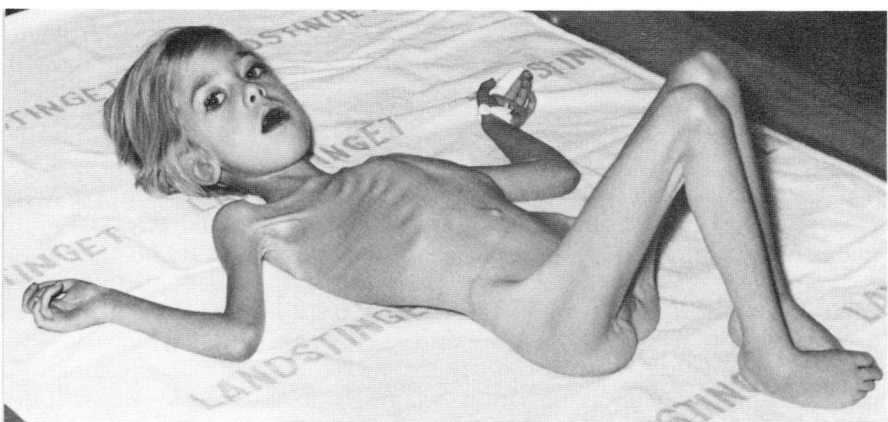

Figure 6.41. A 6-year-old girl with a malignant type of congenital muscular dystrophy. Note the extreme muscular wasting, contractures, and facial weakness

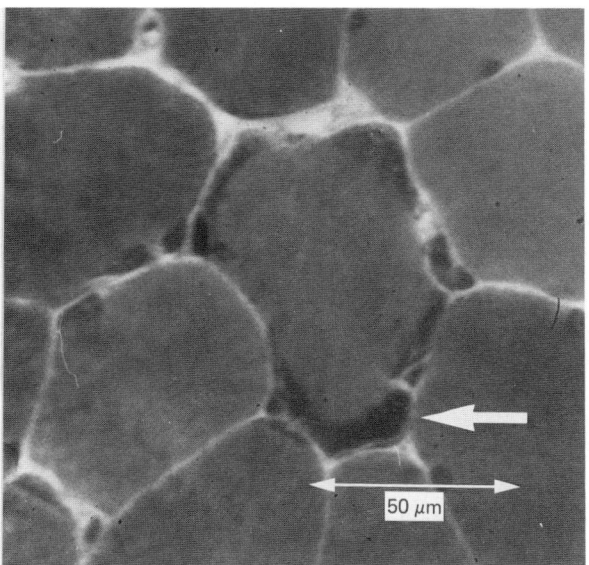

Figure 6.42. 'Ragged-red fibres' in a muscle biopsy from a 14-year-old boy; Gomorri-trichrome staining. The arrow points to the abnormal subsarcolemmal accumulation of material

causing life-threatening disturbances in cardiac conduction; the central nervous system, causing ataxia, extrapyramidal signs, etc.; and the eye, causing retinal abnormalities. The endocrine organs, kidneys, and bone marrow may also be involved. For this multisystem disorder the term *mitochondrial cytopathy* has been coined.

Endocrine myopathy
Endocrine myopathies, seen in hypo- and hyperthyroidism, hypo- and hyperpara-thyroidism, Cushing's syndrome, and acromegaly, are rare in childhood. In children, endocrine symptoms and signs dominate the clinical picture, even when muscle symptoms are present, whereas the opposite may occur in adulthood.

Long-term treatment with high doses of corticosteroids may produce proximal weakness as a side effect; this has been reported more commonly after the use of the fluorinated corticosteroids.

Metabolic myopathy

Glycogenosis   At least four types of glycogenosis may involve the skeletal muscles and cause weakness and hypotonia. All types appear to be hereditary with autosomal recessive inheritance. The lack of enzyme is apparent on histochemical staining of a muscle specimen. The glycogen storage can be demonstrated on a muscle piece fixed in absolute alcohol. The enzyme that is lacking can be identified on a frozen section. In type II, or Pompe's disease, the enzyme α-1,4-glucosidase is lacking. In the originally described cases there were severe cardiac and muscular symptoms from early infancy, and death occurred within the first year of life. Glycogen was stored in the skeletal and heart muscles with characteristic ECG abnormalities, enlargement of the heart, and cardiac failure. Several patients have recently been described with milder symptoms, mainly confined to skeletal muscles, and a clinical picture indistinguishable from muscular dystrophy.

In type III glycogenosis the enzyme amylo-1,6-glucosidase is lacking. Abnormal amounts of glycogen are stored in the liver and in skeletal muscles. The clinical muscle symptoms appear to be milder than in type II. A deficiency of the enzyme phosphofructokinase has also been described, causing increased fatigability with weakness and stiffness of muscle groups subjected to vigorous or prolonged exertion but no abnormalities at rest.

In type V, or McArdle's disease, the enzyme muscle phosphorylase is lacking. Symptoms start insidiously in late childhood or early adulthood with stiffness, pains, and weakness in muscles after prolonged exercise. In early childhood, findings are normal at rest but permanent weakness may eventually develop. The metabolic defect causes an inadequate breakdown of glycogen, the normal source of energy in the working muscle. A typical finding is therefore a lack of the normal increase of lactate in venous blood from a working muscle.

Carnitine deficiency may cause muscular weakness and wasting, i.e. symptoms indistinguishable from other forms of slowly progressive muscle disorders. Muscle fibres contain vacuoles which on special staining are shown to be filled with fat drops. An abnormally low carnitine content can be demonstrated in muscle tissue, plasma, and liver. The diagnosis is important as patients may improve after the administration of carnitine and treatment with corticosteroids.

Carnitine palmityl transferase deficiency is seen only in males who, from childhood, complain of aching pains in muscles, particularly after physical exercise and fasting. Reduced carnitine palmityl transferase activity may be demonstrated in leucocytes or cultured fibroblasts.

In all types of metabolic myopathies *myoglobinuria* may occur, particularly during an acute exacerbation of the disorder. Myoglobinuria may also be seen in any type of primary muscle disease, e.g. Duchenne muscular dystrophy. Paroxysmal myoglobinuria is thus not a disease but a symptom, occasionally present in several primary muscle disorders, particularly those known to have a metabolic background.

Hereditary metabolic myopathy with paroxysmal myoglobinuria due to abnormal glycolysis   This is a metabolic defect with autosomal recessive inheritance. It has its onset in childhood with attacks of muscle pain, muscle weakness, tachycardia, and dyspnoea precipitated by exercise. The attacks are sometimes accompanied by red urine. Hypertrophy of the calf muscles is seen early in the course. The physical findings are otherwise normal in young patients between attacks, but eventually permanent weakness develops. The course is chronic with exacerbations and remissions. The metabolic defect is an abnormally low consumption of oxygen by working muscles, leading to a high oxygen content in the venous blood and an accumulation of acid metabolites in the muscles. These metabolites may damage the cell membrane and cause a leakage of all substances, including myoglobin and all muscle enzymes, from the muscles. They also induce vasodilatation with increased circulation, which accounts for the systemic symptoms. If this syndrome is suspected, a catheter should be placed in the femoral artery and one in the femoral vein; blood collected during exercise should be examined for oxygen saturation, acid-base balance, and lactate content. A high serum activity of muscle enzymes and the presence of myoglobin in the urine supports the diagnosis. The only known treatment is to avoid, as far as possible, the precipitating factors, mainly physical exertion.

Dermatomyositis and polymyositis

Neither a septic myositis nor a specific one, such as trichinosis, will be considered here, as the clinical picture in both of these disorders is dominated by various general symptoms rather than by muscle symptoms.

Polymyositis and dermatomyositis belong to the group of disorders called collagenosis, which is considered to be an autoimmune condition. Myositis may be part of a more widespread disorder, e.g. rheumatoid arthritis, polyarteritis nodosa, or disseminated lupus erythematosus. The description here will be confined to dermatomyositis and polymyositis. The muscle symptoms and signs are the same, whether or not skin symptoms are present. In a rare case the onset is acute and the weakness may then within a few days confine the patient to bed and even necessitate assisted ventilation. With such an acute onset the muscles are usually tender and doughy; the patient may have fever, a high white blood cell count, and increased sedimentation rate; the urine may be red from myoglobin. Usually the onset is more insidious with slowly increasing weakness and fatigue. The trunk, neck and proximal limb muscles are usually affected first and most severely. The throat muscles may be involved, causing difficulty in swallowing. If the patient has no skin symptoms or their significance is overlooked, there is a risk that the disorder will be misdiagnosed as a degenerative disorder. Occasionally the fatigue and weakness have been misinterpreted as a psychic reaction to stress.

Some children with myositis have more inflammation in the tendons and the connective tissue between the muscle bundles than in the muscle fibres. These children complain more of stiffness than of weakness of muscles and of tight tendons. They may, for example, be unable to sit on the floor with their legs stretched out in front of them because of tight hamstring muscles and tendons. The tight tendons may cause limitation of movements in other joints, e.g. elbows, finger joints, or jaw joint, with no involvement of the joint itself.

In childhood, dermatomyositis is much more common than polymyositis. The skin symptoms are usually a dry, slightly scaly, non-itching rash in a butterfly distribution on the face (*see Figure 6.43a*, between pp. 100–101), on finger knuckles (*see Figure 6.43b*, between pp. 100–101), and often also on the knees and elbows.

A bluish tinge around the eyes or over the upper eyelid only (*see Figure 6.44*, between pp. 100–101) is a typical sign of dermatomyositis; it may appear without other skin signs and should therefore be carefully looked for.

Some special investigations are helpful. The serum enzymes are usually increased to a degree proportional to the acuteness (but not to the severity) of the disease. Electromyography reveals myogenic abnormalities and usually also spontaneous activity. Histological examination of muscle tissue reveals inflammatory infiltrates (*see Figure 6.7,* page 168). All these investigations are urgent; the histopathological findings usually provide the necessary confirmation of the diagnosis.

A diagnosis is urgent as myositis is one of the few treatable muscle diseases and treatment seems to be more effective the earlier it is started. In a child with symptoms of a muscle disease, the possibility of myositis must always be considered and actively excluded before the diagnosis of an untreatable condition is established. When a differential diagnosis is impossible, the patient is given the benefit of the doubt and treatment is tried for a limited period.

The drug therapy in myositis is corticosteroids in large enough doses for a long enough time. The initial daily dose of prednisolone is 1.5–2 mg/kg, divided into three or four daily doses. Some weeks may elapse before a clinical response is apparent; it may be preceded by a decrease in the elevated ASAT (aspartate aminotransferase) level. When the first signs of improvement appear, an attempt is made to give the total daily dose as one dose in the morning before 8 a.m. If improvement continues an attempt is made to combine the doses from 2 days into one dose every second morning before 8 a.m. If this is done too soon the patient may react with increased symptoms, and occasionally fever, during the day without treatment. If this happens one must go back to daily administration and make a new attempt some weeks later. The advantage of the every-second-day schedule is a reduction in side effects, particularly growth retardation. When the patient seems to be stabilized after several weeks on an every-second-morning schedule the total dose can be reduced. This must be done slowly and the serum enzymes, particularly ASAT, must be checked, as an increase in the serum level of this enzyme may precede a clinical relapse. Steroid therapy *may* have to continue for several years before it can be completely withdrawn.

If corticosteroids have no effect or if side effects outweigh the beneficial effect, immunosuppressive therapy may be tried. In adults azathioprine is the drug most commonly used; it has been reported as effective also in children. Other immunosuppressive drugs have been reported to have a beneficial effect, but as the number of children with myositis is small, it is difficult to assess their relative value.

Physiotherapy is a necessary complement to drug therapy. In the acute stage it must be cautious, and its purpose is to prevent contractures. With improvement the training can become increasingly active. Overtraining must be avoided; massage is forbidden. Bed-rest is avoided except in the very acute phase.

Calcifications of the connective tissue between muscle bundles is a common complication of myositis in children (*Figure 6.45*), although it does not occur in all cases. It is not known why some children escape this complication. No known treatment can prevent calcifications or has any influence on them. They can be felt from the outside and may limit joint movements; occasionally they become tender. They may ulcerate the skin and produce slow-healing ulcers. Over the years they tend to improve. They can be seen on X-ray of the soft tissue of the limbs.

The prognosis of myositis is good compared with other muscle diseases and better in children than in adults. However, death may occur in the acute stage from severe muscular destruction and respiratory paralysis, or it may be due to chronic progressive muscular weakness and complicating respiratory infections. Inflammation of blood vessels, seen in the connective tissue of the muscles, may also involve other vessels, particularly in the gastrointestinal tract, and bleeding from this area may be the cause of death. This may occur irrespective of treatment with corticosteroids. Treatment probably increases the survival rate and definitely improves the function of muscles in surviving patients. Some patients may also

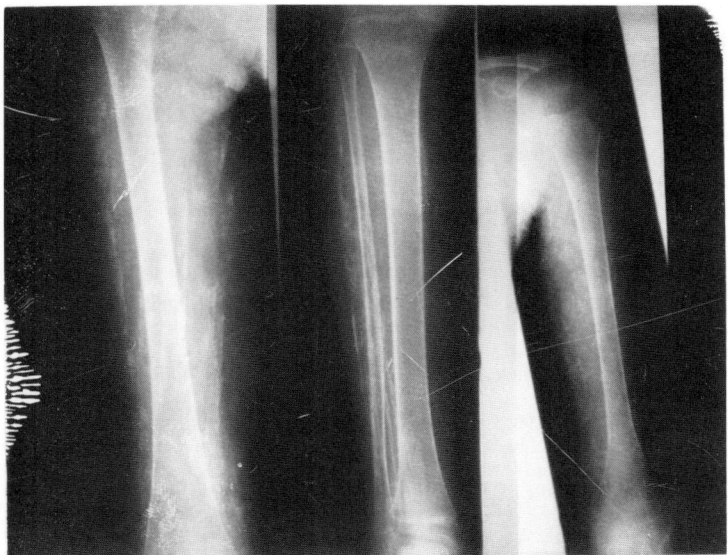

Figure 6.45. Intramuscular calcifications in the thigh muscles, lower leg muscles, and upper arm muscles of a 13-year-old girl who has had dermatomyositis since the age of 8 years

remain handicapped because of permanent muscle weakness, contractures, or complications of the calcifications. As a rule, however, this long-lasting disease results in only mild or no functional impairment.

Myositis ossificans progressiva is described in Chapter 7 (*see* page 217).

Miscellaneous

In a few hypotonic infants and children it is impossible to establish a firm diagnosis, even after extensive investigation. Some of them have a progressive disease whose true nature will eventually be disclosed. However, a few hypotonic infants show a steady improvement, and follow-up reveals no specific findings in them. The term *benign congenital hypotonia* has been created for this group of children. It denotes an *undiagnosed* condition, *not a disease*. It must not be used until the child has been followed-up for some years and has been thoroughly investigated for other causes of muscular hypotonia.

In *Table 6.1* (*see* pages 156–157) most of the conditions discussed in this chapter are schematically summarized and special studies of interest are indicated.

References

BETHLEM, J. (1980) Myopathies. Amsterdam: Elsevier/North Holland Biomedical Press

BETHLEM, J., ARTS, W. F. and DINGEMANS, K. P. (1978) Common origin of rods, cores, miniature cores and focal loss of cross-striations. *Archives of Neurology* (Chicago), **35**, 555–566

BLENNOW, G., GAMSTORP, I. and ROSENBERG, R. (1968) Encephalo-myelo-radiculo-neuropathy. *Developmental Medicine and Child Neurology*, **10**, 485–490

BONUCELLI, C. M., STETTON, G., LEVITT, R. C., LEVIN, L. S. and PYERITZ, R. E. (1982) Prader–Willi syndrome associated with an interstitial deletion of chromosome 15. *Johns Hopkins Medical Journal*, **151**, 237–242

BUCHANAN, D. C., LABARBERA, C. J., ROELOFS, R. and OLSON, W. (1979) Reactions of families to children with Duchenne muscular dystrophy. *General Hospital Psychiatry*, **1**, 262–269

CAVANAGH, N. P. C. (1980) The rôle of thymectomy in childhood myasthenia. *Developmental Medicine and Child Neurology*, **22**, 668–674

DIMAURO, S., TREVISAN, C. and HAYS, A. (1980) Disorders of lipid metabolism in muscle. *Muscle & Nerve*, **3**, 369–388

DUBOWITZ, V. (1980) *The Floppy Infant*, 2nd edn. Clinics in Developmental Medicine No 76. London: William Heinemann Medical Books

DUNN, H. G. (1968) The Prader–Labhart–Willi syndrome. Review of the literature and report of nine cases. *Acta Paediatrica Scandinavica*, suppl. 186

EGGER, J., LAKE, B. D. and WILSON, J. (1981) Mitochondrial cytopathy. A multisystem disorder with ragged red fibres on muscle biopsy. *Archives of Diseases in Childhood*, **56**, 741–752

ENGEL, A. G., LAMBERT, E. H., MULDER, D. M. and GOMEZ, M. R. (1981) Recently recognised myasthenic syndromes. *Annals of the New York Academy of Sciencies*, **377**, 614–639

FIRTH, M., GARDNER–MEDWIN, D., HOSKING, G. and WILKINSON, E. (1983) Interviews with parents of boys suffering from Duchenne muscular dystrophy. *Developmental Medicine and Child Neurology*, **25**, 466–471

FUKUYAMA, Y., OSAWA, M. and SUZUKI, H. (1981) Congenital progressive muscular dystrophy of the Fukuyama type – clinical, genetic and pathological considerations. *Brain & Development*, **3**, 1–29

GAMSTORP, I. (1956) Adynamia episodica hereditaria. *Acta Paediatrica* (Uppsala), suppl. 108

GAMSTORP, I. (1982) Non-dystrophic myogenic myopathies with onset in infancy or childhood. *Acta Paediatrica Scandinavica*, **71**, 881–886

GAMSTORP, I. and SARNAT, H. (eds) (1984) *Progressive Spinal Muscular Atrophies*. International Review of Child Neurology Series. New York: Raven Press

HARPER, P. S. and DYKEN, P. R. (1972) Early-onset dystrophia myotonica. Evidence supporting a maternal environmental factor. *Lancet*, **ii**, 53–55

HECKMATT, J. Z., LEEMAN, S. and DUBOWITZ, V. (1982) Ultrasound imaging in the diagnosis of muscle disease. *Journal of Pediatrics*, **101**, 656–660

HENRIKSSON, K. G. (1980) Polymyositis: diagnosis, prognosis and treatment. Linköping University Medical Dissertations, No 100, Linköping, Sweden

JOHNSEN, T. (1976) A new standardized and effective method of inducing paralysis without adminstration of exogenous hormone in patients with familial periodic paralysis. *Acta Neurologica Scandinavica*, **54**, 167–172

KORNFELD, M. S. and SIEGEL, I. M. (1980) Parental group therapy in the management of two fatal childhood diseases: a comparison. *Health & Social Work*, **5**, 28–34

MERCHLINE, M., RIDDLESBERGER, J. R. and KUHN, J. P. (1983) The role of computed tomography in diseases of the musculoskeletal system. *Journal of Computed Tomography*, **7**, 85–99

MUNSAT, T. L. (1980) The classification of human myopathies. In *Handbook of Clinical Neurology*, Chapter 7. Amsterdam: North Holland Publ. Co.

O'BRIEN, T. A. and HARPER, P. S. (1984) Course, prognosis and complications of childhood-onset myotonic dystrophy. *Developmental Medicine and Child Neurology*, **26**, 62–67

OOSTERHUIS, H. J. G. H., LIMBURG, P. C., HUMMEL-TAPPEL, E. and THE, T. H. (1983) Anti-acetylcholine receptor antibodies in myasthenia gravis. Part 2. Clinical and serological follow-up of individual patients. *Journal of Neurological Sciences*, **58**, 371–385

OUVRIER, R. A., MCLEOD, J. G., MORGAN, G. J., WISE, G. A. and CONCHIN, T. E. (1981) Hereditary motor and sensory neuropathy of neuronal type with onset in early childhood. *Journal of Neurological Sciences*, **51**, 181–197

PEARN, J. (1978) Genetic studies of adult infantile spinal muscular atrophy (SMA type I). *Journal of Medical Genetics*, **15**, 414–417

ROTT, H. D. and MULZ, D. (1983) Duchenne's muscular dystrophy: carrier detection by muscle ultrasound. *Journal de Génétique Humaine*, **31**, 63–65

SMITH, I., ELTON, R. A. and THOMSON, W. H. S. (1979) Carrier detection in X-linked recessive (Duchenne) muscular dystrophy: serum creatine phosphokinase values in premenarchal, menstruating, postmenopausal, and pregnant normal women. *Clinica Chimica Acta*, **98**, 207–216

THOMPSON, C. E. (1982) Infantile myositis. *Developmental Medicine and Child Neurology*, **24**, 307–313

YOUNG, R. S. K., GANG, D. L., ZALNARAITIS, D. L. and KRISHNAMOORTHY, K. S. (1981) Dysmaturation in infants of mothers with myotonic dystrophy. *Archives of Neurology*, **38**, 716–719

WESTERBERG, B. (1982) Neuropediatric aspects of hereditary peripheral neuropathies in childhood. Dissertation Göteborg Medical Faculty. Graphic Systems AB, Göteborg, Sweden

YUNUS, M., MASI, A. T., CALABRO, J. J. and FEIGENBAUM, S. L. (1981) Primary fibromyalgia (fibrositis): clinical study of 50 patients with matched normal controls. *Seminars in Arthritis and Rheumatism*, **11**, 158–170

ZISFEIN, J., SIVAK, M., ARON, A. M. and BENDER, A. N. (1983) Isaacs' syndrome with muscular hypertrophy reversed by phenytoin therapy. *Archives of Neurology*, **40**, 241–242

7

Abnormal muscle stiffness and/or muscle pains

In conditions characterized by abnormal muscle stiffness, the joints show an increased resistance to passive and active movements. The cause may be a non-neurological disorder, which is usually painful, e.g. a fracture, dislocation, osteomyelitis, eosinophilic granuloma in the bone, other bone tumours, or arthritis. These conditions are not discussed here. Stiff muscles have a tendency to become tender and to ache (to a lesser extent this is true also for weak muscles). In all conditions discussed in this chapter (and partly also in the previous chapter) some patients describe their chief complaint as aching pain. Children have a particular tendency to label all unpleasant sensations as painful. The localization of neurological conditions that cause muscle stiffness may be the central nervous system, the peripheral nerves, or the muscle fibres, or it may be unknown.

The central nervous system

Upper motor neurones and connections

SPASTICITY

In spasticity the stiffness increases on abrupt movements and diminishes eventually on slow constant stretching. Muscle reflexes are hyperactive and abnormal reflexes, e.g. the Babinski sign, are present. The lesion is localized mainly in the corticospinal tract, which originates in the ganglion cells of the motor cortex and ends at the synapse to the anterior horn cells. A lesion anywhere along this tract will cause spasticity and weakness. The lesion may be unilateral, causing a *spastic hemiparesis*. It may be bilateral, causing a *spastic diparesis* (arms less affected than legs), *spastic tetraparesis* (arms equally or more affected than legs), or *spastic paraparesis* (only legs affected); the lesion in the last-mentioned situation is usually localized in the spinal cord. Parasagittal tumours, which in adulthood may cause spastic paraparesis, are extremely rare in childhood. The increase in muscle tone usually affects some muscle groups more than others, producing a characteristic posture of the affected limb (*see* pages 279–286).

Spasticity is thus a symptom that helps to localize a lesion in the central nervous system. The occurrence of this symptom gives no information about its cause. The common causes of spasticity in childhood are discussed in Chapters 9, 12, 13, 15, 17, and 18.

RIGIDITY

Rigidity is a tough steady resistance, equal in extensor and flexor muscles, to all movements, abrupt and slow. The resistance may yield in short steps to a slow even stretching, thus producing the symptom called *cogwheel phenomenon*. The increased stiffness persists unchanged after repeated movements in the same joint; thus it cannot be 'worked off'. All active movements are slow and sparse. Abnormal posture of the limb is common. The reflexes are normal, unless the picture is complicated by a lesion in the corticospinal tract. Rigidity may affect only one limb or one side of the body, but in childhood it is usually bilateral. The lesion causing rigidity is localized in the basal ganglia and their connections. Rigidity is thus a symptom that indicates a certain localization of a lesion but tells nothing about its cause. The common causes of rigidity in childhood are discussed in Chapters 12, 13, 16, 17, and 18. A lesion in the same area may also cause involuntary movements (*see* Chapter 11); this symptom often occurs together with abnormal muscle rigidity. A lesion is seldom localized strictly to the basal ganglia and their connections; rigidity is therefore often found together with other movements disorders, e.g. ataxia and spasticity.

DRUG-INDUCED STIFFNESS

Some phenothiazine derivates used for the relief of nausea and vomiting may cause rigidity. This side effect is often marked after the administration of prochlorperazine, which may cause intense symptoms after only one standard dose, particularly in children. In a person sensitive to prochlorperazine, symptoms may start within a couple of hours after the first dose and last for a day, provided no further dose is given. If the administration of the drug is continued, symptoms increase and do not disappear until the drug is stopped. The symptoms are muscle stiffness and a peculiar posture of the head, sometimes of the arms, and occasionally of the legs. The head is forcefully turned towards one side and kept in an unnatural and often uncomfortable position. The hands and arms may be stretched out in a stiff and peculiar way. The muscles are stiff and offer resistance to passive and active movements. The stiffness may increase during acute painful attacks, which force the head and arms into a still more abnormal and painful position.

This dramatic clinical picture may cause considerable diagnostic difficulties, if its connection with prochlorperazine medication is not appreciated. The two common misdiagnoses are encephalitis and tetanus. Patients taking prochlorperazine usually show a false positive Phenistix and ferric chloride reaction of the urine. This can be used as a diagnostic test of the condition in situations when a history is unavailable, and in others as a sign which should alert the physician to ask the correct questions. Although the condition is unpleasant and usually painful, it is self-limiting; sedation may help the patient through the uncomfortable hours. Other phenothiazines may occasionally produce the same type of symptoms, although less dramatically.

Lower motor neurones and connections

TETANUS TOXIN

The toxin produced by the tetanus bacilli causes muscle stiffness, which has its likely localization in the anterior horn cells and their connections in the spinal cord. The tetanus bacilli must enter the body through a wound, which may, however, be small or localized such that it escapes notice. After an incubation period of 5–21 days, the patient becomes irritable and restless and has increased muscle tone and increased muscle reflexes. Within 1–2 days, these symptoms are followed by attacks of painful, involuntary muscle contractions. The attacks increase in frequency, duration, and severity. They are provoked by any stimulus, such as a sudden light or sound, touching the patient or attempts to feed him. Facial muscles are almost always involved, giving the typical signs *risus sardonicus* and *trismus*. Respiratory muscles are also involved; respiration is impaired, and the patient becomes cyanotic and anoxic. Mortality is high in untreated patients.

Accomplished and maintained immunization prevents tetanus. If an unvaccinated person contracts a wound that is suspected to be infected with tetanus, a prophylactic dose of tetanus antitoxin will prevent the disease. When given after symptoms have started, the antitoxin is effective in binding the circulating tetanus toxin but has no influence on the toxin already attached to the central nervous system. The treatment is diazepam in a continuous intravenous infusion. The dose usually required is around 0.5–1.5 mg/kg per hour; it must be adjusted individually to keep the patient symptom-free and comfortable. Only rarely is such a high dose needed that respiration is impaired; if so, assisted ventilation is necessary and must be available. Excellent nursing care is also important. The patient must be kept in a quiet room and cared for with gentle slow movements; a sudden sound or an abrupt touch may elicit new painful spasms. Treatment usually has to be continued for some time, ranging from several days to a few weeks. Only in exceptionally severe cases is the old treatment (curarization, artificial respiration, and feeding through a gastrostomy) necessary; in such cases convalescence is slow. With modern treatment the prognosis is good and sequelae are rare.

Tetanus may infect the newborn infant through the umbilicus. Symptoms are severe and mortality is high in untreated infants. The same treatment as outlined above considerably improves the prognosis.

The peripheral nerves

NEUROMYOTONIA

The aetiology of the condition termed *neuromyotonia* (Mertens) or *continuous muscle fibre activity* (Isaacs) is unknown. The main symptom is a strong resistance to all passive and active movements; the latter are performed slowly, and relaxation after a contraction is difficult. The stiffness can be poorly 'worked off', percussion myotonia is not present, and the stiffness does not respond to a large dose of quinine, thus differing from 'myogen' myotonia (*see* page 213). On electromyography the typical myotonic bursts are not seen. The activity consists of continuous motor unit activity, which does not disappear in spite of good cooperation from the patient, who tries to relax the muscle. It is present simultaneously in agonists and antagonists. The stiffness of the muscle and the continuous activity on the electromyogram (EMG) do not disappear on blockage of the nerve with a local anaesthetic but do disappear on curarization, which blocks neuromuscular transmission at the end-plate.

This condition responds to phenytoin or, usually better, to carbamazepine, two drugs that are known to stop repetitive firing in peripheral nerves and are used, for example, in trigeminal neuralgia. The effect is sometimes dramatic, and the patient remains well as long as he continues to take the drug. The dose is the same as, or slightly lower than, that used in epilepsy (*see* pages 112–113). The ultimate prognosis in neuromyotonia is not yet known.

The muscle fibres

MYOGEN MYOTONIA

Myotonia, which is better called *myogen myotonia* to distinguish it from the more recently described neuromyotonia (*see above*), has been proved to be localized in the muscle fibres, as it persists even after curarization. Myotonia can best be described as an inability to relax the muscle rapidly after a contraction. When the patient makes a fist, he cannot open the hand again quickly (*Figure 7.1*); if he closes his eyes tightly, it is some time before he can open them again; if he looks upward

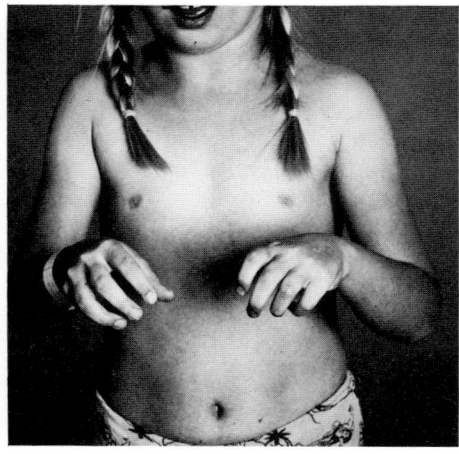

Figure 7.1. Myogen myotonia – this 8-year-old girl with dominantly inherited myotonia congenita has been asked to make a tight fist and then open her hands rapidly. The picture illustrates her inability to do so

and then downward, the eyelids do not follow the downward movement of the eyeballs, and a white crescent of sclera is seen between the eyelid and the iris (*Figure 7.2*); a crying infant maintains the expression of crying for several seconds after he has actually stopped crying. The muscles offer resistance to passive movements in all joints in all directions; this resistance disappears after repeated movements. The patient complains of stiffness of all muscles, possibly mixed with pain; it is most pronounced at the first contraction after a rest and prevents his free movements. It decreases after a few contractions, and can thus be 'worked off'. When the patient gets up from a chair and starts to walk, he walks slowly with an abnormal gait and stiff legs; the gait improves after a few steps, and becomes normal after a variable period, at most several minutes. The first clenching and opening of the fist is difficult; the tenth time the movement is repeated it may be normal. After a few minutes of rest, the stiffness returns. This is the usual relationship between myotonia and movements, although on rare occasions the opposite may be noticed, i.e. increased stiffness after repeated movements – *myotonia paradoxica.* Cooling of the muscles always increases the stiffness. It may be impossible for a patient to 'work off' the stiffness if he is cold.

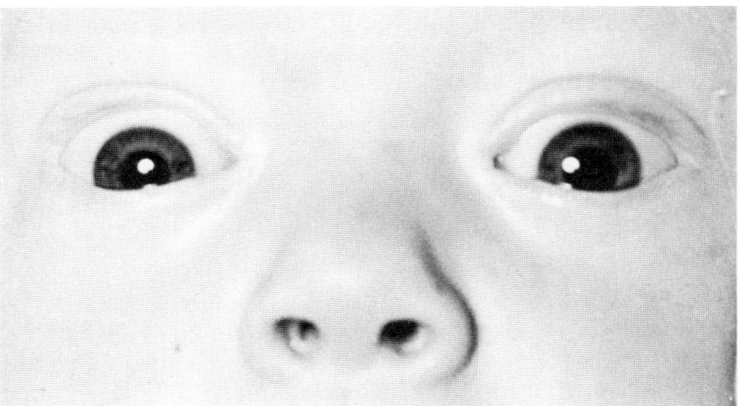

Figure 7.2. Myotonia of the eyelids in a 6-month-old infant

Myotonia can be demonstrated clinically also by tapping the muscles with a small percussion hammer – *percussion myotonia.* In a patient with severe myotonia, the tapping of any muscle will cause a dimple or a furrow, which persists for several seconds and then fades away. Since a thick subcutaneous fat layer may obscure this reaction, the thenar eminence and particularly the tongue are good muscles to examine for percussion myotonia. The patient is asked to extend his tongue on a tongue depressor and the tongue is tapped with the percussion hammer; this produces a dimple which persists for several seconds (*Figure 7.3*). If no myotonia

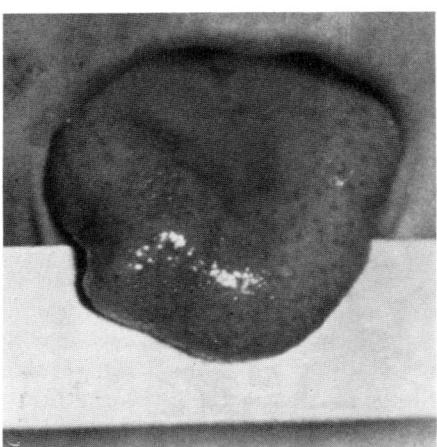

Figure 7.3. Percussion myotonia of the tongue in a 7-year-old girl

can be found in the tongue, it is unlikely that any other clinical examination will reveal myotonia. In an infant or small child with a good subcutaneous fat layer and no desire to cooperate in the examination of the tongue, myotonia can best be observed in the facial and extraocular muscles (*see* page 213); other clinical methods usually fail. The most sensitive method of demonstrating myotonia is electromyography (*see* page 47).

Myotonic dystrophy
Myotonia is a symptom found in several muscle diseases. In myotonic dystrophy (*see* page 194) stiffness is seldom a complaint of the patient, who may not have noticed it. In infants and young children hypotonia and weakness dominate the clinical picture and mask the myotonia, which is often only demonstrable on electromyography.

Myotonia congenita
The clinical picture of myotonia congenita is dominated by myogen myotonia as described on page 213. Myotonia congenita is a genetically determined disease that is usually due to an autosomal dominant gene, as in the family described by Thomsen in 1876. Autosomal recessive inheritance has also been reported. In general the clinical picture is the same, regardless of the mode of inheritance, but it differs in a few details. Myotonia is easy to demonstrate clinically and electromyographically both in dominant and recessive myotonia congenita. In the dominant type, the symptoms are first noted in early infancy and are generalized; in the recessive type, symptoms are seldom noted before 4–6 years of age and usually start in the legs. As a rule, the symptoms are more severe in the recessive than in the dominant type. The myotonia is usually sufficiently severe in both types to be a nuisance to the patient and to limit, for example, his free choice of a profession, but it does not prevent him living an essentially normal life. Many, but not all, patients with myotonia congenita also have unusually large muscles. Myotonia and muscular hypertrophy are the only symptoms of the disease and are nonprogressive. Myotonia is present in both warm and cold surroundings, but is usually more severe if the patient is cold. The administration of potassium may increase the myotonia.

In the dominant type, myotonia is usually detected by the mother in the infant's face during the first 6 months of life. One of the parents and members of his or her family have the disorder and their experience facilitates the detection and correct interpretation of the infant's symptoms. The family also knows about the relative benign nature of the condition and this knowledge diminishes their worries.

In the recessively inherited type the parents are usually unaware that anything is wrong until the child is 4–6 years of age. This delay is probably partly due to the fact that the family has had no previous experience of the disorder. Myotonic symptoms appear first in the legs and spread during the following years to the rest of the body. No other progress is noted. An increased incidence of malposition of the joints, particularly club feet, is seen. The recessive type usually causes more concern; possibly the myotonia is more severe than in the dominant type, but to a great extent this impression is due to the lack of experience of the disorder in the family. For the physician the diagnosis is more difficult when the family history is negative, and the parents may not get an explanation for their child's symptoms. A diagnosis is crucial, as the only way to lessen the parents' concern is to explain the symptoms, give the disease a name, and honestly assure the family that the disease, though lifelong, is not progressive and will not handicap the child.

Myotonia often increases during puberty and pregnancy, otherwise it stays essentially the same throughout life. The patient usually learns to manage his difficulties better in adulthood than during childhood. The muscular hypertrophy, which causes the patient no trouble, develops during childhood and then does not develop further.

In myotonia congenita, unlike myotonic dystrophy, there is no element of progressive muscular weakness and wasting, cardiac disease, eye abnormalities, endocrine disturbances, or dementia. The life expectancy is the same in patients with myotonia congenita, both dominant and recessive, as in normal individuals.

The administration of extra potassium should be avoided in myotonia congenita. A low-potassium diet has been used with some success, but it is difficult to realize for any length of time. ACTH, corticosteroids, procainamide, and quinine relieve myotonia for a limited time in many patients. However, these drugs have side effects which are too serious, at least in children, to justify their use for the purely symptomatic treatment of a nonprogressive, scarcely handicapping, condition. Improvement of myogen myotonia has also been reported following treatment with phenytoin, carbamazepine, and acetazolamide in the same dose as used in epilepsy (*see* pages 112, 113 and 116), but in most patients the effect is insignificant.

Paramyotonia congenita
In paramyotonia congenita, a disease inherited as an autosomal dominant trait, the myotonia is generally milder than in myotonia congenita. The patient may have no symptoms at all when he is warm but becomes abnormally stiff on cooling of the muscles. Thus, he may notice stiffening of the limb muscles and particularly facial muscles in cold weather, and may experience swallowing difficulties when eating ice cream. This stiffness disappears quickly in warm surroundings. If the patient is exposed to more intense cooling, he may become not only stiff but also weak. This weakness may last for minutes or hours and may disappear only on thorough warming, as in a hot bath. Weakness can be provoked *only* by cooling. Muscle stiffness is a less dominating symptom in this disease than in myotonia congenita (*see also* page 183).

On clinical examination myotonia may be found, when carefully looked for, even in warm surroundings, and can usually be demonstrated electromyographically. Cooling of the muscles facilitates its demonstration both clinically and electromyographically. Muscular hypertrophy is not present. Symptoms may worsen during puberty and pregnancy. The patient's activity is limited only slightly by the disease. Some patients respond to treatment with acetazolamide.

Chondrodystrophic myotonia
Chondrodystrophic myotonia (Aberfeld, Schwartz–Jampel syndrome) is a rare syndrome, which is probably inherited as an autosomal recessive trait. Children with this syndrome usually present with stiffness in their second year of life and myotonia can be demonstrated electromyographically. They have a small mouth, small eyes, and usually dislocated hips. Their physical development is impaired with growth retardation that becomes apparent when the child is a couple of years old. Their mental development is normal. The condition is not progressive. Only symptomatic treatment is available. At least two reported patients have been followed-up into adulthood; both (boy and girl) passed through a normal puberty and reached an adult height of 150–152 cm.

Adynamia episodica hereditaria
Myotonia may occasionally be found in adynamia episodica hereditaria but the patient seldom complains of stiffness (*see* page 183). The clinical picture of this disease is dominated by attacks of weakness and abnormal sensitivity to the administration of potassium.

MYOSITIS OSSIFICANS PROGRESSIVA

This is a rare disorder which has its onset in infancy or early childhood. The first symptoms usually appear in the neck and shoulder girdle, where the muscles become stiff and the joints immobilized because of the abnormal formation of bone within the muscles. The abnormal bone can be seen and felt as hard knots in the muscles and as true exostoses attached to skeletal structures (*Figure 7.4*). In the beginning the course may be undulating, i.e. tender swellings may appear within the muscles, remain for a few weeks, and then slowly subside. The patient may also have a low-grade fever. At this stage the clinical picture is confusing and diagnosis

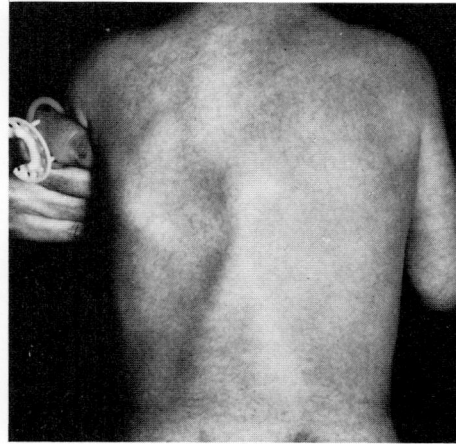

Figure 7.4. The back of a 1-year-old girl with myositis ossificans, showing the tough infiltrations of the subcutaneous tissue, which lead to a generalized stiffness of all movements of the back

is difficult. After some weeks or months the swellings may return in the same place or in a different muscle. Eventually the permanent formation of bone within the muscles is established. The process slowly spreads from the shoulders to the elbows and along the back to the hips and knees; only rarely are more distal structures involved. The patients become severely handicapped and finally bedridden. Growth and physical maturation are delayed, and teeth abnormalities are common. Death is usually due to a respiratory tract infection and occurs, as a rule, during early adulthood. No metabolic defect has been revealed; no treatment is available. The cause is unknown. The occurrence of the disease has been reported in identical twins and in father and child. However, the occurrence of more than one case in a family is an exception. If the disease is genetically determined, inheritance must be due to an autosomal dominant gene, practically all cases being caused by a new mutation.

PRIMARY FIBROMYALGIA

This is a vaguely delineated syndrome, probably belonging to the group of collagenoses. It is rare in childhood but may occur. The syndrome consists of pains in the muscles and around joints (which are usually not involved), particularly at tendon insertions. Physical exhaustion increases the pain, but so also does prolonged rest, when the muscles become stiff and ache. The most characteristic finding is *trigger points,* which are small, constant, intensely tender points in the muscles or at tendon insertions. They may be found in any muscle, but are possibly more common around the shoulders and in the trapezius muscle. Histological examination of a biopsy specimen taken at a trigger point shows an even distribution over the whole cross-section of fibres, which appear moth-eaten. Other objective findings are scarce: neurological examination, joints, and laboratory studies are usually normal. Patients as a rule also complain of symptoms from other systems: the incidence of headache and of colon irritability is increased, constant fatigue is a common complaint, and sleep difficulties with a lack of deep non-REM sleep are particularly common. Patients with these various complaints and scarce objective findings are easily misunderstood and thought to be neurotic, which may impair their ability to cooperate in treatment.

The first step in any therapeutic regimen is to recognize the disorder and its somatic aetiology, which presumably is the patient's lack of deep sleep. This may lead to constant tension in the muscles, from which the syndrome may develop. Suitable hypnotics should therefore be prescribed for a limited period, which may be repeated. Well-balanced physiotherapy is important. The patient must learn to relax his muscles and to find the balance between too much and too little muscular exercise; swimming in warm water is particularly helpful. The acceptance of the disorder as a primary *somatic* condition is the first measure (possibly with *secondary* neurotic symptoms due to constant pain and fatigue). The physician's knowledge and honest reassurance to the patient that the condition is unpleasant but not dangerous are perhaps the most important aspects of treatment.

Localization unknown

STIFF-MAN SYNDROME

This is a rare syndrome of unknown and probably heterogeneous aetiology. The characteristic clinical feature is a severe fluctuating muscle stiffness, which may be severe enough to immobilize the patient. The condition is often painful. The EMG usually shows continuous activity of the motor unit type, often indistinguishable from the findings in neuromyotonia (*see* page 212); some of the patients reported as cases of stiff-man syndrome may have had the condition that has been termed neuromyotonia. Only a few cases with onset in childhood are on record; most reported cases have occurred in middle-aged persons. A therapeutic trial with phenytoin or carbamazepine is justified; some patients may get symptomatic relief from diazepam. The prognosis varies.

ARTHROGRYPOSIS MULTIPLEX CONGENITA

Arthrogryposis multiplex congenita is a heterogeneous syndrome characterized by joint deformities that are apparent at birth (*see* page 340).

Plan of examination in patients with abnormal muscle stiffness

Spasticity is recognized without difficulty on clinical examination alone; hyperactive muscle reflexes and the presence of abnormal reflexes are easily demonstrated. Rigidity is also easy to evaluate clinically, particularly if the cogwheel phenomenon is present. The conditions that may cause spasticity and rigidity are discussed in Chapters 9, 11, 12, 13, 15, 16, 17 and 18. In cases of rigidity with acute onset, muscle pain, and abnormal posturing, the cause may be the administration of drugs, particularly prochlorperazine; a false positive Phenistix or ferric chloride test is usually found in these conditions.

X-ray examination of the muscles may reveal calcifications characteristic of myositis ossificans progressiva. Computerized tomography and ultrasound examination of the limbs may reveal more details about abnormalities in the muscles. X-ray examination of skeletal structures and joints is essential to exclude non-neurological causes of muscle stiffness, particularly when it is painful.

In cases of painful muscle stiffness occurring in attacks that increase in frequency, duration, and severity over hours and days, the possibility of tetanus must be kept in mind. Tightly closed jaws and a risus sardonicus are typical though not pathognomonic findings. When tetanus is suspected it is important to look for a possible route of entry through a wound and to enquire about immunization.

The neurological examination should also include clinical tests for myotonia (*see* pages 213–214). In doubtful cases, electromyography may be helpful in analysing muscle activity. A therapeutic trial may also be useful, since myogen myotonia (the type of myotonia seen in, for example, myotonia congenita) responds to a large dose of quinine, neuromyotonia responds to phenytoin or carbamazepine, and the stiff-man syndrome may respond to diazepam.

References

BECKER, P. E., KNUSSMAN, R. and KUHN, E. (1977) *Myotonia Congenita and Syndromes associated with Myotonia: Clinic-Genetic Studies of the Nondystrophic Myotonias.* Stuttgart: Goerg Thieme Publishers

EDWARDS, W. C. and ROOT, A. W. (1982) Chondrodystrophic myotonia (Schwartz–Jampel syndrome): Report of a new case and follow-up of patients initially reported in 1969. *American Journal of Medical Genetics*, **13**, 51–56

ISAACS, H. and FRERE, G. (1974) Syndrome of continuous muscle fibre activity. *South African Medical Journal*, **48**, 1601–1607

JOHNSEN, T. and FRIIS, M. L. (1980) Paramyotonia congenita (von Eulenberg) in Denmark. *Acta Neurologica Scandinavica*, **61**, 78–87

MERTENS, H. G. and ZSCHOCKE, S. (1965) Neuromyotonie. *Klinische Wochenschrift*, **43**, 917–925

SANDER, J. E., LAYZER, R. B. and GOLDSOBEL, A. B. (1980) Congenital stiff-man syndrome. *Annals of Neurology*, **8**, 195–197

SATOYOSHI, E. and YAMADA, K. (1967) Recurrent muscle spasms of central origin. *Archives of Neurology* (Chicago), **16**, 254–264

8

Localized weakness

Any lesion of the central nervous system, the peripheral nerves, or the muscles can cause local weakness. Non-neurological disorders such as arthritis, osteomyelitis, or a ruptured tendon may also produce localized weakness and atrophy. Low-grade osteomyelitis is probably the most common cause of muscular atrophy confined to one limb with no apparent neurological symptoms or signs. After a traumatic rupture of the Achilles tendon, plantar flexion of the foot is impossible and gives the false impression of weakness of the gastrocnemius muscle. No neurological symptoms or signs are present; a gap in the tendon can usually be palpated, and local tenderness, oedema, and bleeding are present. Some typical clinical pictures characterized by local weakness due to neurological disorders will be reviewed.

Spastic weakness

The spastic cerebral palsy syndromes, besides causing spasticity, also cause weakness of the affected limb (*see* pages 281–286).

Flaccid weakness

Weakness of muscles innervated by cranial nerves

Bilateral weakness confined to the extraocular muscles is seen in ocular myopathy, ocular myasthenia, and the congenital muscle disorders due to mitochondrial abnormalities (*see* page 198). Attacks of unilateral weakness are characteristic of ophthalmoplegic migraine (*see* pages 323–324).

WEAKNESS OF FACIAL MUSCLES

Bilateral facial weakness is a characteristic finding in some of the generalized muscle diseases (*see* pages 193, 194 and 198).

Bell's palsy
Unilateral peripheral facial paralysis, Bell's palsy, usually has an acute onset, preceded for some time (several hours to a day) by discomfort and paraesthesia in

the face. It may occur for no apparent reason or follow a viral infection, a common cold, or tooth extraction. The weakness involves the whole of one side of the face, and there is a difference between the two sides in the patient's ability to wrinkle his forehead, close the eye, lift the corner of the mouth, whistle, or close the lips tightly (*Figure 8.1*). The patient often complains of a 'dead' feeling in the face, but testing reveals no impairment of sensation. The cause of Bell's palsy is not known, and

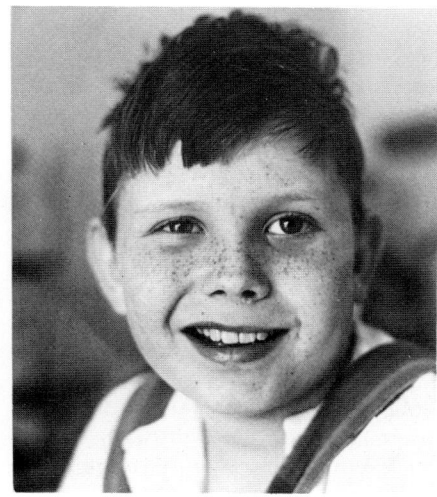

Figure 8.1. A 9-year-old boy with left-sided peripheral facial weakness

probably varies in different cases. Several patients have pleocytosis of the spinal fluid; a viral meningoencephalitis is likely. Mumps, polio, and herpes zoster may all cause pleocytosis and Bell's palsy. Middle ear infection may also be a cause; the ear, nose, and throat region must therefore be examined in a case of Bell's palsy. Lumbar puncture should be performed in the acute phase; if done later it gives no useful information. Electromyography reveals lack of motor unit potentials as the only abnormality in the acute phase (*see* page 47). Fibrillation potentials do not appear until a couple of weeks after the onset. The conduction velocity of the facial nerve also remains normal, at least for a few days; these examinations thus yield little information in the acute phase.

The prognosis of Bell's palsy in childhood is excellent. Practically all patients recover within a couple of weeks without treatment. It is important to protect the eye while it cannot be closed. Treatment of an ear infection, when present, is also necessary. No other measures are indicated. Steroids have no place in the treatment. Electrical stimulation of the facial nerve is highly unlikely to have an effect. In the exceptional case of true Bell's palsy in childhood which does not recover spontaneously, an operation may be considered. It involves the transplantation of free autogenous muscle, e.g. extensor digitorum brevis or palmaris longus, to the face, using the normal contralateral muscle as the source of reinnervation of the transplant.

If the child does not recover within a few weeks, the diagnosis of Bell's palsy must be questioned and the investigation extended to exclude rare causes of facial weakness in a child, such as a tumour arising in the cerebellopontine angle and perhaps constituting part of Recklinghausen's disease (*see* page 373).

Melkersson's syndrome

An episode of peripheral facial weakness in a child may be the first evidence of Melkersson's syndrome, which consists of recurrent attacks of peripheral facial paralysis, facial oedema, and often a furrowed tongue. The first attack of peripheral facial paralysis, which is indistinguishable from Bell's palsy, usually occurs during the second decade, but it may occur during the first one, and as a rule precedes the facial oedema. Familial cases are on record; no other aetiological factor is known.

Nerve damage during delivery

The facial nerve may be damaged during delivery, in which case the infant is born with a facial weakness. This weakness is seldom severe and the infant can usually close the eye. Almost all of these patients recover within a couple of weeks or at most a few months. As a rule, no treatment is necessary.

Möbius' syndrome

A congenital bilateral weakness of the muscles innervated by the sixth and seventh cranial nerves is the typical finding in Möbius' syndrome. The facial weakness is apparent at birth, and the bilateral lip weakness impairs the infant's ability to suck; feeding difficulties are a common finding. The weakness of the extraocular lateral rectus muscle is present at birth, and becomes more evident with increasing age (*Figure 8.2*). Muscles innervated by other cranial nerves may also be involved; weakness of other extraocular muscles and of the tongue and throat muscles may be present. Muscles innervated by the fourth and eleventh nerves always seem to be spared. The cause of the syndrome is unknown; familial cases have been reported. The symptoms of Möbius' syndrome have been ascribed to a presumed congenital

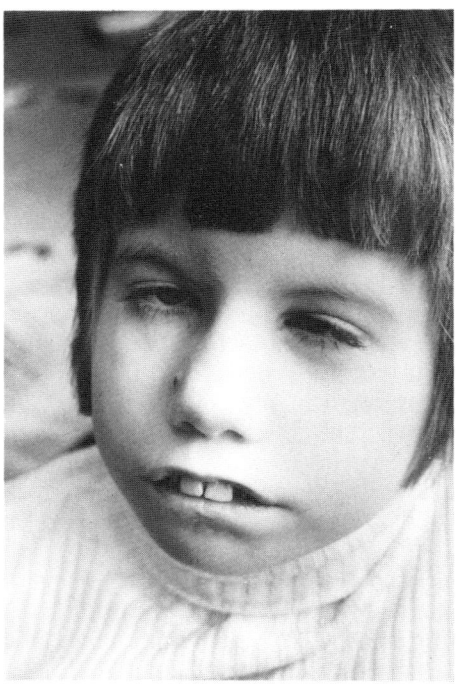

Figure 8.2. A 6-year-old girl with Möbius' syndrome

aplasia of the nuclei of the affected cranial nerves. However, as the intrinsic eye muscles function normally, even when there is complete paralysis of all extrinsic muscles innervated by the third nerve, the more likely interpretation of the findings is a congenital absence of muscles; this view is supported by anatomical findings. Malformation of the hands and feet, an abnormally small hand on one side, and absence of the pectoral muscles are common associated malformations in Möbius' syndrome. The symptoms do not progress. Only symptomatic treatment, e.g. operation for the squint, can be given.

Weakness of the upper extremity

INJURY TO THE BRACHIAL PLEXUS DURING DELIVERY

A lesion of the brachial plexus may occur during delivery. It is more common when the infant is born in the breech presentation and especially so if there are difficulties with the aftercoming head, so that traction must be applied to the shoulders. Other obstetric situations in which the shoulder region is subjected to traction or pressure may also cause a lesion of the brachial plexus. In some of these cases there is a fracture of the clavicle or the humerus; however, this may also occur with no apparent nerve damage. In most cases the lesion is a stretching of the nerve trunks and its blood vessels with some bleeding and surrounding inflammatory reaction. In more severe cases there may be rupture of the nerve trunks or even avulsion of the roots from the cord. In the latter situation, signs of a cord lesion are usually present (*see* pages 162–163).

Erb–Duchenne type
The most common brachial plexus injury during delivery is the Erb–Duchenne type, in which the fifth and sixth cervical roots or the trunk formed by their union are damaged. The muscles most commonly and most severely affected are the deltoid, the supraspinatus and infraspinatus, the teres minor, the biceps, and the brachioradialis muscles; other shoulder muscles may also be involved. The

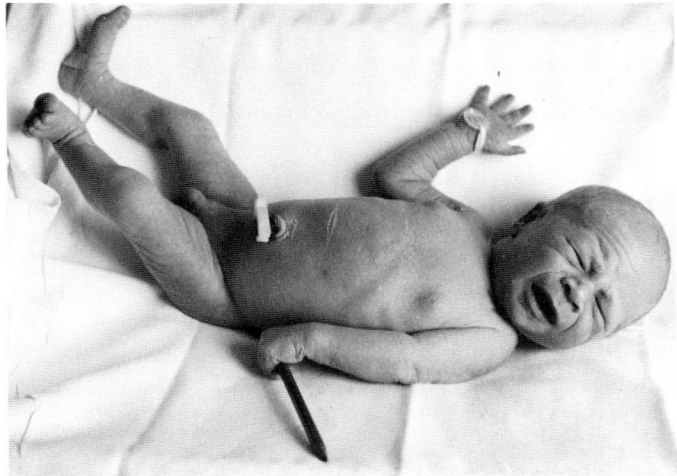

Figure 8.3. A newborn boy with a birth injury to the upper part of the left brachial plexus (Erb–Duchenne type). Note the normal handgrip on the affected side

newborn infant keeps the arm adducted, with the elbow extended and pronated (*Figure 8.3*), occasionally to such an extent that the palm of the hand is turned outward. The infant cannot abduct or elevate his arm or bend it or supinate it at the elbow. The function of the intrinsic muscles of the hand is good. The arm hangs limply at the child's side and does not take part in the movement when a Moro reflex is elicited (*Figure 8.4*). Muscular atrophy is not apparent until at least a few weeks after birth, and even then it is often concealed by the infant's good layer of subcutaneous fat. Sensation is never grossly impaired; finer details cannot be tested. The biceps and the brachioradialis reflexes are absent; the triceps reflex is present and usually normal. Erb–Duchenne palsy is seldom bilateral, and signs of involvement of the spinal cord are rare.

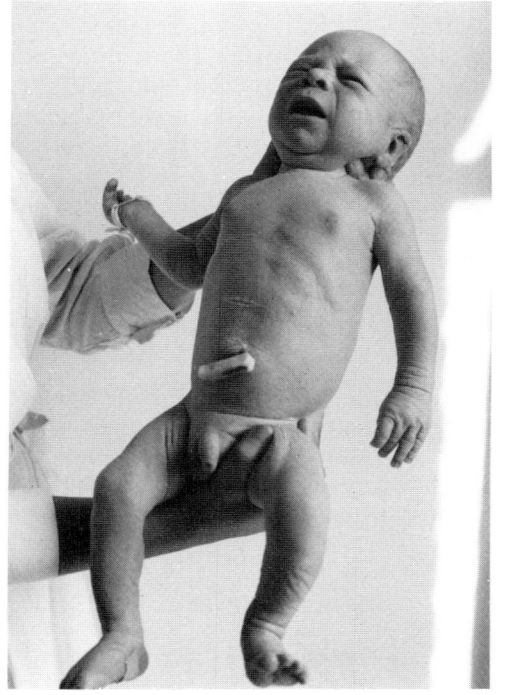

Figure 8.4. Asymmetrical Moro reflex in a newborn boy with a left-sided brachial plexus lesion (Erb–Duchenne type)

The diagnosis is established clinically. It is based on the following observations: the typical posture of the arm, the lack of function of certain muscle groups around the shoulder and the upper arm with preserved function of the hand muscles, the limpness of the arm, and the lack of response from the involved arm on the eduction of an otherwise normal Moro response. Electromyography, performed after a couple of weeks, reveals signs of denervation of affected muscles. The extent of the damage can be better assessed by electromyography than by clinical examination alone. Electromyography may also show evidence of reinnervation before it is apparent clinically and may thus be of help in assessing the prognosis. It is seldom helpful for the diagnosis.

An important differential diagnosis is a fracture of the humerus, usually an upper epiphyseolysis, as the treatment of this condition is different from that of a plexus injury. X-ray examination may not reveal the epiphyseolysis until callus has developed, which takes several days. An infant with signs of an injury to the shoulder should therefore have an X-ray examination of this area about 1 week after delivery.

Prophylaxis is important; with improved obstetric care, severe brachial plexus injury has practically disappeared. Treatment consists of physiotherapy, started as early as possible. The arm is placed and fixed in a position that minimizes traction on paralysed muscles. The correct position is abduction to 90 degrees, external rotation at the shoulder, and flexion to 90 degrees at the elbow; the hand is placed at the level of the head with the palm turned forward (*Figure 8.5*). Gentle passive

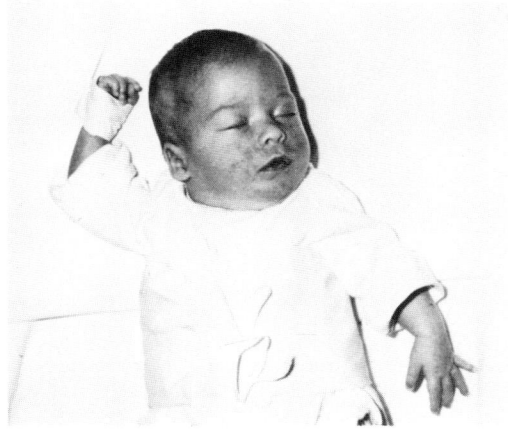

Figure 8.5. A 2-month-old boy with a right-sided brachial plexus lesion (Erb–Duchenne type) and the arm fixed in the desired position

movements through the full range of mobility of the joints without traction are performed several times a day to prevent secondary contractures. As soon as possible the child is stimulated to cooperate with active movements. At this time, fixation of the arm is no longer needed. Complicating fracture of the clavicle may in the beginning require a short period of fixation to relieve the pain, but this has no influence on the ultimate prognosis. Neither operation nor electrical stimulation has a place in the therapeutic programme. The prognosis is fair or good. Improvement is always considerable, but some weakness and atrophy of the shoulder muscles may become permanent (*Figure 8.6*), causing difficulties in hard physical work for boys and cosmetic problems for girls. From a practical point of view, it is important that hand function is preserved in this type of brachial plexus lesion.

Klumpke–Déjérine type

The Klumpke–Déjérine type of brachial plexus lesion is rare in areas where good obstetric care is provided. It may occur during difficult delivery in a face or breech presentation with strong traction in the shoulder region. It involves the seventh and eighth cervical roots and the first thoracic root or the trunk formed by their union. The muscles involved are the intrinsic hand muscles, the triceps muscle, and often, also, the long flexors of the wrist and fingers. The arm is kept flexed at the elbow, and the hand and finger movements are impaired; these latter movements are, however, often difficult to evaluate in a small infant. Shoulder movements are essentially normal. The Moro reflex is asymmetrical as the stretching of the elbow

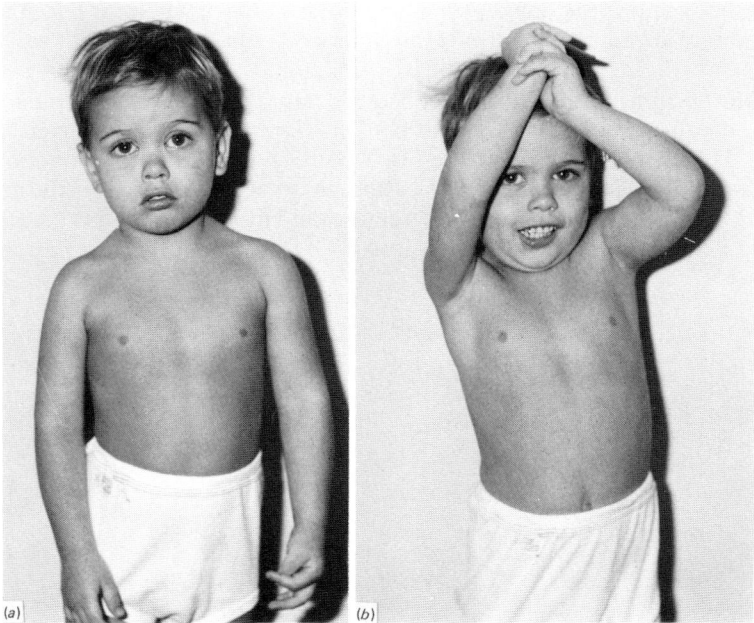

Figure 8.6. A 3-year-old boy with a right-sided brachial plexus lesion (Erb-Duchenne type). Note some atrophy of the shoulder muscles (*a*); the boy cannot elevate his right arm above shoulder level but uses his left hand to lift the right arm (*b*)

and the movements of the hand and fingers are impaired. Atrophy of small hand muscles may be observed after several weeks. Sensation may be impaired in the hand. Trophic disturbances are common. The biceps reflex is present and the triceps reflex absent. Because of the involvement of the first thoracic root and its preganglionic fibres the child often has a Horner syndrome on the side of the arm palsy. A Horner syndrome consists of miosis, ptosis, and enophthalmos; when it is congenital, due to a birth injury, the iris on the side of the palsy usually develops less pigmentation than that on the other side.

The trauma causing the Klumpke–Déjérine type is usually more severe than that causing the Erb–Duchenne type. Avulsion of the roots may therefore be seen; if so, signs of a spinal cord lesion are usually also present. These include evidence of a corticospinal tract lesion with a positive Babinski sign on the side of the arm symptoms, and sphincter disturbances. The Klumpke–Déjérine type may be bilateral, although it is usually more pronounced on one side than on the other.

The treatment is physiotherapy to prevent contractures and provide active training as early as possible. In the acute phase the arm is placed in the same position as described for the Erb–Duchenne type. Some permanent disability is the rule; it is difficult to restore perfect function to the small hand muscles. Sensory disturbances and, when present, signs of a spinal cord lesion increase the difficulties.

Combined type
Damage to the brachial plexus may be more extensive if the birth trauma has been severe. In the newborn period an entire limb may be completely paralysed and

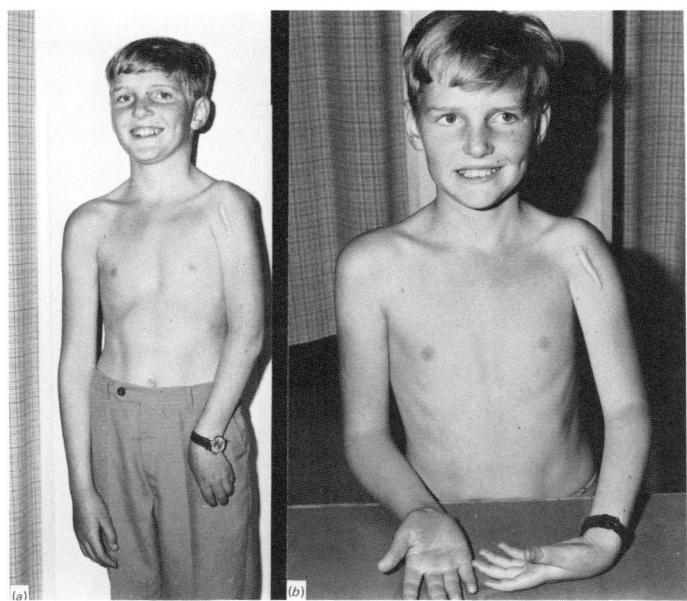

Figure 8.7. An 11-year-old boy with a severe birth injury to the whole left brachial plexus, showing typical position and growth retardation of the arm (*a*), inability to supinate the hand, and severe weakness and atrophy of small hand muscles (*b*)

without sensation; as a rule there is also some evidence of a cord lesion. Treatment is the same as outlined for the Erb–Duchenne type of plexus lesion. Some function usually appears in the shoulder muscles and often in the biceps muscle, whereas hand function and supination remain severely impaired (*Figure 8.7*). Poor sensation persists in the hand. The growth of the whole limb is retarded and the hand usually shows signs of impaired circulation and trophic disturbances.

NEURALGIC AMYOTROPHY FOLLOWING INJECTIONS

An acquired lesion involving the brachial plexus may be seen in older children or young adults for no apparent reason or following an injection of serum or, rarely, an injection of vaccine. The onset is usually acute with radiating pains in the arm and weakness followed by atrophy. When these symptoms follow a serum injection, they usually appear 2–3 days after the onset of the general symptoms of serum sickness, i.e. about 2 weeks after the serum injection. The onset may also be painless; in this situation the patient suddenly discovers that he has weakness and atrophy of his shoulder muscles. Inability to elevate and abduct the arm is the dominating symptom. The treatment is physiotherapy. The prognosis is good in children, as complete recovery within a few months is the rule, although some permanent weakness and wasting may occasionally be seen.

HEREDITARY RECURRENT NEURALGIC AMYOTROPHY

A rare dominantly inherited syndrome of recurrent neuralgic amyotrophy is known. Patients have attacks of shoulder pain followed by weakness (*Figure 8.8*), wasting, hypoactive or absent reflexes, and sensory loss in the arm, and a tendency to recover between attacks. Exceptionally other regions, e.g. the recurrent nerve or the lumbosacral plexus, may be involved, alone or alternating with or combined with involvement of the brachial plexus. The onset may be in childhood. No factors other than inheritance are known; treatment is symptomatic.

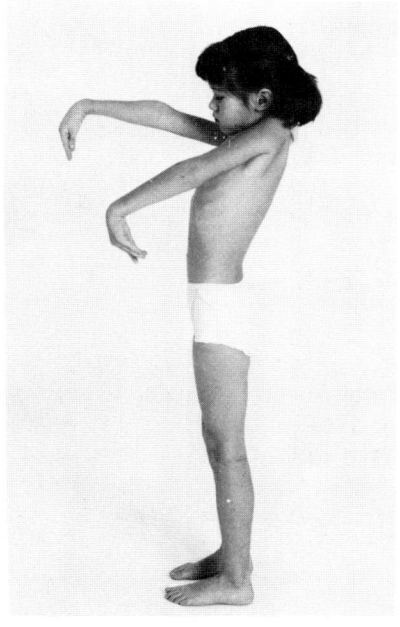

Figure 8.8. A 7-year-old girl with hereditary recurrent neuralgic amyotrophy, demonstrating severe weakness of the wrist extensors a few weeks after the onset of her first attack

CERVICAL RIBS

Cervical ribs may, although rarely, cause symptoms in childhood and adolescence. Symptoms consist of weakness and wasting of the hand muscles. Pain, paraesthesia, and impaired sensation may be present, particularly along the ulnar border of the hand and the forearm. Vascular symptoms, such as blanching or cyanosis of the fingers, may occur and are due to compression of the subclavian blood vessels. The cervical ribs can be seen on X-ray of the cervical spine and the upper part of the thorax. A fibrous band, invisible on X-ray, with the same localization as a cervical rib may exceptionally cause the same symptoms and signs. Treatment is surgical.

CARPAL TUNNEL SYNDROME

The carpal tunnel syndrome is uncommon in childhood; it may occasionally be seen in diabetic adolescents. In this syndrome the median nerve is compressed under the carpal ligament. The first symptom is usually painful paraesthesia in the hand, occasionally radiating up the arm; it may then be misinterpreted as evidence of a lesion of the brachial plexus. It occurs more commonly during the night and may wake the patient. The motor symptoms consist of atrophy of the thenar eminence and weakness of the opposition of the thumb. Neurophysiological examination reveals impaired conduction of the nerve impulse across the wrist in both the motor and the sensory nerve fibres. The injection of corticosteroids under the ligament may relieve the symptoms in a mild case; surgical removal of the pressure on the nerve is the usual treatment. The prognosis is good.

MALFORMATION OF THE CERVICAL CORD

Malformation of the cervical cord may cause peculiar symptoms from the arms and hands, including weakness (*see* page 333).

Weakness of the lower extremity

INJURY TO THE LUMBAR PLEXUS DURING DELIVERY

Weakness of the lower extremities caused by a stretching of the lumbar plexus during a complicated delivery with breech extraction is extremely rare. The lesion may be bilateral. Clinically it cannot be distinguished from bleeding in the lower cord, which may occur in the same type of difficult delivery.

MALFORMATION OF THE LUMBOSACRAL CORD AND THE NERVE ROOTS

Weakness of the lower extremities in the newborn period is often caused by malformations of the lower part of the spinal cord, the roots, and the spine (*see* pages 335–339). When the malformation is obvious and the weakness severe, as in a myelomeningocele, the diagnosis is easy. However, the malformation may not be evident externally, and the infant may originally have only mild or no symptoms, which then slowly progress with the growth of the child. Thus, progressive symptoms may be caused by a congenital malformation; further progression may be prevented by an operation. Impaired sensation and sphincter disturbances are often seen in this situation (*see* Chapter 15).

INJURY TO THE SCIATIC NERVE OR THE SPINAL CORD BY INJECTION

Weakness of one leg may be due to sciatic nerve injury caused by an intramuscular injection given in the buttock. The risk is particularly high in small infants, but this injury may also occur in older children. The sciatic nerve supplies motor nerves to the hamstrings and to all muscles below the knee; a complete lesion thus causes an inability to bend the knee and paralysis of all muscles below the knee. Sensation is impaired in the foot and the outer aspect of the lower leg. The knee jerk is preserved and the ankle jerk is absent. The part of the sciatic nerve forming the lateral popliteal nerve is more superficial and thus more susceptible to injury than the part forming the medial popliteal nerve. A peroneal paresis, causing a foot-drop and a tendency to inversion of the foot, is therefore a typical finding when the injury to the sciatic nerve is superficial. If the injury goes deeper, it also causes weakness of the posterior tibial and gastrocnemius muscles and loss of the ankle jerk; if the whole nerve is damaged, the hamstring muscles are also involved (*Figure 8.9*). Symptoms tend to improve spontaneously, but they seldom regress completely. Physiotherapy may hasten the improvement and prevent fixed contractures. Orthopaedic measures to improve the child's functional ability are important; such measures include stabilizing the foot, correcting the malposition of the foot, and correcting growth retardation of the whole leg, which may occur. However, complete recovery is unusual unless the injury was mild. In the early phase of a severe injury it may be worthwhile to explore the nerve and remove the fibrotic scar tissue surrounding it.

The sequelae of sciatic nerve injury are serious in a child (*Figure 8.9*). The risk of causing such an injury through a gluteal intramuscular injection is greater in a child

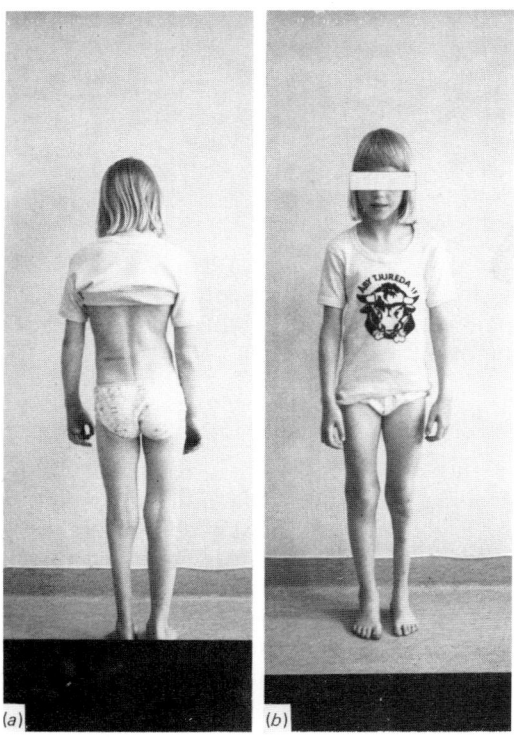

Figure 8.9a and *b*. An 8-year-old girl with the sequelae of a sciatic nerve injury due to a wrongly given injection in the buttock at 4 months of age. Note the severe atrophy of all muscles of the lower leg and the hamstrings

than in an adult, because the available area is smaller and the angle between needle and skin is more critical, and because the child cannot be expected to remain still during the injection. The obvious prophylaxis is to avoid, as far as possible, intramuscular injections in young children, particularly small infants, and to try to find an alternative method of drug administration. When an intramuscular injection *must* be given the quadriceps muscle, though not risk-free (*see below*), is preferred. If there is no possible alternative to using the gluteal region, the injection must be given with great caution and knowledge of the anatomy of the nerve in a small child; an assistant *must* keep the child still.

INJURY TO THE QUADRICEPS MUSCLE BY INJECTION

Because of the risk associated with intramuscular injections in the gluteal area of infants and small children, it is recommended that these injections should preferably be given into the quadriceps muscle. This site, however, also carries a certain though smaller risk Fibrosis of the quadriceps muscle has been described in children, in some as a sequela after intramuscular injections into the muscle. Symptoms originating from an injury in the newborn period usually become apparent when the child is between 6 months and 2 years of age. They consist of a stiff gait, inability to bend the knee, and difficulties in sitting, squatting, and climbing stairs. The patella is higher up on the affected side than on the normal side. On attempted passive flexion of the knee, an indurated quadriceps tendon and muscle may be palpated. The skin may be tightly attached to deeper structures. During the early phase of the condition the quadriceps reflex, muscle bulk, and muscle strength appear normal; later the muscle may atrophy. Treatment consists of surgical removal of the fibrotic tissue and immobilization of the leg in a cast with the knee bent for a couple of weeks, followed by active exercise. The prognosis is good, provided operation is performed before secondary damage of the epiphyseal areas and skeletal growth have occurred.

OTHER CONDITIONS

Peroneal weakness may be the first evidence of polyneuropathy (*see* page 175). It may also be due to pressure on the peroneal nerve at the level of the caput fibulae as seen in crossed-leg palsy, but this is rare in childhood. Oedema, weakness, and in severe cases necrosis of the anterior tibial muscle have been described in viral infections in childhood.

References

ADOUR, K. K., BYL, F. M., HILSINGER, R. L., KAHN, Z. M. and SHELDON, M. I. (1978) The true nature of Bell's palsy: analysis of 1,000 consecutive patients. *Laryngoscope*, **88**, 787–801

CLARK, K., WILLIAMS JR, P. E. and MCGAVRAN III, W. L. (1970) Injection injury of the sciatic nerve. *Clinical Neurosurgery*, **17**, 111–125

DAVID, T. J. and BAUMER, J. H. (1982) Problems of parental bonding and family care in a child with the Möbius syndrome. *Journal of the Royal Society of Medicine*, **75**, 980–982

ERIKSON, A. (1974) Hereditary syndrome consisting in recurrent attacks resembling brachial plexus neuritis, special facial features, and cleft palate. *Acta Paediatrica Scandinavica*, **63**, 885–888

HAKELIUS, L. (1974) Free autogenous transplantation of striated muscle. Dissertation from the Faculty of Medicine, Uppsala, No 196

HARRIS, J. P., DAVIDSON, T. M., MAY, M. and FRIA, T. (1983) Evaluation and treatment of congenital facial paralysis. *Archives of Otolaryngology*, **109**, 145–151

HYDÉN, D., SANDSTEDT, P. and ÖDKVIST, L. M. (1982) Prognosis in Bell's palsy based on symptoms, signs and laboratory data. *Acta Otolaryngologica*, **93**, 407–414

JELLIS, J. E. (1970) Childhood sciatic palsies: congenital and traumatic. *Proceedings of the Royal Society of Medicine*, **63**, 655–656

KNOWLES, J. A. (1966) Accidental intra-arterial injection of penicillin. *American Journal of Diseases of Children*, **111**, 552–556

MASSE, P., POUJOL, J. and BIGAN, R. A. (1965) A propos de trois cas d'enraidissement en extension du genou par fibrose progressive du quadriceps chez l'enfant. *Archives Francaises Pédiatrie*, **22**, 697–705

ROSSI, L. N., VASSELLA, F. and MUMENTHALER, M. (1982) Obstetrical lesions of the brachial plexus. Natural history in 34 personal cases. *European Neurology*, **21**, 1–7

SAUNDERS, F. P., HOEFNAGEL, D. and STAPLES, O. S. (1965) Progressive fibrosis of quadriceps muscles. *Journal of Bone and Joint Surgery* (American), **47**, 380–384

SHAW, E. B. (1966) Transverse myelitis from injection of penicillin. *American Journal of Diseases of Children*, **111**, 548–551

STRICKER, M., MELEY, M. and CHASSAGNE, J. F. (1983) Le syndrome de Moebius. Possibilities chirurgicales. *Revue Oto-neuro-ophtalmologie* (Paris), **55**, 157–161

TOWFIGHI, J., MARKS, K., PALMER, E. and VANNUCCI, R. (1979) Möbius syndrome. *Acta Neuropathologica*, **48**, 11–17

9

Abnormal growth of the head

The head circumference of a healthy, full-term infant at birth is about 35 cm. During the first 6 months it increases by about 8–9 cm, during the next 6 months by about 3 cm, and during the second year of life by about 2 cm. This curve reflects the normal growth of the brain during early postnatal life (*see also* page 31). The growth of the head depends on two factors: the growth of the mass inside the skull, and the elasticity of the skull surrounding the growing mass. If the growth of the mass is abnormally slow or if the skull does not yield in a normal way, the head will remain abnormally small for age; this condition is called *microcephaly*. Asymmetrical yielding may cause an *abnormal shape of the head*. If the growth of the mass is abnormally fast, the skull will usually yield and the head becomes abnormally large for age; this condition is called *macrocephaly* or *megalocephaly*.

Abnormally small head or abnormally shaped head

In these conditions the face of the child grows normally. When the skull remains small it has a low slanting forehead and flat back of the head.

Lack of normal elasticity of the skull

The ability of the skull to give way to pressure from inside depends on the elasticity at the sutures and fontanelles. Premature closure of the sutures and fontanelles, termed *craniostenosis*, reduces the elasticity of the skull and impedes its growth. Its effect depends on which sutures are involved.

CRANIOSTENOSIS

Craniostenosis must be considered when the growth of the skull is slow, when the fontanelle is closed abnormally early, when an abnormal ridge can be palpated over one or more sutures, and when the shape of the skull is abnormal. Skull X-ray reveals the synostosis of sutures. A neurosurgeon must be consulted early, preferably before the infant is 3 months of age, and each case must be assessed individually.

Scaphocephaly
Isolated scaphocephaly is the most common type of craniostenosis. Its cause is premature closure of the sagittal suture, which leads to impaired growth in the width of the skull; the length of the head and the base of the skull grow normally. Affected children thus have a long narrow skull, often described as an upturned boat. The volume of the skull usually remains normal and the development of the brain is seldom impaired. Most patients with scaphocephaly develop normally and have no mental or neurological symptoms or signs, although a few have been reported with evidence of increased intracranial pressure. Surgical treatment is often indicated on cosmetic grounds and occasionally in order to prevent an increase in intracranial pressure and its sequelae.

Brachycephaly and oxycephaly
Brachycephaly arises through symmetrical premature closure of the coronary suture alone (*Figure 9.1*), and oxycephaly arises through symmetrical premature closure of the coronary suture and one more suture. The infant has a short, narrow,

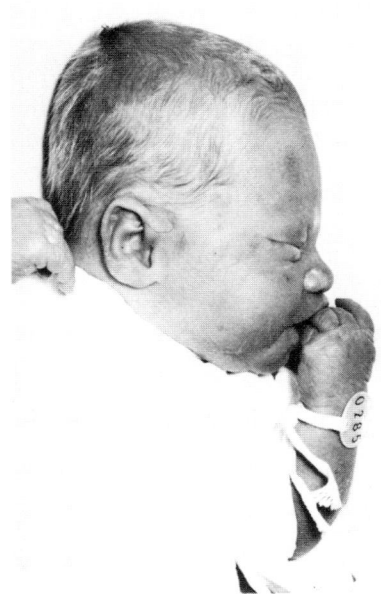

Figure 9.1. A newborn boy with brachycephaly due to synostosis of the coronary suture

tall skull, which grows mainly in height and little in circumference. The base of the skull develops poorly, and the basal cisterns become narrow, possibly obstructing the circulation of the cerebrospinal fluid (*see* page 251). This factor, together with the deficient growth of the skull volume, may cause an increase in intracranial pressure. In infancy this can be diagnosed by the observation of a bulging fontanelle; some infants also vomit and fail to thrive. In older children the symptoms are vomiting and headache. The increase in intracranial pressure, which in some patients is slow and without dramatic symptoms, may eventually cause permanent brain damage with mental retardation, convulsions, and impaired vision due to optic atrophy.

Plagiocephaly

Early closure of the coronary suture on one side causes an asymmetrical skull, termed plagiocephaly. Premature asymmetrical closure of several sutures produces an asymmetrical skull with a variable effect on the growth of its volume. These conditions are rare.

Symmetrical early closure of all sutures

This rare condition causes retarded growth of the skull which is a severe impediment to the development of the brain and causes increased intracranial pressure. It should be suspected in a child with a small symmetrical head, premature closure of the large fontanelle (*see* page 31), and a growth curve of the skull falling well below the normal range. Skull X-ray reveals the closed sutures. Neurosurgical treatment is urgent.

Trigonocephaly

A synostosis of the metopic suture causes trigonocephaly, a malformation of the skull which is usually already apparent in the newborn infant. The eyes are close together, the forehead is narrow with a palpable ridge in the middle, and the shape of the skull seen from above is triangular. The development of the frontal lobes is impaired, and mental retardation is common. The treatment is neurosurgical.

Crouzon's dysostosis craniofacialis

Oxycephaly is one feature of this condition, others being a beaked nose, hypoplastic maxilla, exophthalmos, and strabismus. The craniostenosis is severe and needs early operation to prevent brain damage. The orbits are narrow, and the cause of the exophthalmos; this contributes to the increased risk of optic atrophy, which is seen more often in this condition than in other types of craniostenosis. Craniostenosis may be associated with other malformations, e.g. in Apert's syndrome it is combined with syndactyly of the hands and feet (*Figure 9.2*), and in Carpenter's syndrome with various malformations of the hands, feet, heart, and genitalia.

Intracerebral or porencephalic cyst under pressure

A cyst in one cerebral hemisphere may occasionally contain fluid under sufficiently high pressure to cause asymmetrical growth of the head. The diagnosis is established on computerized tomography of the skull and a shunt may be needed to relieve the pressure (*see Figure 9.3*, between pp. 100–101).

One-sided subdural hygroma

A one-sided subdural hygroma may exceptionally be large enough to cause asymmetrical growth of the child's head. The diagnosis is established on computerized tomography of the head. The treatment is neurosurgical evacuation of the hygroma; removal of the membrane is usually also required.

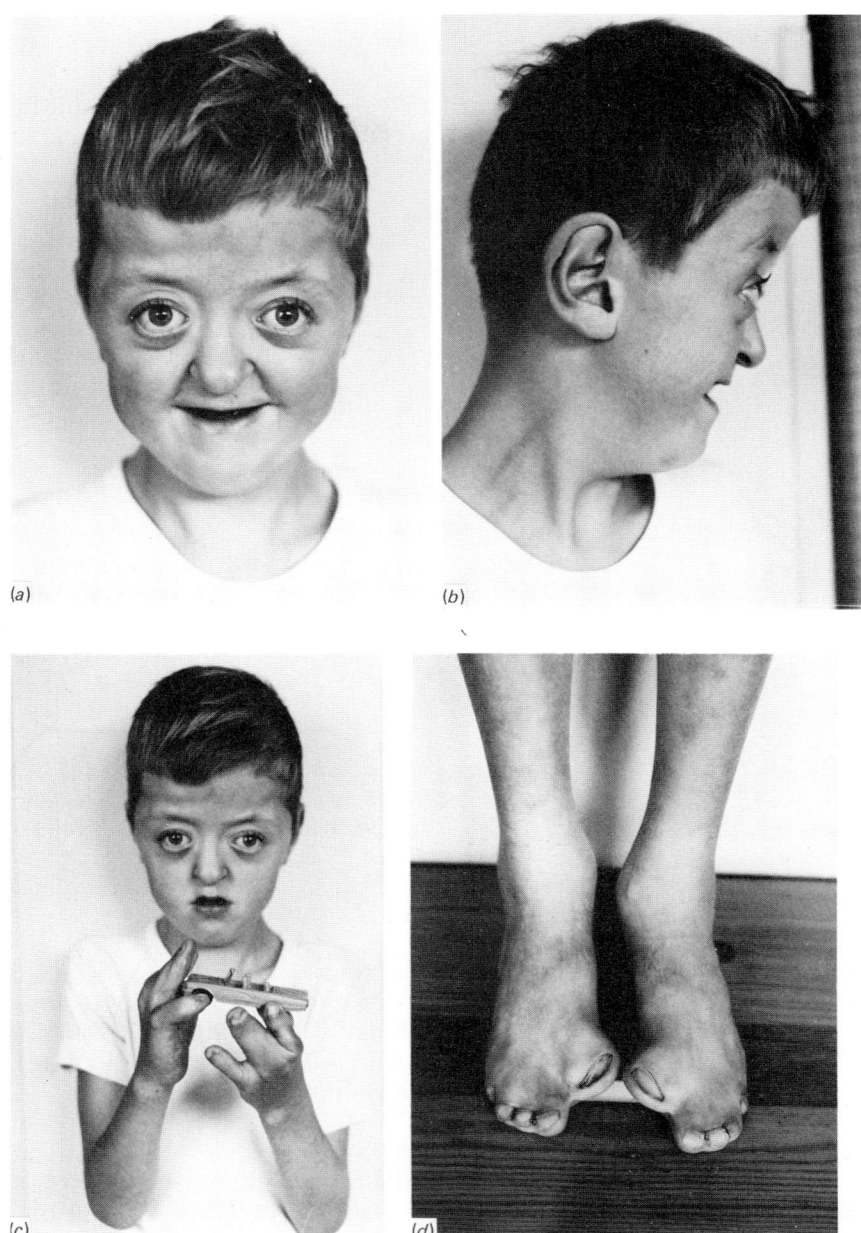

Figure 9.2. A 9-year-old boy with Apert's syndrome. Note the small oxycephalic head and typical facial features with exophthalmos and hypoplasia of the maxilla (*a* and *b*), malformed hands (*c*) and malformed feet (*d*)

Defective growth of the brain

Defective growth of the brain causes slow growth of the skull. The term microcephaly, which means a small head generally, is often used to denote only the condition discussed here, i.e. a small head due to defective growth of the brain (*Figure 9.4*).

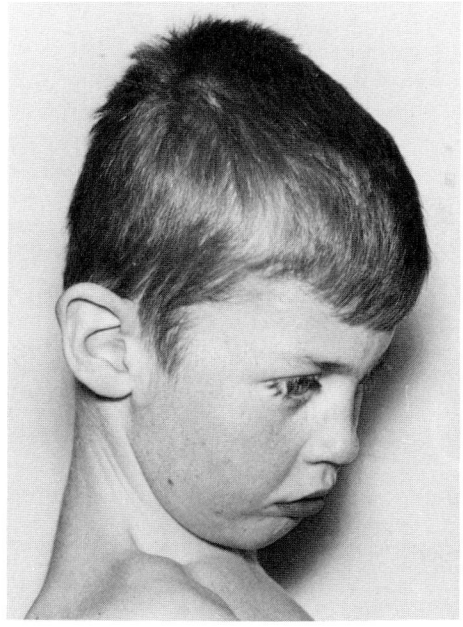

Figure 9.4. A 9-year-old boy with microcephaly and mental retardation for no known reason

MICROCEPHALY

'True microcephaly'
This condition may be inherited; if so, inheritance is recessive and the condition is usually apparent at birth. Mental retardation is evident from an early age, but other neurological symptoms and signs are usually absent. The growth of the brain is slow, and the adult brain weight remains around 500–800 g (normal 1200–1500 g). In some families microcephaly is associated with chorioretinopathy.

Bird-headed dwarfism
A special type of microcephaly, probably inherited as an autosomal recessive, is bird-headed dwarfism, also called *nanocephaly* or the *Seckel type* of dwarfism. These infants are small at birth and remain severely dwarfed. They have a small head; in some cases it is associated with early closure of the sutures. The face is narrow with large eyes, beaked nose, and hypoplastic maxilla and mandible. The patients are mentally retarded but usually less so than is anticipated from the degree of microcephaly.

Prenatal brain injury
Any damage to the fetal brain, e.g. from radiation or infection with rubella, may cause microcephaly. Associated malformations often occur at the same time and in

the rubella syndrome produce a typical constellation of lesions (*see* page 124). Microcephaly may occur as a malformation of the brain for no apparent reason.

Perinatal or early postnatal brain injury
A severe perinatal or early postnatal brain injury may also impede the growth of the brain. Such an injury may be due to anoxia, intracranial bleeding, or meningitis. The acute episode, which causes the brain damage, is usually severe and obvious from the history. Convulsions and neurological symptoms such as a cerebral palsy syndrome (*see* Chapter 12) are often present.

Mental retardation is (in cases of defective growth of the brain) or may become (in cases of lack of skull elasticity) a dominating finding in most individuals with an abnormally small head. Microcephaly is found in many of the conditions described in Chapter 5 and occasionally in cerebral palsy syndromes (*see* Chapter 12). Associated malformations may occur in cases of defective brain growth and in cases of defective skull growth. Signs of increased intracranial pressure are present only in the latter group. The majority of children with a small head belong to the former group, but the few cases that belong to the latter group must be distinguished, as neurosurgical treatment is urgently indicated in this group and may prevent further brain damage. Skull X-ray may be helpful, as it shows closed sutures in this group. However, it is not always easy to decide whether or not the sutures have closed prematurely as patients with defective development of the brain may also show early closure of the sutures. In some cases it is obvious to which group the patient belongs, e.g. a patient with features that are typical of Crouzon's syndrome belongs to the group with lack of skull elasticity, and a patient with a typical rubella syndrome and an appropriate history belongs to the group with defective brain growth. Patients in both groups may have convulsions and neurological signs. When the differential diagnosis is doubtful the patient must be followed-up with repeated clinical examinations, measurement of the skull circumference, and skull X-rays. Any sign of increased intracranial pressure (vomiting, pale discs, swollen discs, bulging fontanelle) is an urgent indication for neurosurgical intervention.

The prognosis is generally poor in patients with an abnormally small head. For the group in which development of the brain is defective, severe mental retardation is the rule, and neurological signs and convulsions are common. Also, early and adequately treated patients in the other group may show some sequelae, such as delayed mental development, convulsions, or impaired vision (except in scaphocephaly, when the skull volume increases normally and the problem is mainly cosmetic). The degree of permanent symptoms and signs depends on the duration and severity of the increased intracranial pressure before treatment.

Benign conditions causing abnormal shape of the head

An abnormally shaped head in the newborn period may also be due to an entirely benign condition, which must be differentiated from the more severe conditions causing abnormal shape of the head, i.e. those in which the abnormal shape is due to lack of elasticity of the skull (*see* page 8).

INTERCALATION OF SKULL BONES

Intercalation of the skull bones is often seen and felt in newborn infants; it has no clinical significance and disappears within a couple of weeks.

CAPUT SUCCEDANEUM

Caput succedaneum is a diffuse swelling over the part of the head that leads during delivery. The swelling consists of oedema and some bleeding into the subcutaneous tissue. It is seen in almost every newborn baby and disappears within a few days.

CEPHALHAEMATOMA

Cephalhaematoma is a well-delineated swelling over the skull, caused by subperiosteal bleeding which raises the periosteum. Its most common localization is over one of the parietal bones, although it may appear over any of the skull bones, and more than one cephalhaematoma may be seen in the same infant. It does not cross a suture. It appears shortly after birth, although it may then be covered by a large caput succedaneum and therefore becomes more marked after a few days. During the first few days it is usually tense and later starts to fluctuate at the top. It appears to be painless and non-tender. It causes asymmetry of the child's head (*Figure 9.5*). The occipital cephalhaematoma is particularly difficult to diagnose, as it may be misinterpreted as an encephalomeningocele (*see* page 329).

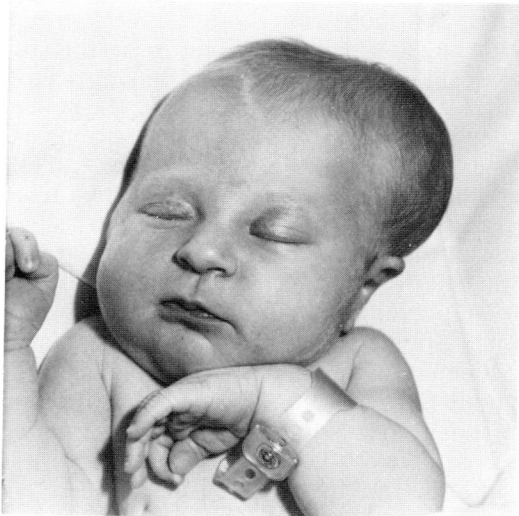

Figure 9.5. A left-sided cephalhematoma in a newborn girl

A cephalhaematoma usually disappears without treatment within a few weeks, but occasionally it may persist for a couple of months. It often leaves a slight thickening of the affected skull bone which may be felt, and can be seen on a skull X-ray. No treatment is needed. Aspiration of the blood does not influence the course and may cause infection and thus be dangerous.

Abnormally large head

Physiological variants

The fetal head constitutes a larger proportion of the whole body the younger is the fetus, thus the head of a prematurely born infant appears large in relation to the body. Small-for-dates term infants whose low birth-weight is due to impaired placental circulation have a normal head size for a term baby, but it appears disproportionately large in relation to the abnormally small body. Head size must thus not be estimated by eye but must be measured and correlated to the age of the infant, preferably the conceptional age when this is known.

The head size can be judged as abnormal on a single measurement only if this measurement is grossly outside normal limits or other signs are present (*see* page 31). Otherwise the head circumference must be measured several times over a period of time so that a curve can be constructed and its slope evaluated. One may find children who from birth and through the first years of life have an abnormally large head; the head circumference in relation to age follows a curve of the same shape and slope as the normal one, but runs constantly above it. In a normally developing infant who has no other abnormal findings, the large head should be considered a *physiological variant with no pathological significance*. The tendency to an increased head size is often inherited; one feels more confident in judging the child healthy and refraining from further investigations if one of the parents also has an abnormally large head.

Abnormal increase in the brain substance

In these conditions the growth of the head is slightly above the normal range, and signs of increased intracranial pressure are only mild. An apparent increase in the brain substance is usually due to a degenerative disease with storage of abnormal metabolic products within the brain cells.

TAY–SACHS DISEASE

In G_{M2}-gangliosidosis, Tay–Sachs disease, abnormal lipids are accumulated within the brain cells, causing an increase in head size and progressive mental, neurological, and ophthalmological symptoms and signs (*see* page 295).

MUCOPOLYSACCHARIDOSES

An abnormal metabolite, possibly the same as in Tay–Sachs disease, is accumulated in the brain substance in acid mucopolysaccharidosis (*see* page 135), causing increased head size; impaired circulation of the cerebrospinal fluid in the basal cisterns (*see* page 251) may also occur in this condition.

CANAVAN'S SPONGY DEGENERATION

The symptoms in Canavan's spongy degeneration of the central nervous system in infancy consist of a slow increase in head size, evidence of slightly increased intracranial pressure, and progressive mental and neurological symptoms (*see* page 304).

FAMILIAL MACROCEPHALY

Macrocephaly with mental retardation and optic atrophy has been reported as a familial disorder, which is probably inherited as an autosomal recessive gene.

ALEXANDER'S DISEASE

This is a rare condition characterized by dementia and an abnormally large head with increased brain substance and normal-sized or slightly enlarged ventricles (*see* page 310).

Abnormal accumulation of fluid within the skull

An abnormally large head is more commonly caused by the abnormal accumulation of fluid within the skull than by an abnormal increase in brain substance.

SUBDURAL HYGROMA

Fluid accumulation outside the brain, i.e. in the subdural space, has been called hydrocephalus externus. As this term is often misunderstood it should be abandoned and replaced by the term subdural hygroma to avoid confusion.

The most common cause of an infantile subdural hygroma is brain injury or anoxia during the neonatal period. In early infancy purulent meningitis may be complicated by subdural hygroma. Thus, the cause is usually an underlying brain disease, definite or alleged, which may by itself produce mental and neurological symptoms. The hygroma will, however, produce slowly progressive mental and neurological signs, and this progression can be stopped by treatment. The incidence of subdural hygroma has decreased considerably, presumably due to improved obstetric and neonatal care and care of infantile purulent meningitis; the introduction of computerized tomography of the skull has also increased the accuracy with which the diagnosis can be established or excluded.

Symptoms and signs
The vague complaints in a case of subdural hygroma consist mainly of failure to thrive, i.e. anorexia, a tendency to vomit, and poor weight gain. A slight delay in psychomotor development is common, and convulsions may occur. An abnormally rapid increase in head size and evidence of mildly increased intracranial pressure, such as a prominent forehead and a full or slightly bulging fontanelle, are often seen; a rapidly increasing head size with signs of severely increased intracranial pressure is an exception. A large one-sided subdural hygroma may cause asymmetry of the skull (*see* page 234). Normal growth of the head is found in many patients with subdural hygroma. Weakness of the extraocular muscles, retinal haemorrhages, pale or swollen discs, and focal neurological signs are occasionally seen.

Diagnostic procedures
Transillumination of the skull is a simple clinical procedure (*see* page 7) which is helpful in the diagnosis of subdural hygroma and which should be performed in every infant with a suspected disorder of the central nervous system. A normal finding on a correctly performed and correctly interpreted transillumination of the skull of a young infant excludes subdural hygroma; an abnormal finding, however, does not prove the diagnosis, as it is seen also in fluid collections of other types, e.g. a porencephalic cyst or an increased subarachnoid space.

The diagnostic method of choice is computerized tomography of the skull which will confirm or exclude the presence of fluid in the subdural space. Other examinations may give some further support to the diagnosis but have less significance. Increased spinal fluid protein (*see* page 52) is seen in some cases of subdural hygroma. The electroencephalogram (EEG) is often abnormal but the abnormalities are nonspecific.

Treatment
The treatment of subdural hygroma is neurosurgical. The hygroma is emptied through a burr-hole, which is placed in the frontal region as this is the usual localization of infantile hygromas. Evacuation of the hygroma is usually sufficient; occasionally its membranes are thick and their removal may be necessary. The insertion of a shunt from the subdural space to the peritoneum is only rarely necessary; the risk of serious complications makes avoidance of this procedure desirable. A small subdural effusion requires no treatment as it is absorbed spontaneously.

Prognosis
The prognosis depends mainly on the severity of the brain injury which occurred simultaneously with the production of the subdural hygroma; the prognosis of the subdural hygroma *per se* is generally good.

HYDROCEPHALUS

Fluid accumulation in the ventricular system is usually termed hydrocephalus or internal hydrocephalus. The term hydrocephalus, which means water-head, could also be used to describe the accumulation of fluid in the empty space that arises in cases of severe brain atrophy; most of these patients have a normal-sized head. This situation, however, is better described as brain atrophy, as that is the primary cause of the accumulation of fluid, which is under normal pressure. The term hydrocephalus is here understood to mean only *expansive hydrocephalus* caused by an accumulation of fluid under increased pressure due to a discrepancy between the flow into the ventricular system and the flow out from it.

Clinical symptoms and signs
The clinical symptoms and signs are due to the increased intracranial pressure. In infants the raised intracranial pressure causes an abnormally rapid increase in the head circumference, a bulging fontanelle, widely separated sutures, engorged veins on the skull (*Figure 9.6*), and the sunset phenomenon (*see Figure 2.7,* page 10). In

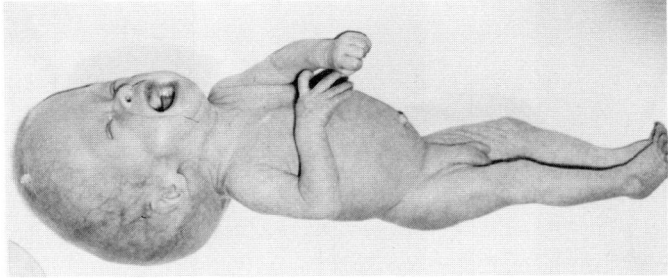

Figure 9.6. A 3-month-old boy with severe expansive hydrocephalus. Note the large head, small thin body, and engorged scalp veins

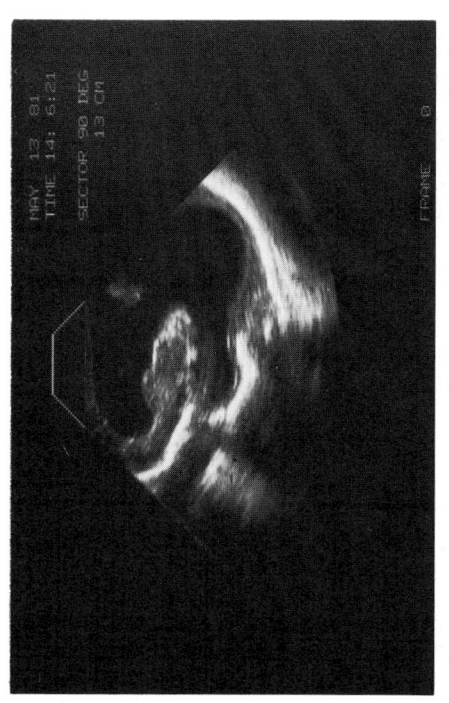
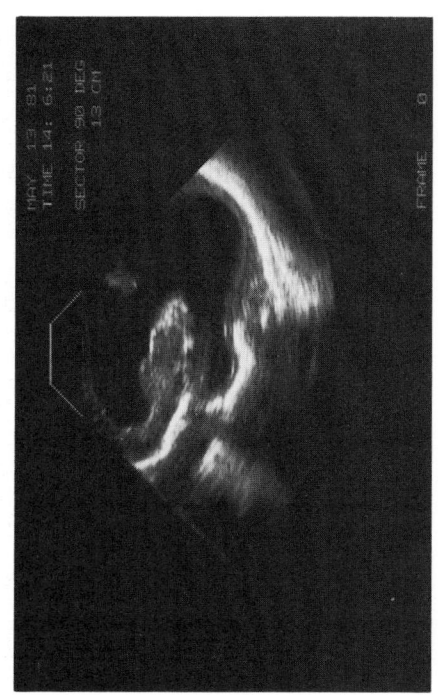
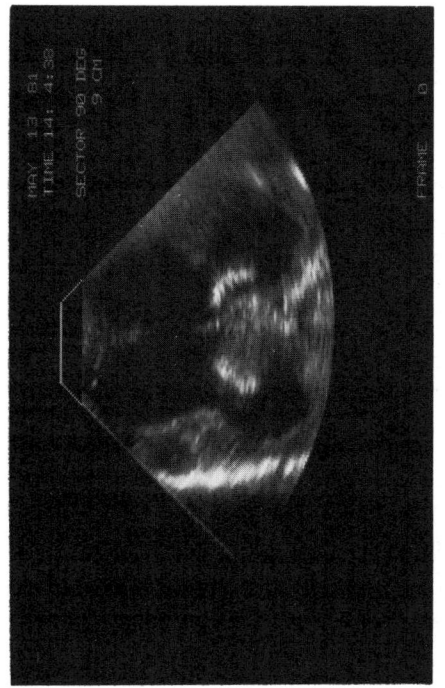
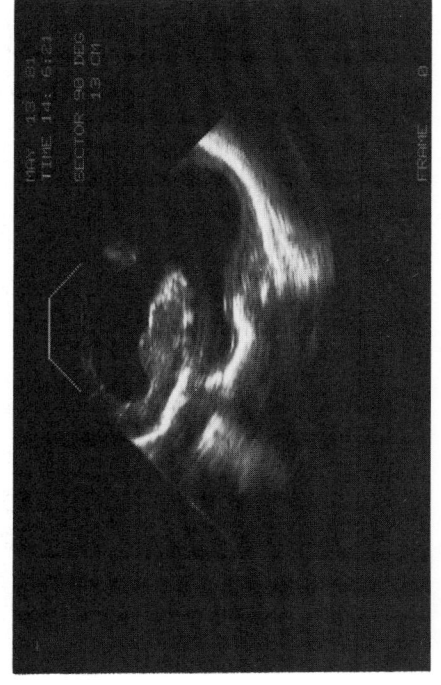

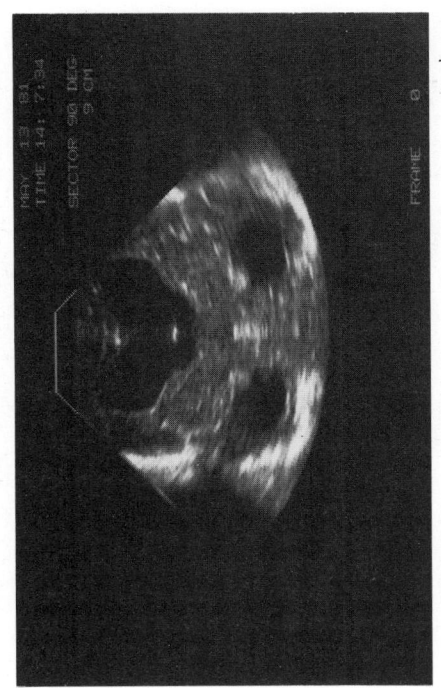

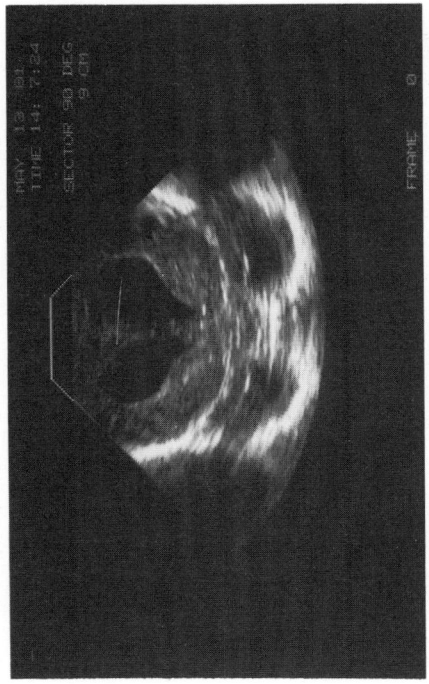

Figure 9.7. Ultrasound examination of the skull of a 1-week-old child with hydrocephalus

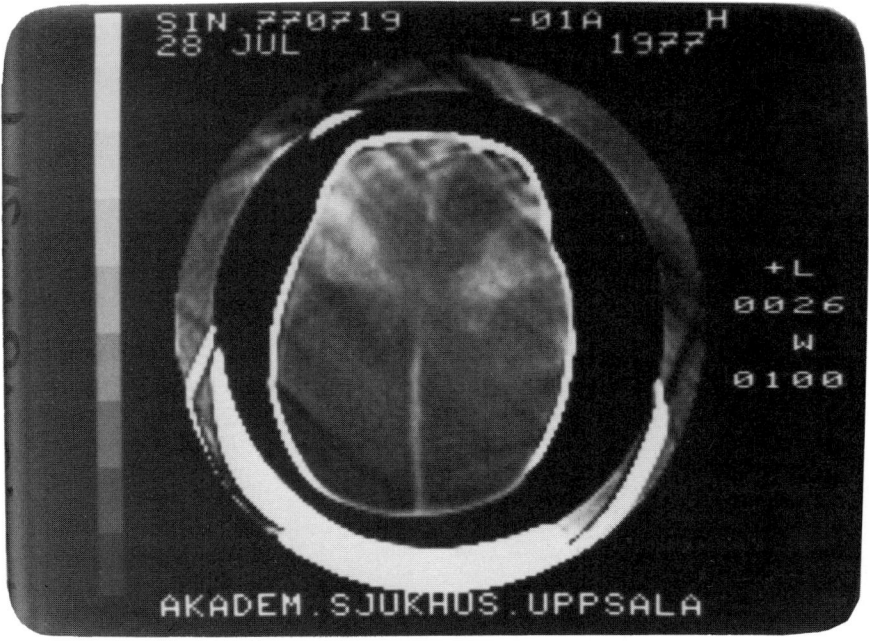

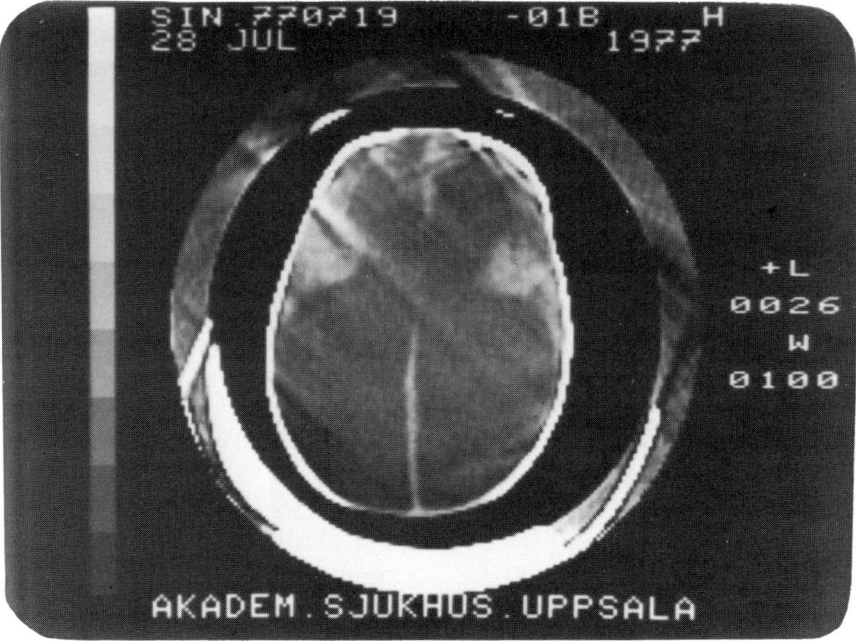

Figure 9.8. Computerized tomography of the skull of a 1-week-old child with severe hydrocephalus for which no cause was demonstrable

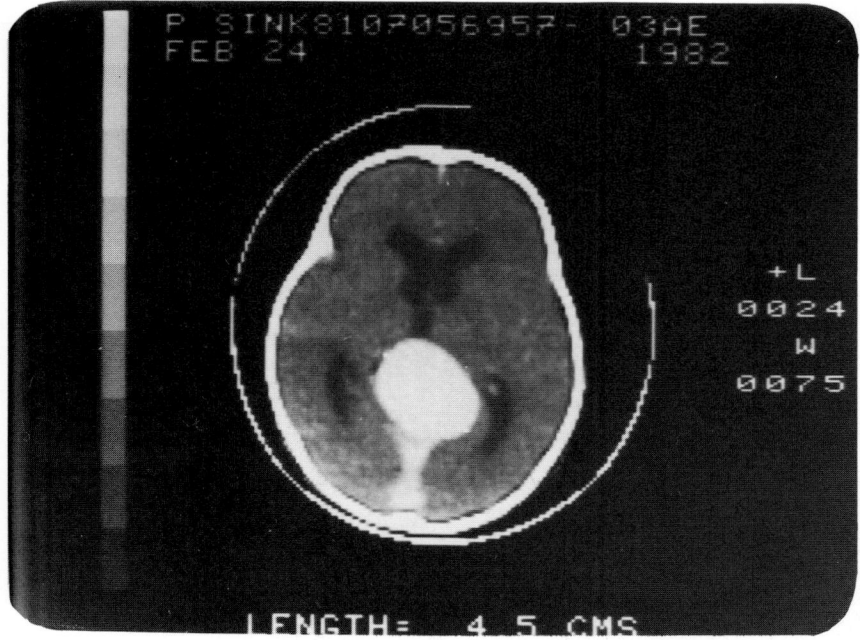

Figure 9.9. Computerized tomography of the skull of an 8-month-old infant with mild hydrocephalus due to a large aneurysm of the vein of Galen (*see also Figure 9.14*)

severe cases bilateral sixth nerve palsy may be present. The optic discs may be pale; swollen discs are rarely seen in infantile hydrocephalus. Provided the cerebral mantle is at least 5–10 mm thick, transillumination of the skull is normal. In most cases of untreated severe infantile hydrocephalus, both mental and physical development is retarded and neurological signs appear, usually spasticity of all four extremities. In less severe cases the fontanelle may be full but not bulging, the separation of sutures may be slight, and the head circumference may be so little outside normal limits that it cannot be judged as abnormal on an isolated measurement; in these cases only repeated measurements will reveal abnormal growth of the skull.

Diagnostic procedures
The two important procedures are ultrasound examination and computerized tomography of the skull. Both reveal the size of the ventricular system, the thickness of the brain mantle, and occasionally the cause of the hydrocephalus. Ultrasound examination is rapid, requires no sedation, and does not disturb a sick infant; it can be repeated at short intervals. It provides good information about the anatomy of the brain when it can be performed through an open fontanelle (*Figure 9.7*). Computerized tomography (*Figure 9.8*) may reveal more details about other malformations of the brain or its blood vessels (*Figure 9.9*), cysts, and tumours (*Figure 9.10*). The two methods supplement each other and should preferably be performed before the treatment is decided. Continuous monitoring of the pressure in the subarachnoid space through an indwelling catheter is, in selected cases, of great value to decide if the child needs treatment. Other diagnostic procedures seldom help in the clinical evaluation of a case of infantile hydrocephalus.

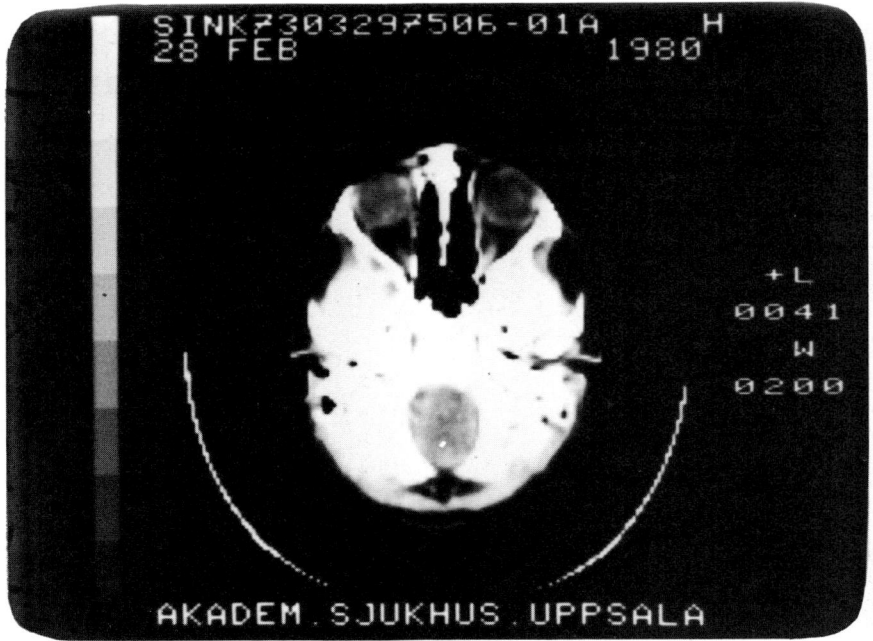

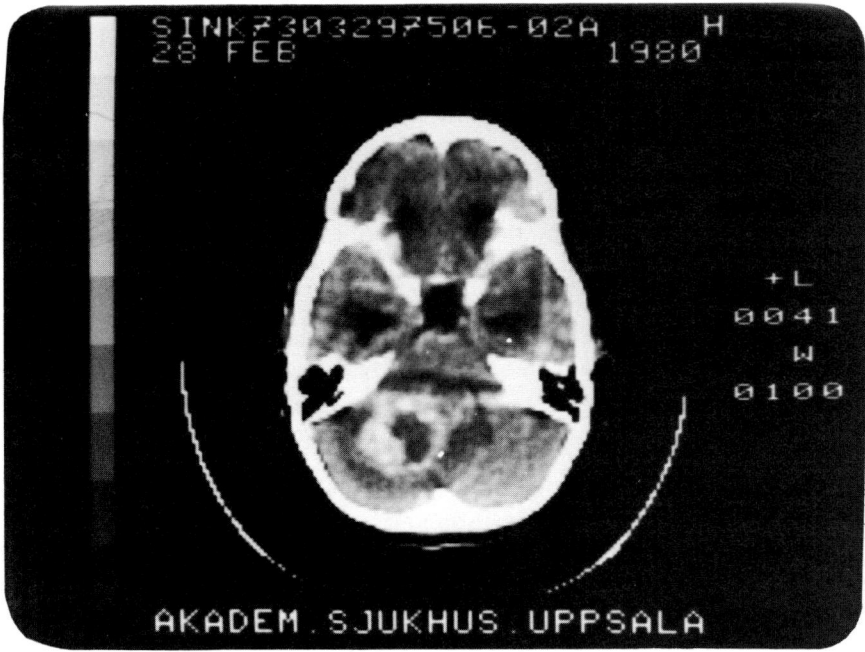

Figure 9.10. Computerized tomography of the skull of a 7-year-old child with hydrocephalus due to a tumour of the posterior fossa

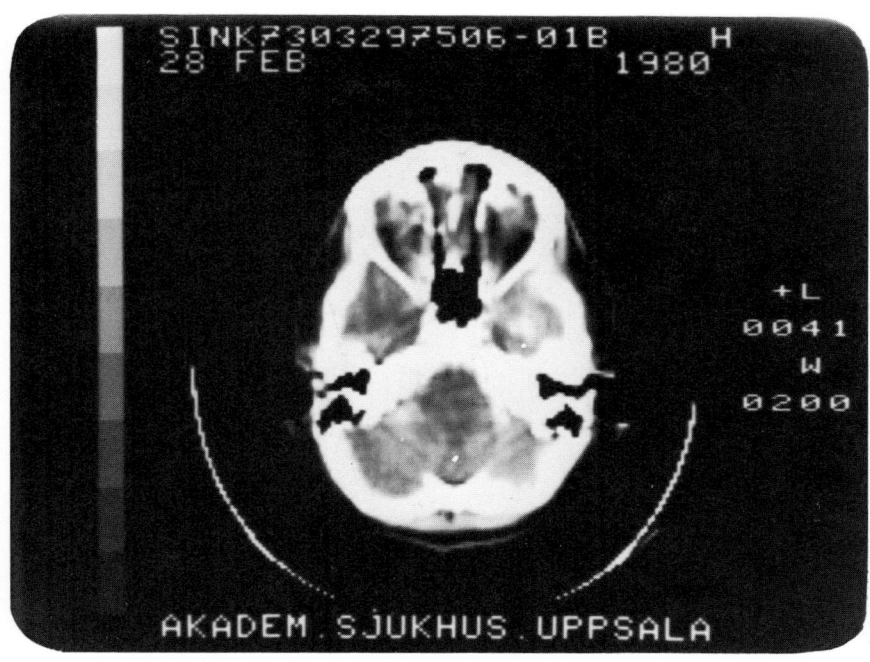

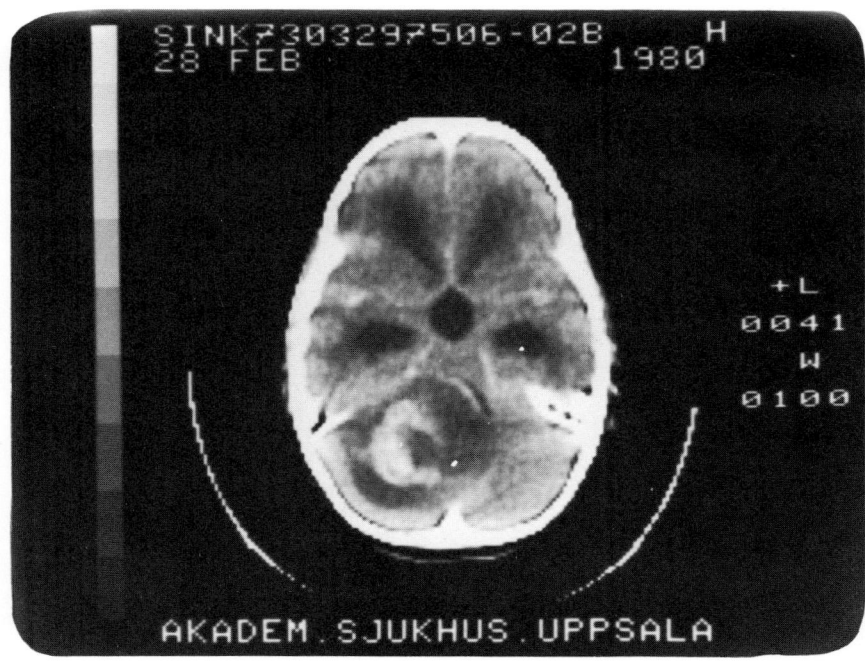

Figure 9.10 (contd)

248

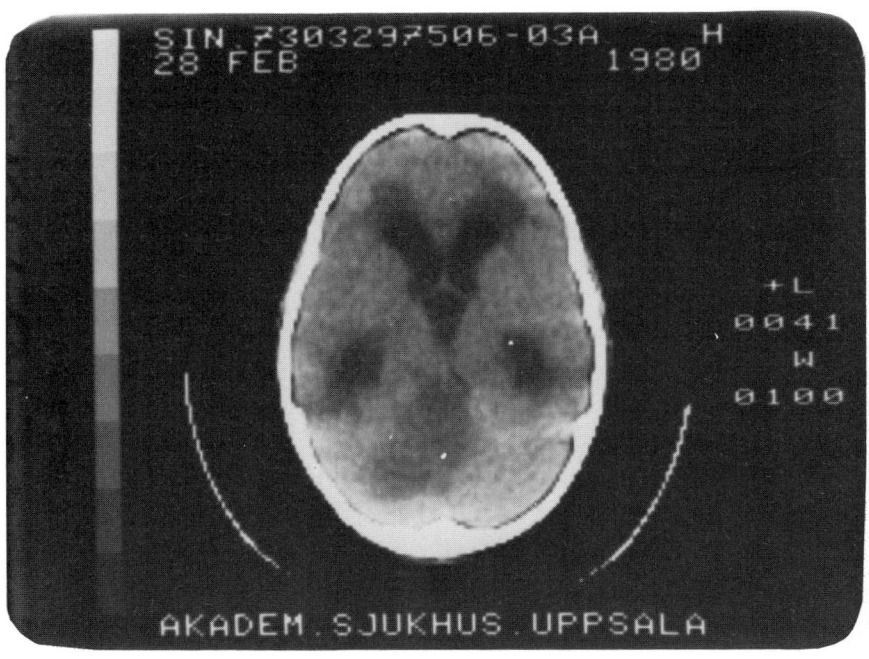

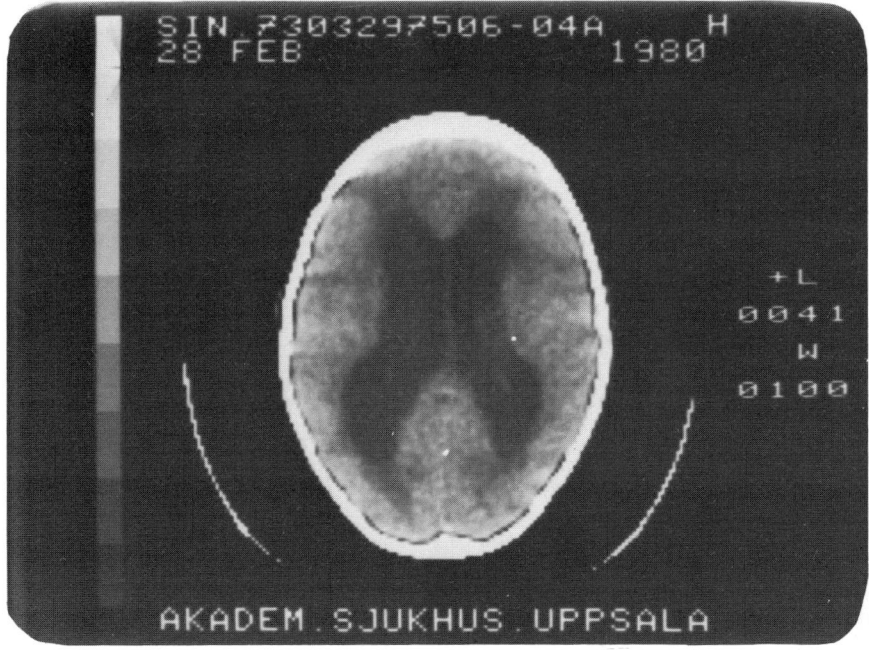

Figure 9.10 (contd)

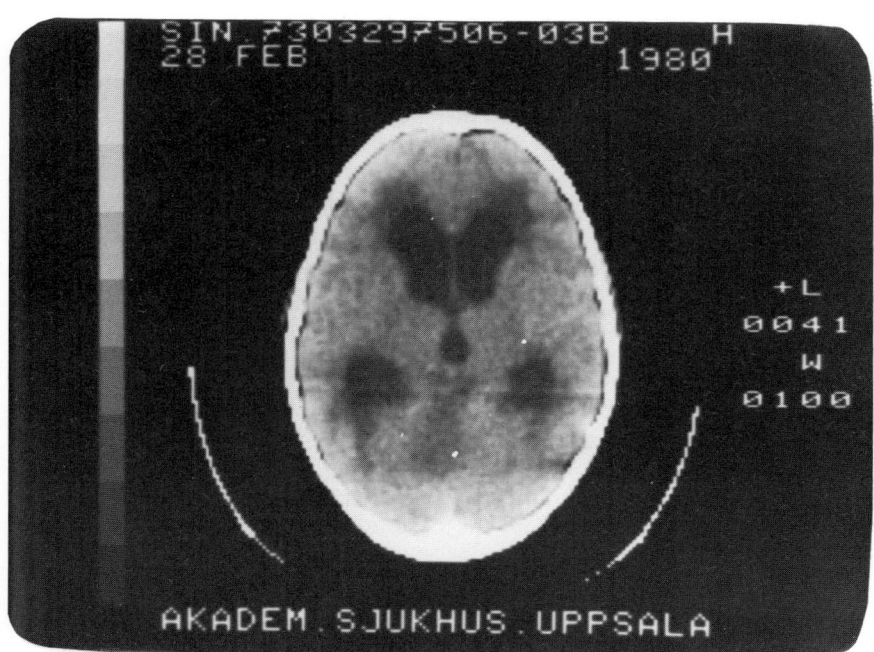

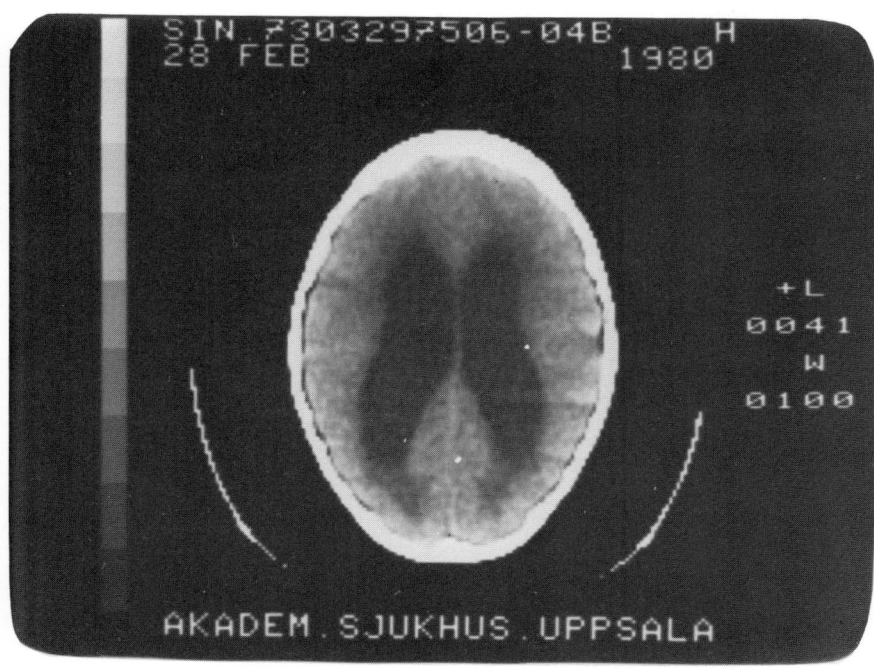

Figure 9.10 (contd)

Production, circulation, and absorption of cerebrospinal fluid

Hydrocephalus is the common end-result of various disturbances of the production, circulation, and absorption of cerebrospinal fluid. It is thus not enough to establish a diagnosis of hydrocephalus; its cause must also be investigated. Cerebrospinal fluid is produced in the ventricular system, probably mainly by the walls of the lateral ventricles, and approximately 25 per cent by the choroid plexus. From the lateral ventricles the fluid passes through the aqueduct to the fourth ventricle, through the foramina of Luschka and Magendie to the basal cisterns and then to the surface of the hemispheres and of the spinal cord, where it is absorbed into the blood. Increased production or any impediment to the circulation or resorption of the fluid will cause an expansive hydrocephalus.

Increased fluid production

Increased production is the likely explanation for the elevated intracranial pressure seen in the acute phase of a purulent meningitis. It may also explain the increased intracranial pressure occasionally seen in vitamin A intoxication, in lead poisoning (*see* page 396), and in some infants during treatment with broad-spectrum antibiotics. A tumour originating from the choroid plexus, i.e. a choroid plexus papilloma, may cause a sufficiently large increase in the production of cerebrospinal fluid to produce hydrocephalus. Plexus papilloma, however, is an extremely rare cause of hydrocephalus.

Impaired circulation or absorption of cerebrospinal fluid

This is the dominant cause of hydrocephalus, and must be investigated according to both the localization of the obstruction and its nature.

Localization of the obstruction   An obstruction of the foramen of Monro causes asymmetrical hydrocephalus, as only one lateral ventricle is affected. The cause is usually a cyst or a tumour.

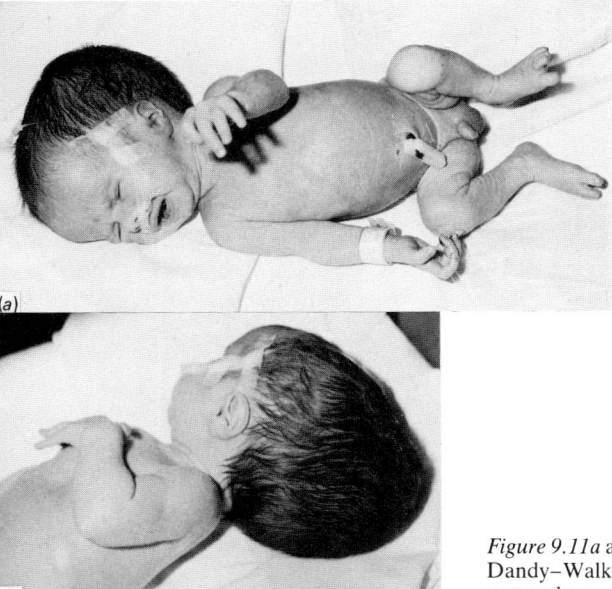

(a)

(b)

Figure 9.11a and *b.* A newborn boy with the Dandy–Walker syndrome. Note the large posterior cyst and severely elongated back of the head

An obstruction of the aqueduct is common in hydrocephalus. The lateral ventricles and the third ventricle are dilated, and the floor of the latter becomes thin and bulging. An obstruction in this region may be due to a primary malformation, to a sequela after inflammation, or to a tumour.

An obstruction of the foramina of Luschka and Magendie causes a dilation of the whole ventricular system and particularly of the fourth ventricle which may expand into a large cyst. The cause may be a sequela after inflammation or a primary malformation with a thin membrane covering the foramina. The latter condition is called the Dandy–Walker syndrome, which also includes cerebellar hypoplasia. The back of the head is enlarged and prominent in patients with this syndrome (*Figures 9.11* and *9.12*) and on transillumination shows a brightly glowing, triangular area.

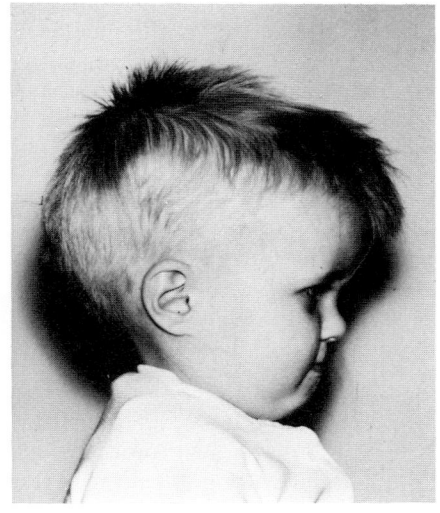

Figure 9.12. A mild case of the Dandy–Walker syndrome in a 2-year-old boy. Note the prominent back of the head

An obstruction of the basal cisterns is the most common localization of the cause of hydrocephalus. It may be due to a malformation that produces disproportion between the size of the base of the skull and the brain; this is seen, for example, in chondrodystrophy and acid mucopolysaccharidosis (*see* page 135). In the Arnold–Chiari malformation the medulla oblongata is enlarged and dislocated through the foramen magnum (*Figure 9.13*), often together with the cerebellum, which causes an obstruction to the flow of cerebrospinal fluid through the basal cisterns. The Arnold–Chiari malformation may rarely be seen as an isolated malformation of the nervous system; as a rule it occurs together with a myelomeningocele (*see* page 335) and is the usual cause of hydrocephalus in that condition.

Inflammation of the meninges due to blood in the subarachnoid space (e.g. arising from a birth injury) or due to bacterial infection of the meninges may cause adhesions that obstruct the flow of fluid through the basal cisterns. Most cases of hydrocephalus that arise peri- or postnatally are produced in this way.

Impaired absorption of cerebrospinal fluid may also be caused by a meningeal irritation and often occurs together with blocked circulation through the basal cisterns. Increased venous pressure impairs the resorption of cerebrospinal fluid

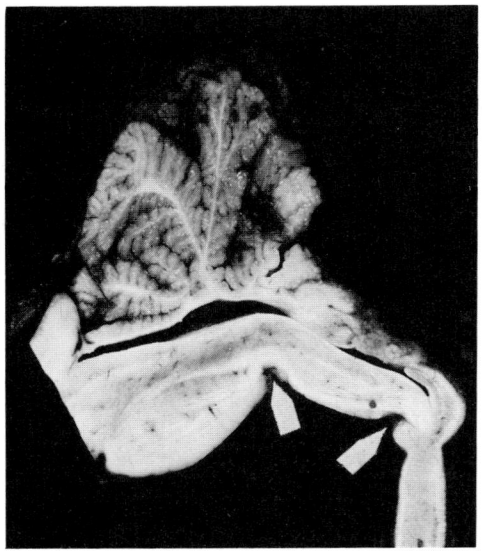

Figure 9.13. A section through the cerebellum and the brain stem in a case of Arnold–Chiari malformation. Note the elongation of the fourth ventricle with caudal displacement of the medulla oblongata and part of the cerebellum into the spinal canal. The upper arrow points to the impression made by the foramen magnum, and the lower one to the transition of the medulla oblongata into the spinal cord

and explains why hydrocephalus may occasionally be seen in congestive cardiac failure. The increase in venous pressure may be local and caused, for example, by a large subdural hygroma, or by an arteriovenous malformation with arterialization of the vein; these conditions may thus be complicated by hydrocephalus. *Figure 9.14* (*see* between pp. 100–101) shows a boy with a mild hydrocephalus caused by a malformation of the vein of Galen (demonstrated on computerized tomography in *Figure 9.9*).

The nature of the obstruction   The obstruction may be due to an anatomic malformation (e.g. aqueductal stenosis, the Dandy–Walker syndrome, or an Arnold–Chiari malformation); to sequelae after inflammation (e.g. bleeding in the subarachnoid space or purulent meningitis); to tumour (e.g. choroid plexus papilloma producing an abnormally large volume of cerebrospinal fluid, or any tumour, particularly in the posterior fossa [*see Figure 9.10*], which obstructs the flow of cerebrospinal fluid); to impaired resorption through a membrane damaged by inflammation; or to increased venous pressure either locally (e.g. caused by a subdural hygroma or an arteriovenous malformation) or generally (e.g. congestive heart failure).

Treatment
If the hydrocephalus is shown to have a treatable cause, it can be removed. However, this is seldom possible; the aim of treatment, then, is to restore the balance between the production and outflow of cerebrospinal fluid. At present, the usual treatment is to insert a subcutaneously placed shunt from the lateral ventricle to the peritoneum with a connecting valve under the skin behind the ear. The purpose of the valve is to regulate the ventricular pressure and allow flow only when it exceeds a certain limit. Different types of valves are available; they open at different pressures, and some individual adjustment of the intracranial pressure may be obtained.

During the time (almost three decades) in which shunt operations have been performed, the technique has improved and the shunt material now used is almost non-irritant. The incidence of shunt complications has decreased considerably, but they have not disappeared completely. The primary operative mortality is negligible. Blockage of the shunt may occur. Blockage of the upper end is unusual but may occur, particularly if the lateral ventricles shrink to slit size, when the shunt end may become attached to the wall. As the child grows the lower end may be pulled out of the peritoneum and end in the subcutaneous tissue, where fluid absorption is poor. The fluid may find its way to the subcutaneous channel around the shunt and expand it. Palpable fluid around the shunt on the chest is a sign of impaired function of the lower end of the shunt. The shunt may become blocked without producing any symptoms or signs; if so, the patient is no longer shunt-dependent. Blockage of the shunt in a shunt-dependent patient will cause a return of increased intracranial pressure and this time, perhaps, in a situation when the sutures and fontanelles are closing. In this situation symptoms start more or less acutely, depending on the severity of the hydrocephalus and the extent of the block. The symptoms consist of headache, vomiting, lethargy, the sunset phenomenon, sixth nerve palsy, and papilloedema with the risk of secondary optic atrophy. Revision of the shunt with restoration of its patency is necessary; in an acute situation it may be urgent. Parents must be well-informed by the physician about this complication and they must be told how to contact the appropriate surgical department in an emergency.

Another complication is infection of the shunt, usually with *Staphylococcus aureus* or *S. albus,* which causes fever and a high white blood cell count. Infection usually also causes blockage of the shunt and a swelling is seen along the shunt channel on the chest. When the shunt is infected this swelling usually becomes red and tender. Before treatment is started, samples must be taken for culture. The signs of infection disappear on treatment with antibiotics, but return again, as soon as the treatment is stopped. An infected shunt must be removed and the increased intracranial pressure reduced to the normal level and maintained there, usually through open drainage, while the infection is treated. Ventriculitis may also be present, requiring the intraventricular application of antibiotics. When the infection has been eradicated, a new shunt can be inserted. A third complication arises when the shunt procedure is too effective, i.e. it reduces the increased intracranial pressure to *below* the normal level, leading to premature closure of the cranial sutures; children with this complication may need an operation for craniostenosis.

The attitude to the management of a shunt in a growing child varies. The policy of some departments is to exchange the lower end of the shunt at fixed intervals, when it can be expected that the child has outgrown his shunt, and before this causes any symptoms. The argument for this policy is that it avoids an acute situation, which may otherwise arise if the shunt suddenly becomes blocked. Other departments wait until symptoms occur. The fact that the statistical risk of shunt problems is highest in the first 3 months after any shunt operation supports the latter policy. Besides, many routine operations may be unnecessary, as spontaneous arrest of the hydrocephalus occurs, even in shunted cases; when a child outgrows his shunt he may no longer be shunt-dependent.

As a rule, it is a good principle never to touch a shunt that gives no problems. This policy requires that the parents are well and repeatedly informed by their physician and that they know whom to contact and where to go if an acute situation should arise.

The ventriculoatrial shunt, used for many years, is now inserted only in the rare case in which there is a contraindication against its placement in the peritoneum. The atrial placement means the presence of a foreign body in the bloodstream and thus a higher risk of complications. If such a shunt becomes infected, the patient develops sepsis with high, spiking fever and positive blood culture. There is also a risk of the formation of thrombi and emboli thrown out in the blood circulation. Some older patients may still have such shunts and may appear with complications. An asymptomatic shunt should not be touched. But if any problems arise which justify an operation on a ventriculoatrial shunt, it should be replaced by a ventriculoperitoneal one, and a shunt made of the newer less irritant material should be used.

Different types of medical treatment have also been attempted, but with little success. Acetazolamide 75 mg/kg per day has been reported to be effective in controlling cases of mild hydrocephalus. However, in these cases the effect of any treatment is hard to evaluate and requires follow-up for many years. Treatment with acetazolamide cannot replace surgery. It may be useful as a temporary measure when for some reason the operation has to be postponed. Its effect in mild cases, when operation is considered unnecessary, is extremely difficult to evaluate.

Not all cases of hydrocephalus need treatment; spontaneous arrest is common. Evaluation of the indications for operation requires long experience. Unoperated patients with hydrocephalus must be followed-up closely. Unnecessary operations must be avoided, but no patient should be allowed to develop evidence of permanent brain injury before the operation is performed.

Course and prognosis

In untreated cases of hydrocephalus mortality is between 50 and 75 per cent, depending on the patient material. In suboptimally treated cases in whom arrest has occurred spontaneously or through an operation at a time when a permanent injury was already present, the patients may show some characteristic symptoms

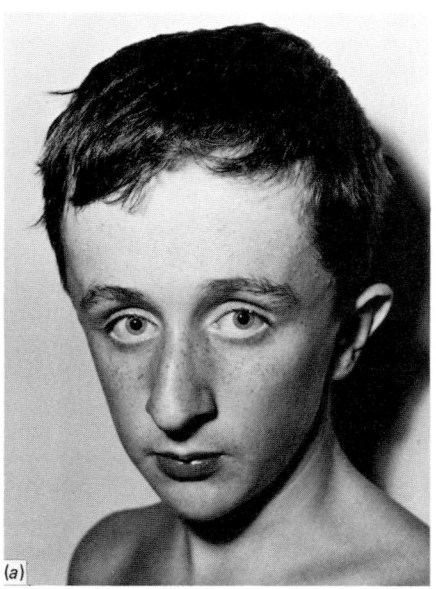
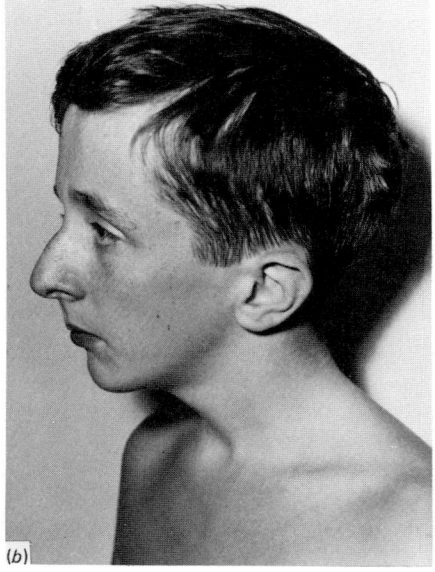

(a)   (b)

Figure 9.15a and *b*. A 14-year-old boy with apparently arrested hydrocephalus and signs. They have a large head (*Figure 9.15*) and often a dysplastic body with a thick fat layer around the abdomen and hips, flat feet, muscular hypotonia, and ataxia with or without spastic diparesis. Precocious puberty may occur. Borderline or mildly retarded mental development is common. Many of these children have mental symptoms described as 'the cocktail party syndrome', i.e. they have a good vocabulary and love to talk but do not listen and thus cannot carry on a conversation. Their good verbal ability contrasts with their poor understanding of the words they use and their inability to follow an abstract logical reasoning.

All patients with an arrested hydrocephalus, occurring spontaneously or through a shunt, carry some risk of *reactivation*. If this occurs, symptoms and signs of increased intracranial pressure (*see* page 241) return, and the patient must be evaluated by a specialist, as he may need a shunt or a revision of the one he already has. The most common cause for reactivation is a skull trauma. This situation must be suspected if a small head trauma causes disproportionately severe symptoms with no evidence of intracranial bleeding.

The prognosis in optimally treated cases of hydrocephalus is good. The majority of these patients show normal physical and mental development, no shunt complications, and no reactivation of the hydrocephalus.

References

ADAMS, C., JOHNSTON, W. P. and NEVIN, N. C. (1982) Family study of congenital hydrocephalus. *Developmental Medicine and Child Neurology,* **24,** 493–498

ANDERSSON, H. and GOMES, S. P. (1968) Craniosynostosis. Review of the literature and indication for surgery. *Acta Paediatrica Scandinavica,* **57,** 47–54

BANKER, B. Q., ROBERTSON, J. T. and VICTOR, M. (1964) Spongy degeneration of the central nervous system in infancy. *Neurology* (Minneapolis), **14,** 981–1001

DONAT, J. F. (1980) Acetazolamide-induced improvement in hydrocephalus. *Archives of Neurology,* **37,** 376

HAGBERG, B. (1962) The sequelae of spontaneously arrested infantile hydrocephalus. *Developmental Medicine and Child Neurology,* **4,** 583–587

HAYDEN, P. W., SHURTLEFF, D. B. and STUNTZ, T. J. (1983) A longitudinal study of shunt function in 360 patients with hydrocephalus. *Developmental Medicine and Child Neurology,* **25,** 334–337

HUTTENLOCHER, P. R. (1965) Treatment of hydrocephalus with acetazolamide. *Journal of Pediatrics,* **66,** 1023–1030

KASARKIS, E. J. and BASS, N. H. (1982) Benign intracranial hypertension induced by deficiency of vitamin A during infancy. *Neurology* (NY), **32,** 1292–1295

KIEKENS, R., MORTIER, W., POTHMANN, R., BOCK, W. J. and SEIBERT, H. (1982) The slit-ventricle syndrome after shunting in hydrocephalic children. *Neuropediatrics,* **13,** 190–194

LIECHTY, E. A., GILMOR, R. L., BRYSON, C. Q. and BULL, M. J. (1983) Outcome of high-risk neonates with ventriculomegaly. *Developmental Medicine and Child Neurology,* **25,** 162–168

LORBER, J. and PRIESTLEY, B. L. (1981) Children with large heads: a practical approach to diagnosis in 557 children with special reference to 109 children with megalencephaly. *Developmental Medicine and Child Neurology,* **23,** 494–504

LORBER, J., SALFIELD, S. and LONTON, T. (1983) Isosorbide in the management of the infantile hydrocephalus. *Developmental Medicine and Child Neurology,* **25,** 502–511

OLSEN, L. and FRYKBERG, T. (1983) Complications in the treatment of hydrocephalus in children. *Acta Paediatrica Scandinavica,* **72,** 385–390

10

Ataxia

Ataxia means a disorder of movement: incoordination, lack of precision and speed of movements, and inability to maintain balance. As the healthy infant has poor balance and poor precision of movements, ataxia cannot usually be demonstrated until the end of the first year of life. Muscular hypotonia, which is a common finding in ataxic patients of all ages, is often the only noticeable neurological sign in young infants who are found to be ataxic towards the end of their first year (*see* page 161).

Different clinical types of ataxia can be distinguished, all of which may be associated with muscular hypotonia. In sensory ataxia the patient has difficulty in appreciating the position of his limbs and the tension of his muscles. All movements are performed better under the control of vision, and incoordination increases when the patient is told to close his eyes. Romberg's test is positive in sensory ataxia, i.e. the patient can keep his balance well with his feet together and his eyes open, but loses it as soon as his eyes are closed. Position sense and vibration sense are usually impaired. Movements are performed slowly and clumsily, particularly if the patient does not keep his eyes on what he is doing. The lesion is localized in the posterior columns of the spinal cord, often also in the dorsal roots and the peripheral nerves.

In truncal ataxia the patient has trouble keeping his balance with his eyes open; his difficulties increase, but only slightly, if he performs the tests with his eyes closed. He walks with a broad-based staggering gait like a person in acute alcohol intoxication. The staggering is particularly apparent if the patient is told to turn around quickly, to walk heel-to-toe on a straight line, or to hop on one foot. All kinds of disturbed gait are better revealed when the child is running than when he is walking. Truncal ataxia may also be observed, when the patient is sitting, as an inability to maintain balance. The patient's difficulties increase if he is asked to cross his legs.

The described difficulties with locomotion are often combined with intention tremor, revealed on the finger-to-nose and heel-to-knee-to-shin tests. In young children, in whom these tests cannot be performed, intention tremor is observed when the patient reaches out for an object, feeds himself, puts his thumb in his mouth, threads pearls on a string, puts small objects through a hole, etc. (*see also* page 28). Truncal ataxia and intention tremor are cerebellar signs and indicate a lesion of the cerebellum or its connections. Adiadochokinesis (*see* page 28) and dysarthric speech are other cerebellar signs. Sensory ataxia and cerebellar ataxia are caused by lesions with different localizations. However, if the lesion is extensive, both types of ataxia may occur in the same patient.

Ataxia is a symptom found in many neurological conditions. In this chapter, diseases with onset in childhood in which ataxia is a dominating feature will be reviewed. Ataxia may also be seen in polyneuropathy (*see* pages 175–179), hydrocephalus (*see* page 255), cerebral palsy (*see* pages 278–279), and conditions characterized by progressive neurological symptoms (*see* Chapter 13). The conditions described in this chapter are divided according to the type of onset of ataxia and the age of the patient at the onset.

Ataxia present from infancy

The findings during infancy are muscular hypotonia and retarded motor development. The infants are floppy and do not learn to sit up until the end of the first year of life. At that age when they try to sit up and reach out for objects, it is apparent that they have poor balance and intention tremor in their hands. Ataxia may thus be suspected but cannot be demonstrated until the infant is about a year old.

Cause

The cause may be prenatal, e.g. a malformation of the cerebellum as seen in the Dandy–Walker syndrome (*see Figures 9.11* , page 250, and *9.12,* page 251). Hydrocephalus is another feature of the syndrome and may also cause the early onset of ataxia without malformation of the cerebellum. The Marinesco–Sjögren syndrome, a genetically determined disease (*see* page 264), causes ataxia of early onset.

A lesion of the cerebellum or its connections may occur in the perinatal period, causing a cerebral palsy syndrome characterized by ataxia alone or in combination with other neurological findings (*see* page 279). A mild and eventually arrested hydrocephalus (*see* page 255), arising in the neonatal period, may cause ataxia of early onset.

Course

Ataxia of early onset often appears to be progressive for a year or two after it has been discovered, but this is probably only because the incoordination becomes more evident as other motor functions develop. On the whole the incoordination remains the same in relation to the child's maturation in other areas of motor function. This means that child achieves new abilities but remains clumsy for his age. Crawling is delayed; when the child eventually learns to crawl, it is done in a peculiar way on hands and knees with the lower legs wagging unsupported up in the air. (*Figure 10.1*). He learns to walk late and has difficulty in learning to run and hop; riding a bicycle and particularly skating may be impossible. In outdoor games he falls behind his peers. At the table he is clumsy and often spills things which brings reproaches. He is accident-prone. Many of these children are restless with a short attention span; some have mild mental retardation. True progression of symptoms does not occur in this group; if such is observed, a tumour (*see* Chapter 17) or a progressive cerebral disease (*see* Chapter 13) must be suspected.

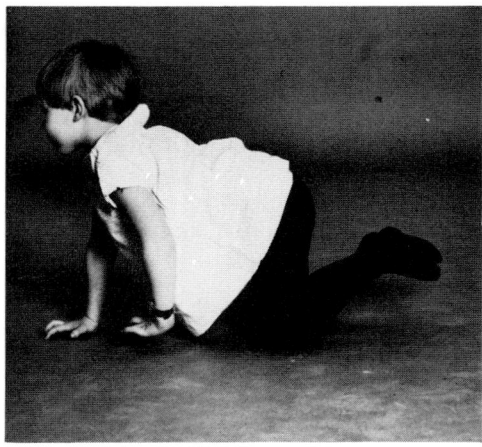

Figure 10.1. A 7-year-old girl with severe ataxia, crawling in a peculiar fashion on her hands and knees with her lower legs unsupported

Diagnosis, treatment and prognosis

The diagnosis is apparent from the history and the clinical findings. The large cyst of the fourth ventricle in the Dandy–Walker syndrome may be demonstrated on transillumination (*see* page 251). Hydrocephalus should be investigated as described in Chapter 9. Laboratory studies are otherwise of little help.

Children with ataxia of early onset are apt to develop secondary neurotic behaviour due to their constant failure in games, in bicycle riding, in skating, at the table, etc. The organic aetiology of the movement disorder is not usually as readily apparent as in other cerebral palsy syndromes. The most important part of the therapy is thus to prevent the secondary neurotic symptoms by informing the family about the organic basis of the child's difficulties. Physiotherapy from an early age is helpful. Most of these children remain clumsy, although with increasing age and maturation they learn to overcome their difficulties and to avoid situations that provoke them.

Ataxia with acute onset during childhood

Ataxia with acute onset during childhood often starts with subjective symptoms of dizziness, nausea, and vomiting. The patients usually show nystagmus, intention tremor, inability to maintain balance in the sitting or standing position, and a staggering gait; difficulties are only slightly enhanced when the patient closes his eyes. Different diagnostic possibilities will be reviewed in relation to the subsequent course.

Rapid improvement

INTOXICATION

Acute onset of ataxia followed by rapid improvement is seen in acute intoxication. Accidental intoxication causing acute ataxia may be seen in children who have been exposed to the vapour of (i.e. inhaled) glue, solvents, or petrol, or who have ingested ethyl alcohol or an overdose of hypnotics, tranquillizers, or antiepileptics.

Differential diagnostic problems seldom arise in this situation provided the history is taken with these possibilities in mind. Diagnostic and therapeutic problems arise, however, when an ordinary dose of an antiepileptic causes ataxia. All antiepileptics may cause ataxia; it is most common after phenytoin and carbamazepine. If a child is on too high a dose of phenytoin it usually takes 5–10 days for the ataxia to develop, and about the same time after stopping or reducing the dose for the symptoms to disappear. Carbamazepine causes some degree of ataxia as an almost unavoidable *initial* side effect during the first weeks of therapy. Slow introduction of the drug diminishes the ataxia which eventually disappears in most patients during continued unchanged treatment (*see* page 113).

Many drugs and poisons and/or their metabolites can be identified by blood and/or urine analysis. This method must be utilized in diagnostically unclear cases.

ACUTE CEREBELLAR ATAXIA

This syndrome is characterized by an acute dramatic onset of ataxia, which is often so sudden that the parents can give the exact date and occasionally the hour of its onset. The disease is most common in toddlers and preschool children but may occur at any age, although onset after puberty is rare. The syndrome is usually considered to be a complication of a viral disease, as it is often preceded by an exanthema, infectious mononucleosis, or infection with polio, Coxsackie, herpes simplex, or ECHO virus; it may, however, occur without any sign of infection.

At the onset affected children have nystagmus, truncal ataxia, and intention tremor. Other structures of the central nervous system may also be involved, giving rise to such symptoms as weakness of the extraocular muscles, weakness of the arms or legs, or reflex abnormalities; ataxia, however, always dominates the clinical picture. The patients are usually nauseated and may vomit; headache and a stiff neck are rarely present. Signs of increased intracranial pressure are not found. The cerebrospinal fluid is usually normal, although pleocytosis (up to 50–100 cells/mm^3) may be found. No laboratory studies or other special examinations are of diagnostic help. The diagnosis is based on the history, the clinical findings, and the course.

Symptoms are stationary for a couple of days or weeks and then subside. Almost all patients recover completely within a couple of months. If the course is more protracted, or if symptoms recur, some other cause of the ataxia must be suspected.

No therapy is necessary in this self-limiting syndrome. Treatment with corticosteroids has been attempted, but its effect, if any, is outweighed by its side effects. It is important to give the parents the correct diagnosis and to inform them about the benign nature of the disorder, as the dramatic onset of the child's symptoms is frightening.

Prolonged or intermittent course

DANCING EYE SYNDROME

The dancing eye syndrome or myoclonic encephalopathy of infants usually has its onset towards the end of the first year of life, but occasionally it starts during the following few years. The onset is acute, with or without a preceding viral infection.

The dominating symptom is a violent nystagmus which involves not only the eyes but also the head. The child thus cannot balance his head, sit up, or stand. Intention tremor is apparent in the arms and legs. The tremor may be so violent that the whole bed is shaken and the child becomes unable to perform any voluntary movement. The jerky movements of the eyes, head, trunk, and extremities disappear during sleep. Neither examination of the cerebrospinal fluid nor computerized tomography of the skull is of diagnostic help. The syndrome has a protracted course, characterized by relapses and spontaneous remissions. It may last for months or years and impair the child's mental development.

A neuroblastoma has been demonstrated in more than half of the patients with the dancing eye syndrome. These patients must therefore be examined carefully for such a tumour. Its removal has led to an improvement or disappearance of the neurological symptoms and signs in most patients. It is usually not possible to demonstrate a definite cause in patients without a neuroblastoma and no causal therapy is available. For these patients the treatment is ACTH 25–80 units per day. Prednisolone 10–40 mg/day can replace ACTH after several weeks or months but is often less effective in the acute phase. The symptoms usually improve or disappear on this therapy but have a great tendency to return when the dose of ACTH or prednisolone is decreased below a certain level. The problem then arises of how to wean the patient from this symptomatic therapy which also produces side effects.

In a child with a neuroblastoma, the prognosis depends on the prognosis for the tumour. In a case without neuroblastoma the prognosis varies but must be considered serious because of the protracted relapsing course.

TUMOURS

A tumour of the posterior fossa must always be considered in children with a fairly acute onset of cerebellar ataxia. In a case of medulloblastoma, signs of increased intracranial pressure precede or occur together with ataxia; in a case of cerebellar astrocytoma slowly progressive ataxia may be the only symptom for several months. The onset is less abrupt than in acute cerebellar ataxia. Clinical suspicion of a cerebellar tumour is an indication for computerized tomography of the skull (*see also* page 365).

MULTIPLE SCLEROSIS

Relapsing ataxia is seen in the rare cases of multiple sclerosis with onset in childhood. Onset before the age of 12 is exceptional, and only a few cases have an onset during the early teens. As in cases with onset in early adulthood the common initial symptoms are attacks of optic or retrobulbar neuritis, ataxia, or regional paraesthesia. The patient must have two separate attacks of symptoms with different localizations before a clinical diagnosis of multiple sclerosis can be established. A slight pleocytosis and/or a slightly elevated protein content may be found in the spinal fluid; these findings are nonspecific and may be absent. Findings that are more specific for multiple sclerosis are an increase of gamma globulin in relation to total protein and to albumin, the presence of bands in the gamma globulin (oligoclonal gammopathy) and the presence of plasma cells. Analysis of the cerebrospinal fluid is important, and must include these special investigations if multiple sclerosis is suspected. The management is the same as in adulthood.

Ataxia with acute onset and an intermittent course may occasionally be seen in Refsum's disease (*see* pages 263–264).

Ataxia with insidious onset during childhood

When ataxia has an insidious onset during childhood, it may be difficult to date its exact onset and to be certain that it has been present from infancy.

Slow progression

Insidious onset and slow steady progression may be seen in cases of cerebellar astrocytoma (*see* page 365). This type of ataxia is seen in several of the conditions described in Chapter 13 in which other progressive neurological and mental signs are also found.

FRIEDREICH'S ATAXIA

The classic progressive ataxia of childhood is Friedreich's ataxia. It is inherited as an autosomal recessive gene. Symptoms start insidiously during childhood, usually during the first decade. The first symptom is unsteady gait which is usually apparent as clumsiness in certain games. The difficulties increase in darkness. If the child is examined at this stage, the common findings are a positive Romberg test, an unsteady gait particularly with the eyes closed, impaired vibration and position sense, and hypoactive or absent muscle reflexes, particularly in the legs, indicating involvement of the posterior columns and posterior roots. Many patients have pes cavus, and this deformity may be present even before any neurological symptoms or signs are apparent. The symptoms progress slowly and steadily: the patient has increasing difficulty in walking, even with his eyes open; nystagmus, intention tremor, and dysarthria appear as evidence of involvement of the cerebellum and its connections. Muscular atrophy, particularly of the lower legs, occurs and indicates involvement of the ventral roots and peripheral nerves. The muscle reflexes disappear. The plantar response becomes extensor, indicating involvement of the corticospinal tract. Skeletal deformities, particularly scoliosis, and flexion contractures of the knees develop. Optic atrophy is usually seen at this stage. The conduction velocity of peripheral nerves is as a rule decreased on the sensory side, whereas the findings on the motor side are variable. The atrophic muscles show electromyographic evidence of denervation. The patients are usually confined to wheelchairs in their late teens or early twenties. Evidence of cardiomyopathy, seen on the ECG (T wave inversion, signs of left ventricular hypertrophy, and extrasystoles) and on ultrasound examination of the heart, is found in about 90 per cent of patients with Friedreich's ataxia. The cardiomyopathy, which may be demonstrable before the neurological signs are apparent, is probably part of the syndrome. An increased incidence of diabetes mellitus is also found in Friedreich's ataxia. The connection between the cardiac, endocrine, and neurological abnormalities is unknown; they all appear to be parts of the same disease. Intellectual function may be impaired late in the disease.

There is no treatment for the disease *per se*. Physiotherapy and technical aids are of some help to the patients. The prognosis is poor; the patients become severely handicapped and death occurs between 20 and 50 years of age.

Several inherited syndromes have been described as variants of Friedreich's ataxia. Conditions included in this ill-defined group all have ataxia as a prominent feature in various combinations with spasticity, optic atrophy, and mental impairment. When a more specific diagnosis can be established, e.g. leucodystrophy (*see* page 302), the condition should not be included under this heading. The clinical picture, course, and prognosis vary from family to family, but there is a great resemblance between affected members of the same family. No treatment is available.

RETINITIS PIGMENTOSA, DEAFNESS AND ATAXIA

In the syndrome in which retinitis pigmentosa is combined with congenital deafness and with vestibulocerebellar ataxia and mental abnormality in a proportion of cases (Hallgren, 1959), the deafness is present from an early age and the retinitis pigmentosa develops during school-age. Almost all the patients with severe deafness also have nystagmus and an unsteady gait; these symptoms are slowly progressive throughout life. Various mental symptoms develop in some patients. The syndrome is inherited as an autosomal recessive gene. No treatment is available. Retinitis pigmentosa and deafness are also found in Refsum's disease (*see* page 263).

ATAXIA TELANGIECTASIA

This condition is inherited as an autosomal recessive trait. Symptoms start in early childhood with slowly increasing cerebellar ataxia. The telangiectases may already be present at 2 years of age but usually first become apparent when the patient is between 4 and 6 years. Their most common localization is on the conjunctiva, where they simulate conjunctivitis; they may also be found in a butterfly distribution on the face, on the ears, on the neck, and in the cubital and popliteal areas.

The patients slowly become increasingly handicapped from their ataxia. Other neurological symptoms such as muscular weakness and wasting may appear; mental development may stagnate or even regress. Physical development and growth are retarded.

Recurrent infection of the nasal sinus and the lungs is another typical feature of the syndrome. The abnormal susceptibility to respiratory tract infection is due to an impaired immunological mechanism. Lack of gamma globulin IgA has been demonstrated in about two-thirds of examined patients with ataxia telangiectasia. Impaired cellular immunity with depletion of lymphoid tissue and lack of development of the thymus is also found. Patients who survive the increasing neurological handicap and the great number of respiratory infections appear to have an unusual propensity to develop neoplasms.

The diagnosis is difficult to establish in young children before the telangiectases are apparent, but when they are present the diagnosis causes no problem. The absence of IgA in the serum supports the clinical diagnosis but its presence does not exclude it. Computerized tomography of the skull may be normal or may reveal an atrophic cerebellum.

No treatment for the disease *per se* is available. Infections must be treated vigorously, and tumours must be treated according to their localization and nature, although the patients appear to be abnormally susceptible to radiotherapy. Gamma globulin seems to be of limited value.

The prognosis is poor. Most patients die during late childhood or early adulthood. At autopsy the cerebellum is found to be macroscopically normal or slightly atrophic; microscopic examination reveals a loss of Purkinje cells, in particular, but also of granular cells and basket cells of the cerebellar cortex. The thymus is found to be absent or very small with a marked decrease in lymphocytes and an absence of Hassall's corpuscles. The relationship between the abnormalities of the central nervous system and those of the lymphatic system is not known.

Intermittent course or stationary symptoms

CHRONIC INTOXICATION

Ataxia with insidious onset, fairly constant symptoms or an intermittent course may be seen in cases of chronic intoxication, e.g. with antiepileptics. Monitoring the dose by determinations of the serum level of the drug diminishes this risk considerably.

HARTNUP DISEASE

This condition is inherited as an autosomal recessive trait. The patients have a pellagra-like itching eruption on the parts of the skin that are exposed to light. Neurological symptoms consist particularly of ataxia, nystagmus, double vision, and increased muscle reflexes. Mild symptoms may be present at all times, but they increase and become severe during attacks, at which time mental symptoms are common (e.g. depression, confusion, hallucinations, and even psychotic behaviour). The disease is one of the group of disorders caused by inborn errors of metabolism, and is probably caused by an abnormality of tryptophane metabolism. An increased excretion of amino acids with a typical pattern, called the 'H pattern', is found in the urine; there is also an increased excretion of indican, indoles, and indole acids. The administration of large amounts of nicotinic acid clears the skin rash and improves the neurological signs but does not influence the abnormal excretion of amino acids.

REFSUM'S DISEASE

The syndrome described by Refsum, which he termed heredopathia atactica polyneuritiformis, is inherited as an autosomal recessive trait. The onset is usually in adulthood but a few childhood cases are on record. The course is chronic, characterized by relapses and spontaneous remissions. During periods of deterioration the patients become more ataxic and show evidence of a new relapse of polyneuropathy; symptoms improve but do not disappear during remissions. The patients have atypical retinitis pigmentosa, pupillary abnormalities, and often cataract and nerve deafness. Cardiac abnormalities are found in some patients. The cerebrospinal fluid protein is increased, and the cell count is usually normal.

The symptoms and signs are caused by an abnormality of lipid metabolism with the accumulation of phytanic acid and an increased level of phytanic acid in the serum. This finding is pathognomonic for Refsum's disease. The increased amount of phytanic acid is to a large extent derived from phytol, which constitutes one-third of the weight of chlorophyll, and from the phytanic acid present in butter and other types of animal fat. A diet low in phytol and phytanic acid, i.e. free of chlorophyll-containing plants and animal fat with a high content of phytanic acid, seems to improve the neurological symptoms of Refsum's disease.

MARINESCO–SJÖGREN SYNDROME

The Marinesco–Sjögren syndrome is genetically determined with autosomal recessive inheritance. It is characterized by ataxia with early onset, in many cases during infancy; severely delayed motor development; mental retardation; bilateral cataracts from an early age, possibly from birth; and short stature. Slowly progressive muscular weakness and wasting has been noted in some patients during early adulthood. Asphyxia in the neonatal period has been reported in some of the described patients with the Marinesco–Sjögren syndrome; if such an episode has occurred and the family history is negative, it is difficult to distinguish between this syndrome and neurological and ophthalmological sequelae due to anoxia. The cataracts are treated surgically and the ataxia with physiotherapy, but there is no available treatment for the disease *per se.*

Management of the ataxic child

The two urgent diagnoses to keep in mind when a child develops ataxia are intoxication and cerebellar tumour, as they require immediate causal treatment. Analysis of blood and/or urine for suspected poisons or their metabolites is of good diagnostic help in doubtful cases. It is usually possible to differentiate a case of acute cerebellar ataxia (peracute onset, no signs of increased intracranial pressure, improvement within a few weeks) from a cerebellar tumour (fairly acute onset, often evidence of increased intracranial pressure, deterioration) on clinical grounds alone, but when the differential diagnosis is in doubt, computerized tomography of the skull must be performed. Examination of the cerebrospinal fluid is often of value, as some of the progressive degenerative diseases in which ataxia is a feature cause increased spinal fluid protein. If there is clinical suspicion of a tumour of the posterior fossa, lumbar puncture must not be performed unless computerized tomography of the skull has first excluded an expansive process. Friedreich's ataxia is diagnosed on careful neurological examination alone; the constellation of sensory ataxia or combined sensory and cerebellar ataxia, absent muscle reflexes, and positive Babinski signs is typical in Friedreich's ataxia but is otherwise rarely seen. Cardiac examination including an ECG and, in doubtful cases, ultrasound examination of the heart is important because of the high incidence of cardiac involvement in Friedreich's ataxia and Refsum's disease. Examination of the fundi reveals optic atrophy in Friedreich's ataxia and atypical retinitis pigmentosa in Refsum's disease. Deafness and attacks of polyneuropathy are typical features of Refsum's disease and should be followed-up by the determination of phytanic acid in the blood.If a skin rash is present the urine must be examined for amino acids, indican, indoles, and indole acids. Telangiectases may simulate conjunctivitis and a skin rash; investigation of the serum level of immunoglobulins may reveal an immunological defect in these patients. The ataxia is treated with physiotherapy. It is important for all the adults around the child to understand and accept that the ataxic child cannot help being clumsy and that blame only increases his difficulties.

References

ALTER, M., TALBERT, O. and CROFFEAD, G. (1962) Cerebellar ataxia, congenital cataracts, and retarded somatic and mental maturation. *Neurology* (Minneapolis), **12**, 836–847

BARBEAU, A. (1978) Metabolic ataxias. In *Taurine and Neurological Disorders,* pp. 403–413, Ed. Barbeau, A. and Huxtable, R. J. New York: Raven Press

BOLTSHAUSER, E., HERDAN, M., DUMERMUTH, G. and ISLER, W. (1981) Joubert syndrome: clinical and polygraphic observations in a further case. *Neuropediatrics,* **12**, 181–191

BRANDT, S., CARLSEN, N., GLENTING, P. and HELWEG-LARSEN, J. (1974) Encephalopathia myoclonica infantilis (Kinsbourne) and neuroblastoma in children. A report of three cases. *Developmental Medicine and Child Neurology,* **16**, 286–294

DUNN, H. G. (1973) Nerve conduction studies in children with Friedreich's ataxia and ataxia-telangiectasia. *Developmental Medicine and Child Neurology,* **15**, 324–337

GOUTIERES, F. (1981) Les ataxies chez l'enfant. Aspects clinique et genetiques. *Journal de Génétique humaine,* **29**, 211–220

HALLGREN, B. (1959) Retinitis pigmentosa combined with congenital deafness; with vestibulo-cerebellar ataxia and mental abnormality in a proportion of cases. *Acta Psychiatrica Scandinavica,* suppl. 138

HARDING, A. E. (1981) Friedreich ataxia, a clinical and genetic study of 90 families with an analysis of early diagnostic criteria and intrafamilial clustering of clinical features. *Brain,* **104**, 589–620

OUVRIER, R. A., McLEOD, J. G. and CONCHIN, C. (1982) Friedreich ataxia. Early detection and progression of peripheral nerve abnormalities. *Journal of Neurological Sciences,* **55**, 137–145

REFSUM, S., SALOMONSEN, L. and SKATVEDT, M. (1949) Heredopathia atactica polyneuritiformis in children. *Journal of Pediatrics,* **35**, 335–343

SANNER, G. (1979) Pathogenetic and preventive aspects of non-progressive ataxic syndromes. *Developmental Medicine and Child Neurology,* **21**, 663–671

SANNER, G. and HAGBERG, B. (1974) 188 cases of non-progressive ataxic syndromes in childhood. *Neuropädiatrie,* **5**, 224–235

THORÉN, C. (1964) Cardiomyopathy in Friedreich's ataxia. *Acta Paediatrica* (Uppsala), suppl. 153

TUCK, P. R. and McLEOD, J. G. (1983) Retinitis pigmentosa, ataxia, and peripheral neuropathy. *Journal of Neurology, Neurosurgery and Psychiatry,* **46**, 206–213

WALDMANN, T. A., MISTI, J., NELSON, D. L. and KRAEMER, K. H. (1983) Ataxia-telangiectasia: A multisystem hereditary disease with immuno-deficiency, impaired organ maturation, X-ray hypersensitivity, and a higher incidence of neoplasia. *Annals of Internal Medicine,* **99**, 367–379

11

Involuntary movements

The various types of involuntary movements are described separately; more than one type, however, may occur in the same patient, and the distinction between different types may be difficult.

Tremor

Tremor is a rhythmical shaking movement which is usually most pronounced in the hands and fingers. It disappears during sleep. Tremor that is present only when the patient makes a deliberate movement is termed intention tremor, and is part of ataxia (*see* Chapter 10). Tremor that is present at rest is caused by a lesion of the basal ganglia or their connections. It may be the patient's only symptom or it may occur together with other disturbances of movement and posture.

Essential tremor

Essential tremor is the term used for the condition characterized by tremor and no or practically no other symptoms. This condition is inherited as an autosomal dominant trait. The onset is usually in childhood or adolescence, although in a few reported families, affected members noted the onset in their fifth or sixth decade. The patient complains of shaky unsteady finger movements. Tremor of the fingers and the hands is found on examination; it is present at rest and increases only slightly on voluntary movements. Nystagmus, head tremor, other disturbances of movement or posture, and other neurological abnormalities are not found. The tremor may remain stationary throughout life or show a slow and mild progression. It is an annoying condition, which impairs the patient's ability to manage cutlery nimbly at the table and to write rapidly and neatly, but otherwise has no influence on his ability to live a normal life. The tremor increases if the patient feels that he is being watched and criticized. The beta-blocking drug propranolol usually has a good symptomatic effect in a dose of 10–40 mg two to four times a day. Propranolol medication can be tried without fear of producing side effects, as these are rapidly reversed on withdrawal of the drug. Sleep difficulties and nightmares are disturbing side effects which may be more unpleasant than the tremor.

266

Tremor combined with other disorders

Tremor may occur together with choreoathetosis (*see below*) and dystonic posture (*see* page 270). It may also occur together with rigidity and constitute a Parkinson-like syndrome. Paralysis agitans or Parkinson's disease is a condition that usually affects middle-aged or older persons. A similar clinical picture with onset in childhood or adolescence has been reported. This picture may arise as a sequela after acute encephalitis; if so, the cause is obvious from the history, and the course is nonprogressive. The patient may show other neurological or mental symptoms, depending on the extent of the brain lesion. This syndrome was typically seen after the epidemic encephalitis lethargica occurring after World War I; although the syndrome is rare today it may still occur as a complication of other types of encephalitis.

The condition termed juvenile paralysis agitans is inherited as an autosomal recessive trait. Its onset is in childhood or adolescence, with tremor followed by rigidity of variable severity and often signs of involvement of the corticospinal tract. The condition is slowly progressive. Other disturbances of movement and posture have been reported in a few patients. The findings at autopsy consist of atrophy and degeneration, particularly of the globus pallidus and its connections, but also of the substantia nigra and the corticospinal tract.

The symptomatic treatment of the Parkinson-like syndromes is principally the same in childhood as in adulthood. It is important to stimulate the patients to as much activity as possible and to train them to independence; physiotherapy is of help in this connection. Drug therapy is given according to the same principles as in adulthood with levodopa as the basic drug. By careful adjustment of the dose, levodopa usually reduces the rigidity but has less influence on the involuntary movements. As in adults the effect tends to abate after several years of treatment. Because juvenile paralysis agitans is rare, experience with other drugs and neurosurgical operations on the basal ganglia remains scarce. All measures used in adults may also be considered for use in children. The prognosis is serious, as the condition is chronic with a tendency to progress and eventually to become less responsive to treatment.

Resting, fine finger tremor is often seen in *progressive spinal muscular atrophy of type 1* (*see* page 171). It is also a typical feature of *hyperthyroidism* (*see* page 389).

Choreoathetosis

Choreoathetosis consists of slow writhing movements of the head, neck, and extremities (athetosis) and of large sudden jerks, usually of the arms and hands (chorea). Because of these uncontrolled movements all intentional activity is disturbed and the patient may have great difficulty in keeping his balance when sitting or standing (*Figure 11.1*). The facial and tongue muscles may also be involved, causing grimacing and dysarthria. If choreoathetosis is the only neurological sign, muscular tone is decreased and the patients do not develop permanent contractures, although they may keep a limb in a fixed unnatural position (*Figure 11.2*). If the lesion also involves the corticospinal tract, spasticity is present and contractures may be a problem. All choreoathetoid movements disappear during sleep. The anatomical localization of the lesion in choreoathetosis is the basal ganglia and their connections.

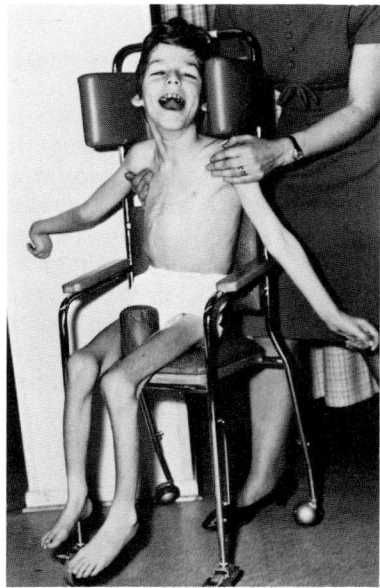

Figure 11.1. Choreoathetosis in a 10-year-old boy. Note the large jerks of the arms, impairing the patient's ability to keep his balance; the abnormal posture of the right hand; and the abnormal co-movements of the face and the tongue

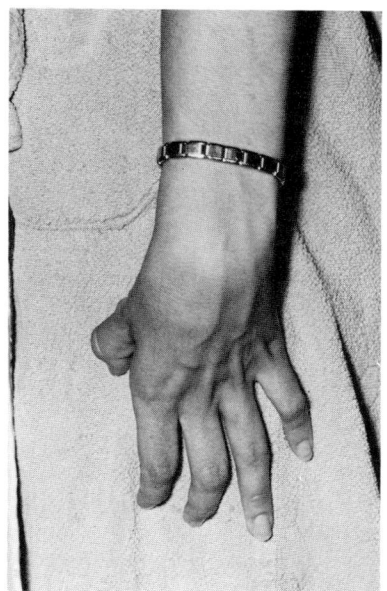

Figure 11.2. Athetosis. Note the abnormal posture of the hand and the tense tendons

Choreoathetosis as a cerebral palsy syndrome

Choreoathetosis may occur as a sequela after a neonatal or early postnatal brain injury and thus constitute a cerebral palsy syndrome (*see* page 278). The border between these conditions and the Parkinson-like syndrome that occurs after early encephalitis (*see* page 267) may be indistinct.

Sydenham's chorea

Chorea minor, Sydenham's chorea, is the neurological manifestation of acute rheumatic fever. It is rarely seen before 5 years of age or after 20 years; its peak incidence is around 10 years of age. It is seen more often in girls than in boys.

Symptoms start gradually with tiredness, irritation, and an inability to sit still. The child's movements become jerky and unsteady – he spills things at the table and his handwriting deteriorates; attention and blame make him worse. His speech may become slurred. Within a couple of weeks the patient's symptoms have increased to such an extent that he constantly performs sudden, purposeless, jerky movements which prevent any intentional action. The term St Vitus' dance has been used for centuries to describe this condition. Neurological examination reveals these involuntary movements and profound muscular hypotonia (*Figure 11.3*) and usually no other signs. Evidence of mild or moderate carditis is often found. Arthritis is seen in some patients; other signs of rheumatic fever are exceptions. A normal or slightly elevated sedimentation rate is the rule. The cerebrospinal fluid is usually normal; a mild pleocytosis is only rarely seen.

The diagnosis is based on the clinical findings; the combination of cardiac and acute neurological signs is characteristic.

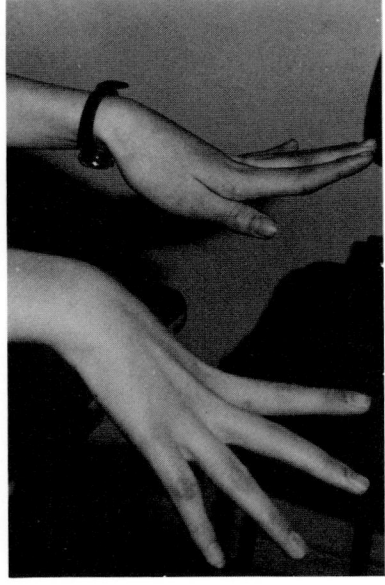

Figure 11.3. Typical posture of the hands of a 13-year-old girl with Sydenham's chorea

The usual course is deterioration over a couple of weeks, stationary symptoms for about a month, and then improvement. As a rule all neurological symptoms disappear within 6–12 weeks, although the tendency for the patient to perform jerky movements when he is tense may continue for several more months. An increased sensitivity to dopaminergic drugs and a tendency to develop side effects during treatment with these drugs seem to persist for several years, possibly lifelong, in some patients after chorea minor.

The treatment is symptomatic. Bed-rest, help with feeding, salicylates, and sedatives make the patient more comfortable during the acute phase of the disease.

Penicillin is given in the acute phase to eradicate the streptococci responsible for the rheumatic infection and continued as prophylaxis against new attacks, as in other cases of rheumatic fever.

Disturbed metabolism of uric acid

Choreoathetosis is a typical finding in the syndrome characterized by an increased level of uric acid in the blood (*see* page 134).

Huntington's chorea

Huntington's chorea is inherited as an autosomal dominant trait. It usually has its onset in adulthood, but in about 1 per cent of cases its onset is during the first decade. The first symptoms are speech difficulties, often in combination with grimacing and other involuntary movements of the face and tongue, mental stagnation and deterioration, and convulsions. Rigidity may be an early symptom or occur later; in cases with severe rigidity, choreoathetosis is mild or absent.

The electroencephalogram (EEG) is usually abnormal, but the findings are nonspecific. No other laboratory studies are of diagnostic help. The diagnosis is thus based on the clinical findings and the positive family history; in a child whose family history is unknown the diagnosis is almost impossible to establish.

The course is progressive with increasing mental symptoms and therapy-resistant convulsions. Either rigidity or choreoathetosis increases and confines the patient to bed. Death occurs either in status epilepticus or from complications of bed-rest. No therapy is available except symptomatic treatment for the convulsions. Autopsy reveals degeneration of both the basal ganglia and the cerebral cortex.

Torsion dystonia

Dystonia musculorum deformans or torsion dystonia is a clinical syndrome with a presumably heterogeneous background. Autosomal dominant inheritance has been described in some families; the family history is, however, entirely negative in many cases. Onset of the condition may occur at any age from infancy to childhood. Most of the cases with onset before puberty seem to occur in children who up to the age of 6–8 years have been healthy and have developed normally. At that age symptoms start gradually and progress slowly over the following years.

Symptoms usually start with slow involuntary twitching movements of a limb, e.g. a consistent inward turning of the foot. These involuntary movements spread to other limbs and to the head and trunk, until the patient is unable to sit or stand, and all intentional activity is prevented. The involuntary movements also engage the facial muscles, causing grimacing and speech difficulties. All involuntary movements disappear during sleep. Convulsions are not part of the syndrome. The mental development is probably always normal, in spite of the grave impairment of the child's ability to communicate verbally.

On examination the involuntary movements are revealed, together with the rigidity which strongly forces limbs into abnormal positions. Muscle reflexes may be difficult to evaluate; they are usually found to be normal when it is possible to get the patient relaxed. A positive Babinski sign may be present.

The diagnosis is based on the clinical picture, as there are no laboratory studies that are of diagnostic help. The course is slowly progressive; the patient becomes increasingly handicapped and finally bedridden. Physiotherapy has little influence on the condition. The benzodiazepines chlordiazepoxide and diazepam may diminish muscle tension and involuntary movements. When effective, the treatment must continue for years to prevent the recurrence of symptoms when the drug is stopped. Levodopa may be tried; a good symptomatic effect has been reported in a few patients, but deterioration has also been seen in some cases. Great improvement has been reported after neurosurgical operations on some of these severely handicapped children.

A clinical picture resembling torsion dystonia may be seen as an acute reversible condition in patients taking prochlorperazine (*see* page 211). Other drugs, e.g. haloperidol, may have the same side effect.

Epilepsia partialis continua

Epilepsia partialis continua is the term used to describe a condition in which a conscious patient has constant painless spasms localized to one muscle group, usually the facial muscles on one side. Unlike all other types of involuntary movements these twitchings *do not* disappear during sleep. Their cause is usually an irritative lesion of the cerebral cortex – often a brain abscess, occasionally a tumour. The EEG is severely abnormal; focal severe slowing or spike activity is recorded from the area predicted from the clinical picture. Computerized tomography of the skull must be performed, possibly supplemented with other neuroradiological examinations.

Myoclonic jerks

Myoclonic jerks may vary in severity from occasional twitchings of a muscle group to severe generalized spasms, which may throw the patient to the ground. They shift in localization from one muscle group to another. Myoclonic jerks are often combined with epilepsy and mental deterioration and are seen in some of the diseases characterized by progressive mental and neurological symptoms (*see* Chapter 13). They may also be part of the syndrome arising after an episode of severe brain anoxia. The involuntary movements disappear during sleep.

Almost all patients with myoclonic jerks have an abnormal EEG. The results of other laboratory studies vary with the cause of the jerks (*see* pages 88 and 300). When no cause is apparent, a complete neurological, ophthalmological and metabolic investigation must be performed. Myoclonic jerks are usually a poor prognostic sign, indicating a condition with a grave prognosis. However, occasionally myoclonic jerks may be seen in epileptic patients with no apparent progression of the disease and no evidence of mental retardation. Drug therapy of myoclonic jerks consists of antiepileptic drugs. Chlormethiazole 0.25–0.5 g one to three times a day has been effective in a few patients; the best therapy in most patients seems to be sodium valproate in combination with a small dose of clonazepam (*see also* pages 114, 115 and 300); some patients improve on this therapy, but only a few become completely seizure-free.

Tics

Tics are involuntary muscle jerks which are usually localized in the face, particularly around the eyes and occasionally involving the neck muscles. They usually recur in the same area, which may be unilateral or bilateral and does not correspond to the distribution of a nerve, a root, a segment, or a localized part of the cerebral cortex. They disappear during sleep. Tics have a psychiatric and not a neurological basis. The neurological examination gives a normal result as do all special investigations including electroencephalography. The treatment of tics is difficult and involves careful and patient psychiatric evaluation and therapy.

Maladie de tic convulsif

The syndrome called Gilles de la Tourette's syndrome, or maladie de tic convulsif, is a condition on the borderline between neurology and psychiatry. The cause is unknown but an organic background is most likely. The onset is usually in childhood. The characteristic features are progressively violent muscular jerks involving the face and shoulders and the subsequent development of spasmodic involuntary noises, which are at first unintelligible but later become coprolalic. The disease thus causes a severe social handicap. All symptoms disappear during sleep. Its prognosis is poor, as the symptoms are usually chronic and often progressive. The diagnosis is based on the typical behaviour of the patient; neurological examination and special investigations including an EEG are usually normal.

The condition is difficult to treat. The best drug is haloperidol which in a dose of up to 12–15 mg/day relieves the symptoms in many patients. However, haloperidol causes extrapyramidal side effects which, at a dose high enough to be effective, may be too disturbing to justify the further use of this symptomatic drug. Other sedatives, antiepileptics, and tranquillizers may be tried but usually have insignificant or no influence on the condition. The course is chronic, often with fluctuations.

Rhythmic head-banging

Rhythmic head-banging is often seen in healthy children in their second and third half-year, particularly when they are bored, tired or irritated. Within certain limits it is thus a normal phenomenon. When excessive in intensity or duration, it may be a sign of mental retardation, emotional problems, or lack of stimulation and thus require further investigation.

Management of the child with involuntary movements

The first question is always: 'Do the involuntary movements disappear during sleep?' All types do so except epilepsia partialis continua; immediate investigation including neuroradiology is urgent in this condition. The various types of involuntary movements can usually be differentiated by observation. The family history, possibly examination also of the parents, is most important in Huntington's chorea and essential tremor, as these conditions are inherited as an autosomal dominant trait; the same is presumably true for some cases of dystonia musculorum deformans. The combination of chorea and carditis is typical of chorea minor,

Sydenham's chorea. Myoclonic jerks occur haphazardly, whereas tics usually recur in the same area which has no neuroanatomical correspondence. The EEG is usually normal in tics and gravely abnormal in myoclonic jerks, often with spikes occurring simultaneously with the jerks. A patient with myoclonic jerks needs a complete neurological, ophthalmological and metabolic investigation; a patient with tics needs psychiatric evaluation and help.

Physiotherapy is not very successful in the treatment of these movement disorders. Antiparkinsonian drugs are as useful in children with paralysis agitans as in adults. Patients with severe dystonia and abnormal posturing may benefit from diazepam. The relief of symptoms by neurosurgical operation has been reported in some patients. Patients with tics, and particularly with the severely handicapping condition Gilles de la Tourette's syndrome, seem to benefit from treatment with haloperidol.

References

BYERS, R. K., GILLES, F. H. and FUNG, C. (1973) Huntington's disease in children. *Neurology*, **23**, 561–569

GORDON, N. (1980) Choreathetosis of genetic origin. *Developmental Medicine and Child Neurology*, **22**, 521–524

HAGBERG, B., KYLLERMAN, M. and STEEN, G. (1979) Dyskinesia and dystonia in neurometabolic disorders. *Neuropädiatrie*, **10**, 305–320

HELLSTRÖM, B. (1982) Progressive dystonia and dyskinesia in childhood. A review of some recent advances. *Acta Paediatrica Scandinavica*, **71**, 177–181

LAKKE, J. P. W. F. (1981) Classification of extrapyramidal disorders. *Journal of Neurological Sciences*, **51**, 311–327

LARSSON, T. and SJÖGREN, T. (1960) Essential tremor. *Acta Psychiatrica Scandinavica*, suppl. 144

MARSDEN, C. D. and HARRISON, M. J. G. (1974) Idiopathic torsion dystonia. *Brain*, **97**, 793–810

OUVRIER, R. A. (1978) Progressive dystonia with marked diurnal fluctuations. *Annals of Neurology*, **4**, 412–417

SACHDEV, K. K., SINGH, N. and KRISHNAMOORTHY, M. S. (1977) Juvenile parkinsonism treated with levodopa. *Archives of Neurology*, **34**, 244–245

SANNER, G. and BERGSTRÖM, B. (1979) Benign torticollis in infancy. *Acta Paediatrica Scandinavica*, **68**, 219–223

SHAPIRO, A. K., SHAPIRO, E. S., BRUNN, R. D. and SWEET, R. D. (1978) *Gilles de la Tourette syndrome*. New York: Raven Press

SLEIGH, G. and LINDENBAUM, R. H. (1981) Benign (non-paroxysmal) familial chorea. Pediatric perspectives. *Archives of Diseases in Childhood*, **56**, 616–621

12

Cerebral palsy

The definitions suggested for cerebral palsy are numerous and can be summarized in the following essential points:

1. The localization of the lesion is in the brain
2. The lesion is permanent and nonprogressive, although the clinical picture may change during life
3. The lesion arises in early life and interferes with the normal development of the brain
4. The clinical picture is dominated by a disorder of movement and posture and impairment of the patient's ability to make voluntary use of his muscles; it may be complicated by other neurological and mental symptoms and signs.

The incidence of cerebral palsy varies in different countries. This variation is to some extent real and depends, for example, on the standard of obstetric and neonatal care and on the incidence of prematurity. To some extent, however, it depends on the reporting and registration of cases, and the incidence increases if mild cases are included. The incidence in the Scandinavian countries is around 1.2–1.5 per 1000 living newborn infants.

Causes of cerebral palsy

The cause of cerebral palsy may be a prenatal, perinatal, or postnatal injury to the brain.

Prenatal causes

INHERITANCE

When more than one case of presumed cerebral palsy is found in a sibship, the primary reaction of the examiner is to doubt the diagnosis, as most of the degenerative cerebral diseases (*see* Chapter 13), which may be mistaken for cerebral palsy at a single examination, are inherited as an autosomal recessive trait and thus often affect sibs. However, autosomal recessive inheritance seems to exist as a rare prenatal cause of true nonprogressive cerebral palsy. The diagnosis of this condition, which as a rule presents clinically as diparesis and ataxia, is difficult to establish, as the patient must be followed-up for many years before a progressive disease can be excluded. The occurrence of more than one case of cerebral palsy in the same family does not prove inheritance of the condition. The cause may be a perinatal brain lesion, since obstetric complications (e.g. premature delivery) may occur more than once in the same mother.

INFECTION

If the mother becomes infected the organism may cross the placenta and infect the fetus, in this way causing a prenatal brain injury. The most common fetal infections are syphilis, toxoplasmosis, rubella, and cytomegalic inclusion body disease. All may cause acute symptoms and signs in the newborn infant, followed by evidence of permanent brain damage later in childhood. The dominating finding is mental retardation (*see* pages 124–125) but movement disorders may also arise.

OTHER COMPLICATIONS DURING PREGNANCY

Complications of pregnancy, such as an anoxic episode, X-ray radiation, and maternal intoxication, may affect the fetus. If such a condition damages the fetal brain, the usual sequela is mental retardation, occasionally combined with cerebral palsy.

Perinatal causes

ANOXIA

The most common cause of cerebral palsy is still a brain injury occurring in the perinatal period although the incidence is decreasing steadily with improved obstetric and neonatal care. Anoxia may occur immediately before or after birth. The risk is increased if the delivery is complicated, for example, by abnormal position of the fetus or disproportion between the maternal pelvis and fetal head leading to prolonged labour.

INTRACRANIAL BLEEDING

The same conditions as cause anoxia may also cause intracranial bleeding. This may consist of heavy bleeding from a venous sinus, usually due to a tear of the tentorium cerebelli. Such a haemorrhage encircles the brain stem, impairing the function of the circulatory and respiratory centres and thus increasing the anoxia. Punctate haemorrhages in the brain substance are often found in anoxia and are probably caused by it. Anoxia and bleeding thus occur together, and it may be difficult to separate the effect of one from the other.

A haemorrhage may also be localized within the brain substance and eventually produce cerebral palsy. A common site of bleeding, particularly in small infants born several weeks before term, is the subependymal white matter surrounding the ventricles (*see Figure 3.23,* page 75). It is conceivable that the occurrence of bleeding or its deterioration may be connected with a sudden increase in blood pressure, which could be a consequence of slightly rough handling of the infant.

Although there is no scientific proof of the connection it is wise to handle these small infants as little as possible, always with great gentleness, and to avoid, for example, eliciting a Moro reflex. A small immature infant with subependymal bleeding usually shows no obvious symptoms or signs, and the high incidence of this occurrence has only become apparent through routinely performed ultrasound examination of the skull of newborn infants born more than 4 weeks before term. A lesion with this localization carries a slightly increased risk of the later development of spastic diparesis (*see* page 284). The subependymal blood may break through to the ventricles. If this happens, the infant usually shows impaired respiration, a bulging fontanelle, and a decreasing haemoglobin value. Intracranial bleeding increases the risk of the development of hydrocephalus and cerebral palsy. However, the great majority of these prematurely born infants, particularly those without intraventricular bleeding, show normal development and only mild or no sequelae.

Blood may enter the subarachnoid space. This may slightly increase the risk of hydrocephalus but does not usually significantly affect the child's further development. An intracranial haemorrhage may be localized to the subdural space, where it may cause cortical injury by pressing on the underlying cortex and interfering with its blood circulation (*see also* page 240).

PREMATURITY

As mentioned above, birth more than four weeks before term carries a slightly increased risk of cerebral palsy, particularly spastic diparesis.

JAUNDICE

Jaundice during the neonatal period may cause permanent brain damage with cerebral palsy. Treatment of neonatal infections, phototherapy of the jaundiced infant, and exchange transfusions are measures that are usually effective in the prevention of brain injury. In the exceptional case in which brain damage is not prevented, the area particularly affected by the bilirubin is the basal ganglia; the type of cerebral palsy produced is usually choreoathetosis, often combined with deafness.

PURULENT MENINGITIS

A purulent meningitis (*see* pages 343–345), which in the perinatal period is usually due to Gram-negative bacteria, may cause brain injury with cerebral palsy as a sequela.

EXPANSIVE HYDROCEPHALUS

Expansive hydrocephalus, arrested spontaneously or through a shunt operation, may cause permanent brain damage and cerebral palsy, usually a combination of ataxia and diparesis. Pale discs due to optic atrophy may occasionally be seen (*see* page 255).

Postnatal causes

Any brain injury that occurs during the postnatal period of brain development may cause cerebral palsy. Examples of such injuries include an accident with physical head injury; meningitis; encephalitis; an infarction due to occlusion of a blood vessel; bleeding for no apparent reason or from an arterial or arteriovenous malformation; or a scar after an operation for a brain tumour.

Clinical picture

The motor disorders associated with cerebral palsy can be divided according to the nature of the dysfunction and to its localization. Nonmotor abnormalities may complicate the clinical picture.

The nature of the motor dysfunction

SPASTICITY

In spasticity there is a constant increase in muscle tone, increased muscle reflexes often with clonus, and a positive Babinski sign. The tonic neck reflex may persist longer than normal but is seldom pronounced, and other neonatal reflexes disappear at the normal age. The hypertonicity is permanent and does not disappear during sleep. The increase in tone is not the same in all muscle groups, causing a typical posture of the affected limbs with a tendency to contractures. The arm is kept adducted, flexed at the elbow and the wrist, the hand is pronated, and the fingers are flexed with the thumb across the palm. The leg is adducted, flexed at the hip and the knee, and the foot is kept in a plantar-flexed position with the sole turned inwards. The lesion causing spasticity is localized mainly in the corticospinal tract. Spasticity dominates in all reported surveys of cerebral palsy; spastic children constitute approximately two-thirds to three-quarters of all children with cerebral palsy.

CHANGING MUSCLE TONE

Infants in whom the muscle tone changes between being abnormally high and abnormally low are usually flaccid during their first few months. They lie in the frog-like position and are easily mistaken for infants with a disorder of the motor unit (*see* Chapter 6) unless the significance of normal or increased muscle reflexes is appreciated. Their motor development is severely delayed. Towards the end of the first year the tendency to change between abnormally high and abnormally low tone starts. When the infants are left alone, they are flaccid and may maintain the frog-like position; when they are disturbed in some way (e.g. examined or handled) they become tense and assume the same posture as described for spastic children. However, since they relax when left alone, and particularly during sleep, they do not develop contractures. The muscle reflexes are normal or moderately increased and clonus is seldom present. Babinski's sign may or may not be present. Characteristic of this type of cerebral palsy is the persistence of neonatal reflexes, sometimes throughout childhood. The tonic neck reflex (*Figure 12.1*) and the Moro reflex are particularly pronounced, but the sucking, rooting, and grasp reflexes may also persist. The lesion is usually caused by severe perinatal asphyxia, occasionally in combination with jaundice; its main localization is in the brain stem. As it often extends to the basal ganglia and the cerebellar connections, the syndrome of changing tone may be combined with choreoathetosis and/or ataxia. This

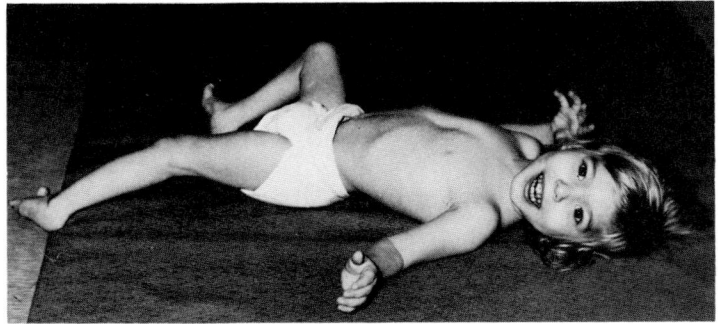

Figure 12.1. A 3½-year-old girl with a cerebral palsy syndrome dominated by changing muscle tone and persisting neonatal reflexes. Note the marked tonic neck reflex

syndrome, which in many other reports is called 'mixed forms of cerebral palsy', constitutes a severe disorder of motor function; the affected child is particularly difficult to train because of the persisting neonatal reflexes. As the child grows older, high muscle tone becomes increasingly dominant; the clinical picture in the adolescent usually shows no trace of abnormally low muscle tone. About 10–25 per cent of children with cerebral palsy have this syndrome.

CHOREOATHETOSIS

Children with choreoathetosis have a movement disorder characterized by disturbing involuntary movements and abnormal posture (*see* page 268). These patients are usually flaccid as small infants and may be misdiagnosed as having a disorder of the motor unit (*see* pages 160–161). The involuntary movements and abnormal posture usually develop during the second half-year. Neonatal reflexes often persist (*Figure 12.2*), and the syndrome of variable tone (*see above*) is often combined with choreoathetosis. Spasticity and ataxia may also be found. The motor handicap is often severe; the abnormal posture (*Figure 12.3*) impairs the normal use of the limbs, and the involuntary movements interrupt any intentional motion. Abnormal co-movements are disturbing; they are particularly common in the facial muscles (*Figure 12.4*). The condition may, however, be milder and confined to the tongue and facial muscles and/or one hand (*Figure 12.5*). Deafness is the nonmotor disorder that most often complicates choreoathetosis (*see* page 288). The main lesion is in the basal ganglia and is often caused by severe jaundice or severe asphyxia during the newborn period. Between 5 and 25 per cent of children with cerebral palsy show choreoathetosis; the figure depends to some extent on whether or not the syndrome of changing tone is distinguished as a separate entity.

ATAXIA

Ataxia is a disturbance of coordination (*see* page 256). Patients with this condition are usually flaccid during infancy and show retarded motor development. Towards the end of the first year, when they start to reach out for objects and may try to sit up, it becomes apparent that they lack balance. The abnormally low muscle tone persists throughout childhood. The children have intention tremor and lack precise

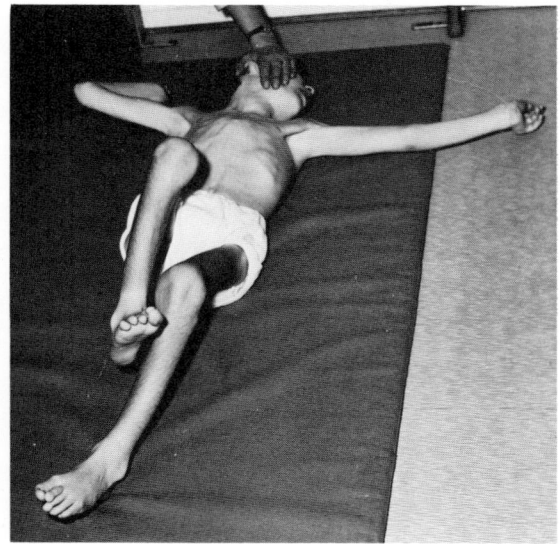

Figure 12.2. A tonic reflex in a 10-year-old boy with the syndrome of changing muscle tone and choreoathetosis

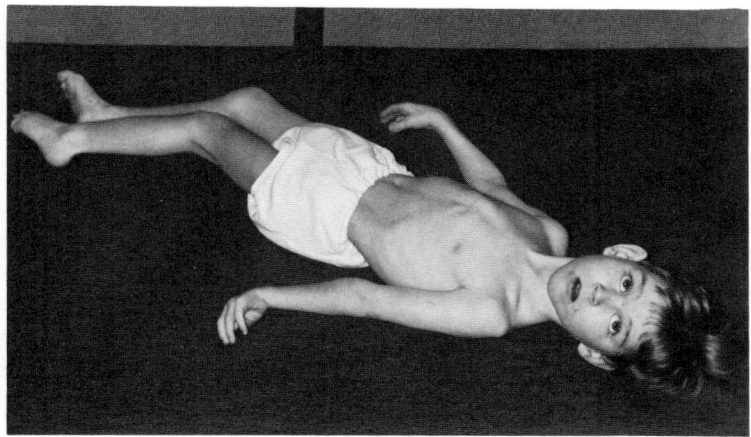

Figure 12.3. An 8-year-old boy with cerebral palsy dominated by choreoathetosis. Note the abnormal posture of the left hand

rapid movements. They learn to walk later than normal and remain clumsy and awkward. Some never learn to walk. They may crawl in a peculiar fashion, which is seen only in atactic children (but not in all of them), resting on their hands and knees and keeping their lower legs unsupported up in the air (*see Figure 10.1,* page 258). They have great difficulty in learning to ride a bicycle or to skate. Muscle reflexes are normal and neonatal reflexes disappear at a normal age, unless the picture is complicated by other types of motor dysfunction. The lesion is localized in the cerebellum and its connections. The reported incidence of ataxia varies between 1 and 15 per cent of children with cerebral palsy, but is usually around 10 per cent.

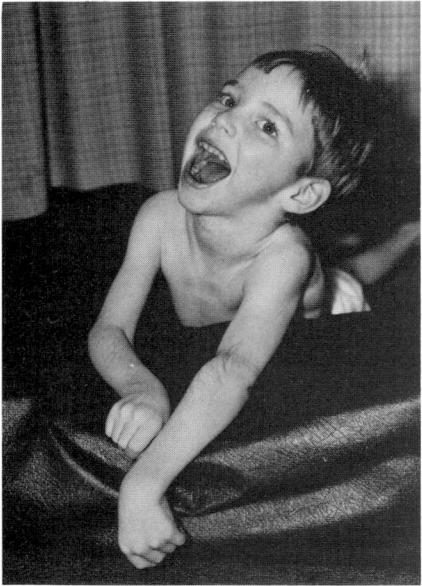

Figure 12.4. An 8-year-old boy with cerebral palsy dominated by choreoathetosis. Note the abnormal posture of the hands and the abnormal co-movements of the facial muscles, particularly the open mouth

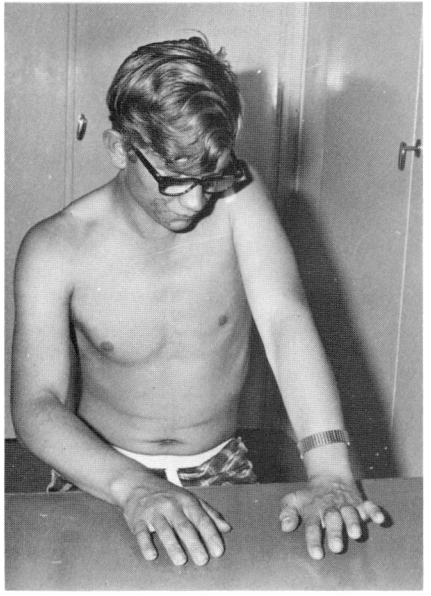

Figure 12.5. A 16-year-old boy with athetosis of the left hand

MIXED FORMS

Choreoathetosis combined with spasticity or with the syndrome of changing tone are the two most common mixed types of motor dysfunction, but all kinds of combinations may occur. Some authors include all patients with the syndrome of changing tone under the heading 'mixed forms', even when these patients have no other movement disorder. The lesion causing a mixed type of cerebral palsy is usually extensive.

The localization of the motor dysfunction

Spasticity may affect one limb only (*monoplegia* or *monoparesis*), an arm and leg on the same side (*hemiplegia* or *hemiparesis*), all four limbs and legs more than arms (*diplegia* or *diparesis*), or all four limbs and arms equal to or more than legs (*tetraplegia* or *tetraparesis*). Monoparesis and triparesis are rare constellations, whereas spastic hemiparesis and diparesis are the two dominating types of cerebral palsy.

HEMIPARESIS

Hemiparesis may be found in a young infant, several months of age, who either has a negative previous history or is known to have experienced an event such as convulsions or asphyxia during the perinatal period. A postnatal cause is found in about one-third to one-quarter of hemiparetic children. The cause may be meningitis, physical brain injury, or the condition called *acute infantile hemiplegia*.

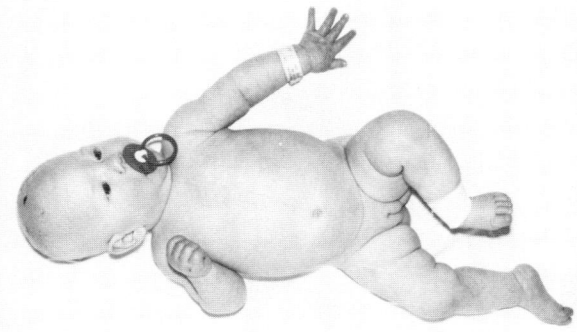

Figure 12.6. A 3½-month-old girl with a severe right-sided hemiparesis, almost hemiplegia. Note the way the girl holds her right hand fisted with the thumb across the palm. Her right leg is also inactive, but the asymmetry is more apparent in the upper than in the lower limbs

This condition occurs in previously healthy children, 6 months to 4 years old, who suddenly fall ill with a high temperature and convulsions; vomiting and diarrhoea often precede these symptoms. When the child regains consciousness after the convulsion, he is found to be hemiparetic. It is likely that the gastroenteritis produces a disturbance of water and electrolyte balance, which together with the high fever provokes and maintains the convulsions. Disturbed water and electrolyte balance with high fever may cause thrombophlebitis of the cortical veins with impaired circulation, and the effect of all these factors may be permanent brain damage. This can probably be prevented in many cases by cautious correction of the electrolyte disturbance, by lowering the temperature, and by rapid control of the seizures (*see* pages 94–95 and 109–111).

A hemiparesis is detectable in a child of 3–4 months of age by watching the child's hand function. At this age normal children start to open their hands and to use them for the active grasping of objects. *Figure 12.6* shows a 3½-month-old infant with a severe hemiparesis, almost hemiplegia; it also shows impaired function of the right leg, but the asymmetry of the hands is more obvious.

As a rule, hemiparetic children show fairly normal general motor development, and most of them learn to walk at a normal age. On examination it is particularly important to observe the movements of the arm when the child is walking or running. In mild cases nothing abnormal may be found in the movement of the child's leg, even when he is running, but the arm comes up slightly in front of the

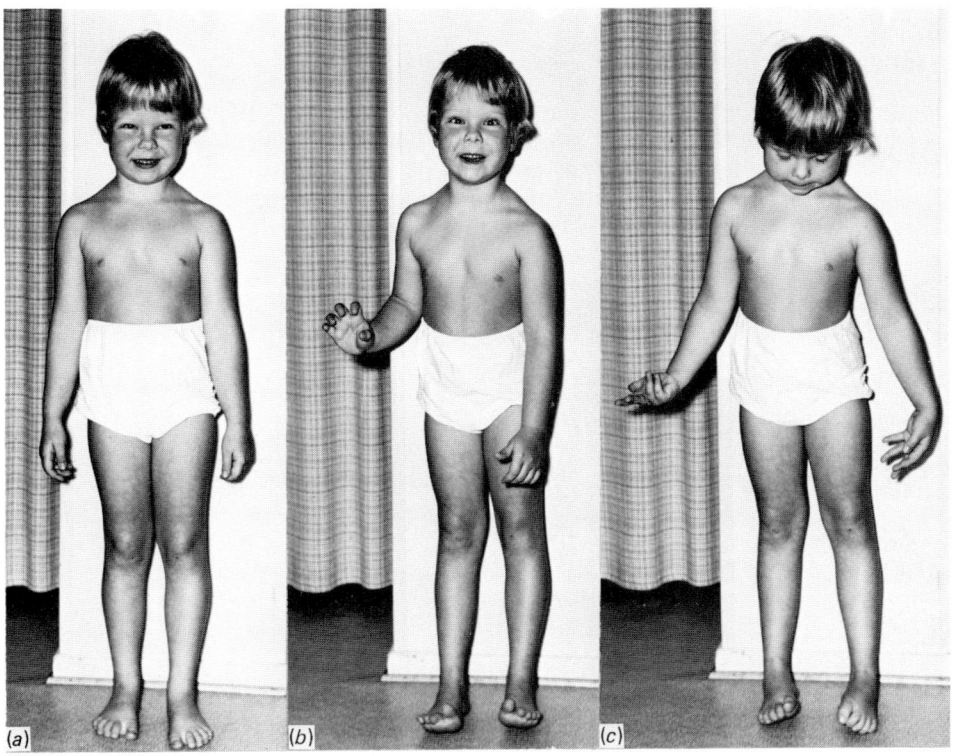

(a)   (b)   (c)

Figure 12.7. A 6-year-old girl with a right-sided hemiparesis. While she is standing nothing abnormal is apparent (*a*); abnormal co-movements of the right hand are seen when she walks on her heels (*b*) and on Fog's test (*c*)

child, with the shoulder adducted and the elbow bent, and takes no part in the normal swinging co-movements (*see Figure 2.36,* page 30). The increased tone is best found on examination of the arm; Grasset's sign (*see Figure 2.28,* page 24) is positive, and the child has trouble keeping both hands in front of him with elbows stretched and palms up (*see Figure 2.29,* page 25). When the child tries to walk on his heels or on the lateral edge of his feet (Fog's test), the arm and the hand on the affected side make characteristic co-movements (*Figure 12.7*). Increased tone and abnormal reflexes are also found in the leg. The growth of the whole side is

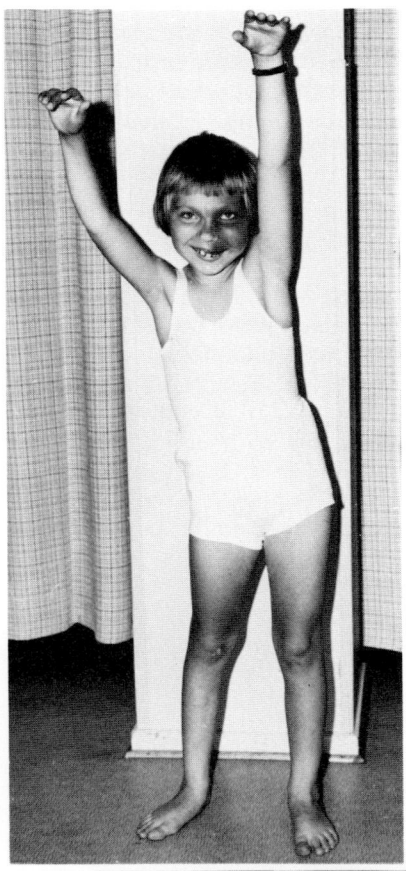

Figure 12.8. Underdeveloped extremities on the right side of a girl with Sturge–Weber syndrome (naevus flammeus on the left side of the face)

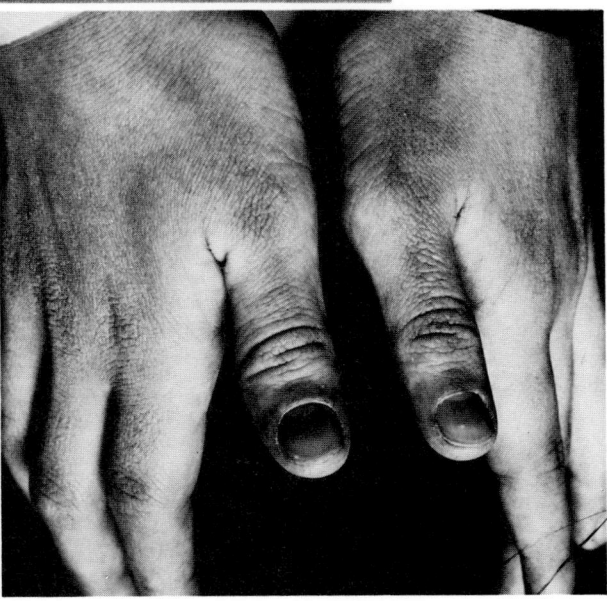

Figure 12.9. The hands of a 16-year-old girl with a slight hemiparesis. Note the difference in nail size between the thumbs

retarded (*Figure 12.8*); this can usually best be demonstrated by comparing hand and foot size on the two sides. The smallest demonstrable evidence of growth retardation of an upper limb is a difference in the size of finger-nails between the two hands (*Figure 12.9*). Impaired sensation may be found. Convulsions are common in hemiparesis.

SPASTIC DIPARESIS

This condition may be seen as a sequela after premature birth. It should be stressed that most infants born before term show entirely normal development, but *if* they show any abnormality, spastic diparesis is the type most commonly seen. Their motor development is retarded. Difficulties in sitting up are usually discovered during the second half-year. These infants have trouble sitting with their knees extended as they have a tendency to fall backwards. Forced bending of the hips produces bending of the back and causes the child to fall forwards. The best way for them to sit is usually in the 'tailor's position', when they can also support themselves with their hands (*Figure 12.10*). On attempting to stand, they stand on

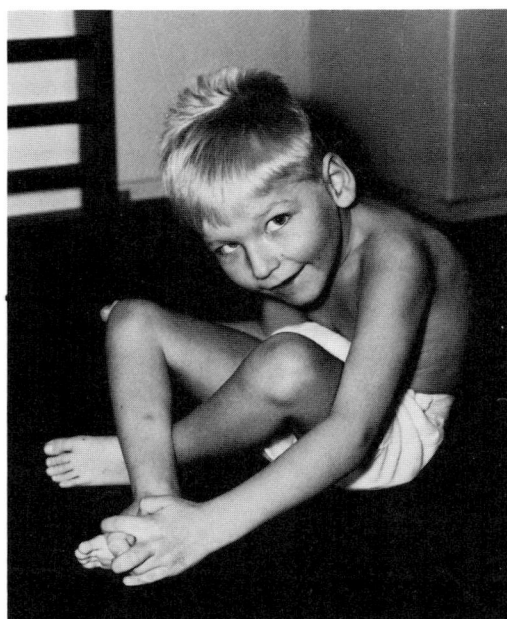

Figure 12.10. A 6-year-old boy with severe spastic diplegia and strabismus sitting in the tailor's position. Note the rounded back when the boy is sitting with his hips and knees flexed

their toes and keep their legs crossed (*Figure 12.11*). Only children with mild diparesis learn to walk at a normal age; most diparetic children either learn to walk only after physiotherapy or never learn to walk. The disturbed motor function of the hands can usually be demonstrated during the child's second year, as his control of small finger movements does not mature in the normal way (*see* pages 18 and 28). Strabismus is a particularly common finding in spastic diparesis (*Figure 12.12*).

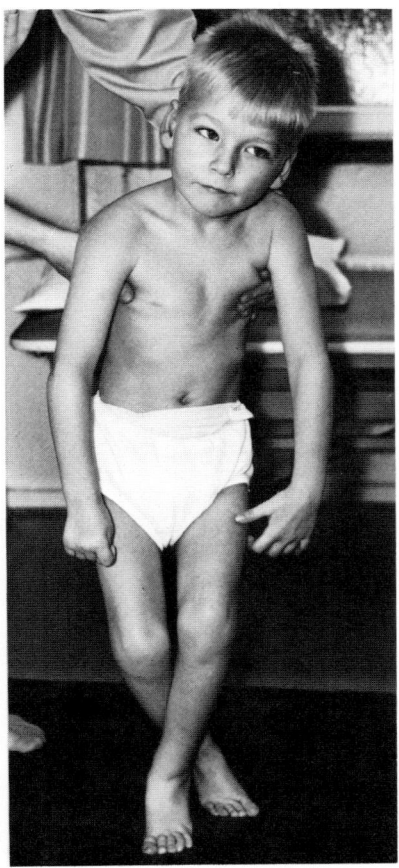

Figure 12.11. A 6-year-old boy with severe spastic diplegia, which is more pronounced on the right than on the left side. Note the typical position of the legs with the hips and knees flexed and the legs crossed; note also the clenched right hand with the thumb across the palm

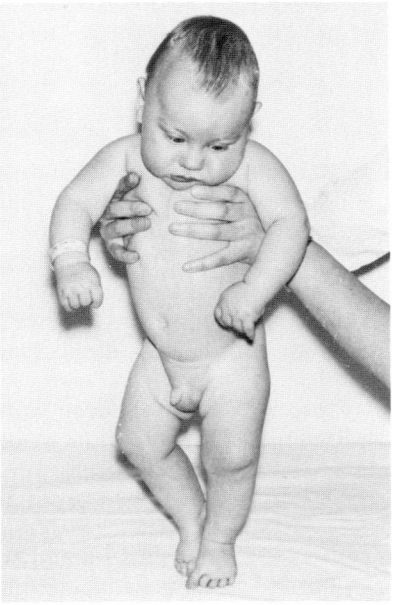

Figure 12.12. A 7-month-old boy with spastic diparesis. Note his tendency to stand on his toes, to cross his legs, and to keep his hands overpronated. This boy was born after 32 weeks of gestation

TETRAPARESIS

In tetraparesis (*Figure 12.13*) all four limbs are affected, the arms at least as seriously as the legs. These children have an extensive brain lesion, usually due to severe perinatal asphyxia or a severe postnatal physical brain injury. Many are mentally retarded; convulsions are common.

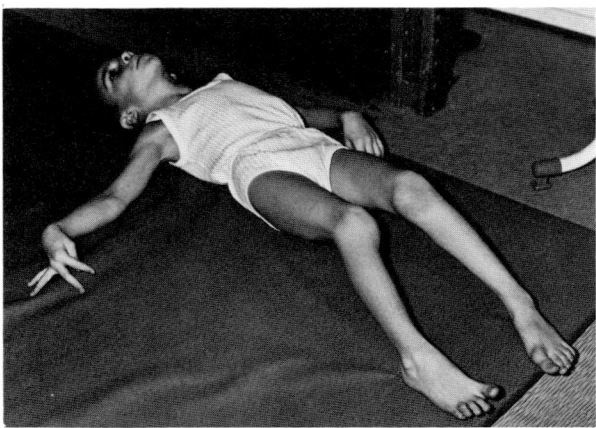

Figure 12.13. A 7-year-old boy with spastic tetraparesis. Note the flexion contractures of the hips and knees and the upturning toe on the right foot

NONSPASTIC DISORDERS

The nonspastic disorders can be divided into unilateral and bilateral cases, according to their localization. A bilateral distribution is much more common than a unilateral one, although the two sides are usually not affected to the same degree.

Nonmotor dysfunction complicating cerebral palsy

IMPAIRED MENTAL DEVELOPMENT

This is found in at least half of the patients with cerebral palsy. Mental retardation of variable degree is found in about one-third of children with cerebral palsy and particularly in the groups spastic tetraparesis, severe spastic diparesis, and ataxia. Mental development must always be assessed with great caution in young children with retarded motor development, as their general ability may be much better than is revealed by their movements. The motor handicap must always be well understood and trained to the child's full potential before his intellectual development is evaluated.

Other types of impaired mental development may also be seen in children with cerebral palsy. Some of them demonstrate the syndrome of short attention span, lack of concentration, restlessness, and unpredictable behaviour. This syndrome may be combined with mental retardation or occur in a child with normal intellectual development.

Extreme slowness of movements and thinking, often together with immature behaviour, may be found in retarded or intellectually normal patients with cerebral palsy. This defect may constitute a severe problem for the adult patient in his adjustment to work.

Children with a handicap from an early age are at risk of becoming overprotected and spoilt. It is so much easier to help the handicapped child for whom a true compassion is felt than to teach him to do things for himself. In this way the child's own urge to become independent may be lost, and his handicap becomes more severe than corresponds to his neurological deficit.

In mild cases of cerebral palsy, particularly mild ataxia, there is a risk that the organic cause of the child's difficulties will be overlooked and he will be considered a slow, clumsy, awkward child who cannot behave at the table, has trouble learning to draw and write, and cannot keep up with his peers in games. Blame and reproaches may cause the child to develop a neurosis which, when added to the clinical picture, may further impair the child's ability to function.

CONVULSIONS

Convulsions complicate the clinical picture, particularly in tetraparetic and hemiparetic children. An electroencephalogram (EEG) must be performed in these conditions; a hemiparetic child with an EEG showing distinct epileptic potentials may need to be started on antiepileptic treatment even before clinical convulsions have occurred. The management of convulsions is discussed in Chapter 4.

GROWTH RETARDATION

Retarded growth is seen in all kinds of movement disorders, since normal muscle activity is an important stimulus to skeletal growth. The greatest practical significance of growth retardation is demonstrated in hemiparesis; the unequal hand, foot, and nail size serves as an important diagnostic sign; an unequal length of the legs must be corrected in order to avoid secondary scoliosis.

IMPAIRED SENSATION

Impaired sensation is most commonly found in cases of hemiparesis, and then more often on the hand than on the foot. Disturbances of sensation are usually vague and difficult to demonstate; they are best revealed as impaired two-point discrimination and/or impaired stereognosis. The difficulties of training motor function increase if sensation is disturbed. The development of an abnormal body image is particularly common in children who show disturbances of both motor function and sensation.

EYE SIGNS

Eye signs are found in at least one-quarter of children with cerebral palsy. The most common finding is convergent strabismus, which is seen particularly in children with spastic diparesis. Refractive errors are found more often in children with cerebral palsy than in healthy children. Cataracts are seen, particularly in children who have had a stormy perinatal period with asphyxia. Scars after choreoretinitis are seen in children who have had a fetal infection. Optic atrophy is not a feature of cerebral palsy caused by perinatal complications.

IMPAIRED HEARING

Impaired hearing is found in about 5–10 per cent of all children with cerebral palsy. As a rule the hearing defect is of the neurogenic type, affecting particularly the perception of high tones, thus seriously impairing the child's ability to understand words. A hearing defect is found most commonly in children with choreoathetosis, and occasionally in the syndrome of changing muscle tone.

SPEECH DIFFICULTIES

Speech difficulties may be due to a moderate or severe hearing defect or to mental retardation. In choreoathetosis, in particular, the involuntary movements may also affect lip and tongue muscles and severely disturb the child's control of these muscles; excessive and persistent drooling is often found in this type of speech difficulty. Poor control of tongue and lip muscles is rarely seen as the only manifestation of cerebral palsy. Aphasia may complicate the picture in patients with a late-appearing spastic weakness of the dominant side and occasionally in patients with other types of cerebral palsy. A combination of two or more of these factors may occur. It is therefore not surprising that a large proportion of children with cerebral palsy show speech difficulties.

Differential diagnosis

Certain clinical situations must alert the physician to the possibility that the child's difficulties may not be caused by cerebral palsy. Only symptomatic treatment can be given in cerebral palsy; conditions for which a causal therapy is available must therefore not be overlooked. Although no treatment is yet known in most of the degenerative diseases of the central nervous system, a correct diagnosis in such cases is of practical importance to the family, as most of these diseases are hereditary, whereas inheritance is rarely seen in cerebral palsy. The family can thus be counselled on the risk of further children developing the same symptoms.

Positive family history

A positive family history is always a warning sign. True cerebral palsy may presumably occur as an autosomal recessive trait, particularly a mixed type of ataxia and mild spastic diparesis. The same mother may have more than one prematurely born child who develops cerebral palsy or other obstetric complications at more than one delivery. However, the occurrence of neurological signs in sibs should always alert the physician to the possibility that they may be caused by a degenerative disease (see Chapter 13) and not cerebral palsy.

No history implying a cause of cerebral palsy

The absence of a history of acute brain injury does not exclude cerebral palsy. The examination to exclude other diagnostic possibilities must, however, be more thorough than when an obvious cause is known from the history. In this connection it must be stressed that a likely cause of cerebral palsy does not prove that the child has this condition. Also, a child who has had a stormy neonatal period may later develop a progressive degenerative disease or a brain tumour, for example.

Progressive symptoms

Progressive symptoms, although compatible with a diagnosis of cerebral palsy, should cause this diagnosis to be questioned. Evidence of an extending process, i.e. the occurrence of new neurological symptoms and signs, excludes cerebral palsy and points to a growing lesion or a degenerative disease; the investigation of such a case must include computerized tomography of the skull (*see* pages 57 and 60–69).

Optic atrophy

Optic atrophy, which is a common finding in several degenerative lesions (*see* pages 294 and 301–305), is rarely seen in cerebral palsy, unless its cause includes a period of increased intracranial pressure.

Hemiparesis

The possibility that a hemiparesis may be caused by a neurosurgically accessible lesion, such as a subdural haematoma, a subdural hygroma, or a porencephalic cyst under pressure, must be kept in mind and the indications for computerized tomography of the skull kept wide.

Ataxia

Although ataxia is consistent with a diagnosis of cerebral palsy, it occurs also in many other conditions, and other possibilities must be kept in mind. Only cerebellar ataxia is seen in cerebral palsy; if sensory ataxia is present, a degenerative disease of the spinal cord and/or the peripheral nerves (*see* pages 261 and 177–179) is the likely explanation. Cerebellar ataxia is also seen in several of the progressive degenerative disorders described in Chapter 13. It may be even more important to remember that the cerebellar astrocytomas of childhood (*see* page 365) grow slowly and may for years produce a very slowly increasing cerebellar ataxia as the only finding, before signs of increased intracranial pressure eventually appear.

Paraplegia

The term paraplegia has deliberately been omitted in the description of the cerebral palsy syndromes. By spastic paraplegia is meant spasticity and weakness of the legs only, when even a careful examination reveals no signs of impaired function of the arms and hands. Although pure paraplegia may be caused by a brain lesion and thus be considered a cerebral palsy syndrome, this is rarely the case. In adults, pure paraplegia is as a rule caused by a lesion of the spinal cord, and the same is true in childhood. If careful neurological examination of a child reveals symptoms and signs from the legs only, a lesion of the spinal cord must be considered and excluded before a diagnosis of cerebral palsy is accepted.

Special examinations

Special examinations are desirable in children with suspected or proven cerebral palsy. All children with cerebral palsy must have a thorough eye examination. Vision and hearing should be tested as early as possible, as defects of these senses greatly influence the training and education of the child. Examination of the cerebrospinal fluid must be performed at least once in all children with findings suggesting cerebral palsy. If this diagnosis is correct, the cerebrospinal fluid is found to be normal. An increased spinal fluid protein must always prompt further investigation, as it is not seen in cerebral palsy but may occur in cases of intracranial tumour, subdural hygroma, and progressive degenerative diseases; a normal finding does not, however, exclude such conditions.

An EEG is desirable, particularly in patients with hemiparesis or tetraparesis because of the high risk of convulsions in these conditions.

Psychological testing of children with cerebral palsy is generally of great help in order to advise the best way to teach them. Their intellectual ability is often underestimated by school authorities and overestimated by the doctor and the physiotherapist who have for a long time cared for the patient; objective psychological testing is therefore often necessary. It must not be performed until the child's motor handicap has been well trained, and when it is done due consideration must be given to this handicap. Also, children with normal intellectual function may have specific learning difficulties; correctly individualized teaching gives the child a fair chance of the best possible development.

Special metabolic studies should be performed according to the same principles as discussed for mental retardation (*see* pages 151–152).

X-ray of the spine is important in patients who have a pure paraplegia or monoplegia of one leg. The possibility of a spinal cause for these conditions is often overlooked. Electromyography may reveal denervation of leg muscles and thus prove the involvement of peripheral motor neurones (anterior horn cells, anterior roots, peripheral nerves) and also map out the level and distribution of the abnormality. A myelogram may be desirable in selected cases.

The indications for ultrasound examination and computerized tomography of the skull should be kept wide, as these methods are of great help in excluding other, possibly treatable, conditions that may be the cause of the child's symptoms and signs. The clinical situations in which the diagnosis of cerebral palsy (i.e. a condition accessible to symptomatic but not causal therapy) must particularly be questioned are reviewed in the previous section (*see* pages 288–289).

Treatment

The fact that no causal therapy is available in cerebral palsy must not lead to therapeutic nihilism, as intense and well-planned symptomatic therapy can greatly improve the condition of the child.

Habilitation

The basis of treatment is the training of disturbed function, and in this area the physiotherapist has the main role. Physiotherapy must start as soon as impaired motor function is diagnosed. In a young infant it involves placing the patient in such positions that contractures and an abnormal pattern of movements are prevented as much as possible; the older infant can be tempted to perform certain movements, and the older child can be given verbal instructions. Throughout childhood, and particularly in the young age-group, most of the treatment is given with the help of the parents. Ideally, the physiotherapist treats the child several times a month and also checks the daily programme performed by the parents. The physiotherapist is part of a habilitation team which consists of specialists such as physicians, psychologist, social worker, speech therapist, and specialized teacher. Every member of the team is an expert in his area of habilitation; the parents are experts on their own child and are the most important members of the team. When the child is a couple of years old, it becomes vital for him to have contact with other children, preferably as a member of a small group of healthy children. It is practically always possible to arrange the life-style of a child with cerebral palsy in such a way that he grows up in his own family, and receives his training from the habilitation team on an outpatient basis and his education through day nursery, playschool, or school with special arrangements for him, possibly including a personal assistant. Many children with cerebral palsy benefit greatly from short periods of institutionalized care. These periods consists of a few weeks of intense training and stimulation of the child once or twice a year or every second year; the arrangement also gives the family a rest from the continuous responsibility. In this way, institutions for physically handicapped children can offer them and their families great help, while retaining integration and family care as the basic principles.

Whenever possible, physiotherapy should continue throughout childhood and adolescence. It can never harm the patient. However, the shortage of physiotherapists enforces a reduction of the time spent with a patient whose general and motor development obviously improves little in spite of intense and long-term treatment.

Orthopaedic surgery

An orthopaedic surgeon must work in collaboration with the habilitation team. Different types of special shoes, calipers, and technical aids may be of help to the child; they should be chosen and used under the guidance of the physiotherapist. One aim of physiotherapy is to prevent contractures, but this is not possible in all patients, some of whom may develop fixed contractures in spite of early and intense treatment. Orthopaedic operations may then be of great benefit to the patient. In general it can be said that intense physiotherapy must precede and follow any operation. Surgical procedures are of value only in patients with continuous hypertonus, i.e. spasticity; patients with other types of cerebral palsy, particularly those with the syndrome of changing tone, may deteriorate after operation. It is usually easier to correct impaired function of the legs than of the arms. Operations on the legs can often be performed during preschool and early school years, whereas operations on arms and hands are preferably delayed until the second decade.

Adduction of the hips can be corrected by exeresis of the obturator nerve or by tenotomy of the adductor tendon. Extension of the tendons of the medial hamstring muscles can also diminish the adduction. Transposition and extension of other tendons and osteotomy may be of value in correcting internal rotation and flexion contracture of the hip. The surgical treatment of hip adduction can be started when the child is around 3 years of age; other operations are usually performed at a later age.

Flexion contraction of the knee can be treated by transposition of the tendons of the knee flexors to the femur condyles. This operation carries a certain risk of producing overstretching of the knee and instability of the trunk. An equinus position of the foot can be treated by extension of the gastrocnemius, by detachment of the gastrocnemius heads from the femur condyles, or by lengthening the Achilles tendon. A valgus position of the foot can be corrected by arthrodesis.

Surgical treatment should start with the proximal joints, as correction of the hip may also have a beneficial influence on the foot. If the child has bilateral difficulties, the same procedure should be performed on both sides within a short space of time, as the child cannot utilize improved function on one side only. Different types of operations should be separated by a period of intense physiotherapy, and the child must be re-evaluated before a new procedure is planned. Many other surgical methods are available. The best results are obtained when there is good collaboration between the orthopaedic surgeon and all members of the habilitation team; each child is evaluated individually, and the orthopaedic surgeon uses the methods in which he is most experienced.

In hemiparetic children it is important to try to correct a difference in the length of the legs. Growth-stimulating operations can be performed on the poor leg at any age during childhood. An attempt to retard the growth of the good leg can be made during the preadolescent growth spurt.

The transplantation of tendons in the arm may also be of value to correct an abnormal position. However, the influence of this procedure on the fine motor function of the hand and fingers is small.

Drug therapy

Effective antiepileptic drug therapy is important in all children with cerebral palsy and convulsions (*see* page 287). Attempts to treat the increased muscle tone and involuntary movements with various tranquillizers have on the whole been disappointing. If the child's main symptom is rigidity a trial with levodopa is justified and may be successful. Other patients with increased muscle tone and involuntary movements may, though rarely, benefit from diazepam or baclofen.

Special training and treatment

Defects of eyesight and hearing and speech difficulties require the help of the appropriate specialists and therapists, who should then be included in the habilitation team. Stereotactic neurosurgical operations may help children with cerebral palsy, particularly if the clinical picture is dominated by choreoathetosis. The value of these operations is debated, as the results are variable; a few well-selected patients may benefit greatly from such operations.

Education

The child with cerebral palsy must be taught according to his intellectual level, whenever possible in an ordinary school and together with children without a motor handicap. He must be provided with special help and technical aids. For some handicapped adolescents the stress of competing with nonhandicapped class-mates may become too great; special classes for physically handicapped children should therefore be available and the option of transferring to a boarding-school should exist, particularly for teenagers. The general rule is integration of handicapped and nonhandicapped children; this is advantageous for both groups and avoids the early separation of a handicapped child from his family and normal surroundings.

Parental cooperation

An honest realistic attitude towards the parents and their membership on an equal level in the habilitation team around the child are necessary conditions for helping the child and his family to adjust to his handicap. The risk of overprotecting the severely handicapped child and of neglecting the organic cause in the mildly affected child must be kept in mind. The whole family – not only the child – needs continuous support and must feel that no aspect of the child's difficulties is neglected.

Prognosis

In Scandinavia and Britain the incidence of persons with full working capacity (i.e. as adults) among patients registered as cases of cerebral palsy is estimated to be about 20–25 per cent; partial working capacity is found in roughly the same proportion. About 30–50 per cent of all patients diagnosed as cases of cerebral palsy need to be cared for in institutions for the mentally retarded.

The prognosis is best in mild cases of uncomplicated hemiparesis and diparesis. The capacity for work decreases with increasing motor difficulties. Complications such as mental retardation, epilepsy, and defects of hearing and vision play an important part, however, and are perhaps even more important than the motor handicap in limiting the patient's working capacity.

References

CHRISTENSEN, E. and MELCHIOR, J. C. (1967) Cerebral palsy. A clinical and neuropathological study. Clinics in Developmental Medicine No. 25. London: Heinemann

DALE, A. and STANLEY, F. J. (1980) An epidemiological study of cerebral palsy in Western Australia, 1956–1975. II: Spastic cerebral palsy and perinatal factors. *Developmental Medicine and Child Neurology,* **22,** 13–25

GOUTIERES, F., CHALLAMEL, M.-J., AICARDI, J. and GILLY, R. (1972) Les hémiplégies congénitales. *Archives Franchaises Pédiatrie,* **29,** 839–851

GUSTAVSSON, K.-H., HAGBERG, B. and SANNER, G. (1969) Identical syndromes of cerebral palsy in the same family. *Acta Paediatrica Scandinavica,* **58,** 330–340

HAGBERG, B., HAGBERG, G. and OLOW, I. (1975) The changing panorama of cerebral palsy in Sweden 1954–1970, I. *Acta Paediatrica Scandinavica,* **64,** 187–192

HAGBERG, B., HAGBERG G. and OLOW, I. (1975) The changing panorama of cerebral palsy in Sweden 1954–1970, II. *Acta Paediatrica Scandinavica,* **64,** 193–200

HAGBERG, B., HAGBERG, G. and OLOW, I. (1976) The changing panorama of cerebral palsy in Sweden 1954–1970, III. *Acta Paediatrica Scandinavica,* **65,** 403–408

HAGBERG, B., SANNER, G. and STEEN, M. (1972) The disequilibrium syndrome in cerebral palsy. *Acta Paediatrica Scandinavica,* suppl. 226

KYLLERMAN, M. (1981) Dyskinetic cerebral palsy. Academical Dissertation, Medical Faculty, Göteborg, Sweden

LADEMANN, A. (1978) Postneonatally acquired cerebral palsy. *Acta Neurologica Scandinavica,* suppl. 65

LAGERGREN, J. (1981) Children with motor handicaps. Epidemiological, medical and socio-paediatric aspects of motor handicapped children in a Swedish county. *Acta Paediatrica Scandinavica,* suppl. 289

ROBINSON, R. O. (1973) The frequency of other handicaps in children with cerebral palsy. *Developmental Medicine and Child Neurology,* **15,** 305–312

STANLEY, F. J. (1979) An epidemiological study of cerebral palsy in Western Australia, 1956–1975. *Developmental Medicine and Child Neurology,* **21,** 701–713

13

Diseases characterized by progressive neurological and mental symptoms and signs

The conditions described in this chapter are characterized by progressive neurological and mental symptoms and signs. They are mainly hereditary and degenerative with a proven or postulated metabolic basis. Diseases which may at some time during their course show progressive symptoms are also discussed in Chapter 4 if the dominant symptoms are convulsions; in Chapter 5 if mental retardation dominates the clinical picture; in Chapter 6 if weakness is the main symptom; in Chapter 10 if ataxia prevails; in Chapter 11 if the chief complaint is involuntary movements; in Chapter 15 if a malformation exists; in Chapter 16 if the symptoms are caused by infection; and in Chapter 17 if a tumour is the known cause of the symptoms.

In many cases it may be difficult to differentiate between a stationary and a progressive disorder, particularly if the progression is slow. Also, the child's own development continues during a disease; in a case of stationary mental retardation the development is abnormally slow but constant, whereas in a progressive condition this velocity subsides with time although it may be a considerable time before this is apparent. A very severe stationary condition may effectively block any development. A delay in psychomotor development becomes easier to observe and demonstrate with increasing age of the child. All these considerations must be taken into account by the physician when trying to decide whether a condition is stationary or progressive.

The conditions described in this chapter are not reviewed in a strictly logical order, based on their biochemical mechanism, as this is not known for several of them. The order is therefore arbitrary, and based on clinical findings as far as possible. The conditions are divided into groups as follows:

1. Those in which early symptoms are dominated by evidence of a grey matter disease (i.e. mental deterioration, convulsions, or macular abnormalities).
2. Those in which early symptoms are dominated by evidence of a white matter disease (i.e. spasticity, ataxia, optic atrophy, and possibly involvement of the peripheral nervous system).
3. Those which cannot be classified.

It must be stressed that *no disease affects strictly either the grey or the white matter*; only in the early phase of the disease is one system affected more than the other. Thus, all grey matter diseases eventually also produce symptoms and signs from the white matter and vice versa.

Conditions with early main manifestations caused by grey matter dysfunction

G$_{M2}$-gangliosidosis

This biochemical defect causes the normal G$_{M2}$-ganglioside to be stored in an abnormally large amount, mainly in the nervous tissue, causing a ballooned appearance of the ganglion cells (*Figure 13.1*). This abnormal storage is due to the

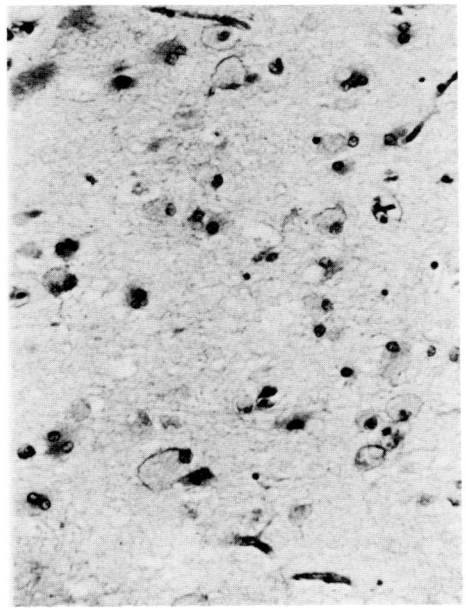

Figure 13.1. A section from the frontal lobe cortex in a case of Tay–Sachs disease. Many nerve cells have disappeared. The remaining nerve cells have a distinct border and are ballooned with the nucleus placed excentrically. Note also the increased number of glia cells with a small, round dark nucleus

low activity of an enzyme, hexosaminidase, which exists in three different forms, A, B and S. In *Tay–Sachs disease* there is a lack of hexosaminidase A and S, and in *Sandhoff's disease* of hexosaminidase A and B. Both conditions are inherited as autosomal recessive traits and have a similar clinical picture. The infants appear healthy at birth; after several weeks they start to become irritable and particularly sensitive to sound, showing an exaggerated startle response to any sound, whereas they seem increasingly uninterested in visual stimuli. Psychomotor development stagnates at around 4–6 months of age, the infants cease to give visual contact and to fix and follow with their eyes, which show large wandering movements, indicating that the child is becoming blind. At this time the typical cherry-red spot is usually seen. The ganglion cells of the retina are involved in the same process as those of the brain; as the retinal ganglion cells are concentrated in the macula, its normal reddish colour is lost and it appears grey. However, the fovea contains no ganglion cells, and this spot therefore has a bright red colour which contrasts with the otherwise greyish macula.

The head often grows too rapidly, due to the abnormal storage of material in the brain which causes an increase in the brain substance. Seizures, often of the myoclonic type, start as a rule at around 6 months of age. The EEG findings are grossly abnormal, often of the type called hypsarrhythmia (*see* page 92). The child's condition deteriorates and he loses all contact with his surroundings. Death usually occurs during the second year, but survival until 4 years of age is known. Only the nervous system is involved in Tay–Sachs disease, whereas children with Sandhoff's disease also show moderate hepatosplenomegaly. At least 80 per cent of children with Tay–Sachs disease are of Jewish, mainly eastern Europe, ancestry.

The lack of enzymes can be demonstrated in tears, blood serum, white blood cells, and cultured fibroblasts. Healthy gene-carriers can also be identified, as their enzyme level is roughly half-way between that of sick infants and of healthy non-gene-carriers. The amniotic fluid can be analysed also, providing a useful method for prenatal diagnosis.

During the last decade the issue has been confused by reports about the lack of hexosaminidase in a great variety of neurological conditions. Thus, low activity has been described in some patients with late-infantile, juvenile, or adult onset of progressive encephalopathies, atypical spinocerebellar ataxia, Friedreich's ataxia, progressive spinal muscular atrophy, and also in a few adults with no neurological symptoms or signs. The interpretation of these findings is unclear.

Generalized gangliosidosis (synonyms: generalized G_{M1}-gangliosidosis or type 1 G_{M1}-gangliosidosis)

This condition is inherited as an autosomal recessive trait. At birth the infants already show coarse facial features, frontal bossing, depressed nasal bridge, and oedema of the face and extremities. The infants fail to thrive and their psychomotor development is severely retarded from the beginning. Hepatosplenomegaly is the rule. A cherry-red spot may be seen in the fundi, but is not an obligate finding. Seizures usually start at around 6 months of age; death during the second year is the rule. These children also have features similar to those with the Hurler syndrome (*see* page 135) with involvement of the bones, causing kyphoscoliosis, short broad hands, and flexion contractures of the elbows and knees.

The brain, bones, liver, and spleen show an abnormal storage of G_{M1}-ganglioside and mucopolysaccharide, possibly also an oligosaccharide containing mannose. The enzyme beta-galactosidase is missing. Methods are available for prenatal diagnosis. No effective treatment exists.

Variants have also been described with later onset, slower progression, and less involvement of skeletal structures.

Cerebral G_{M1}-gangliosidosis or type 2 G_{M1}-gangliosidosis

Children with this disorder usually appear healthy and develop normally up to the age of 6–14 months, when development stagnates and eventually deteriorates. Seizures and an abnormal sensitivity to sound are common. The children usually show no non-neurological symptoms or signs. The neurones of the brain are filled with lipids; in the lamina propria of a rectal biopsy, foam cells are found filled with PAS-positive material. Beta-galactosidase is decreased in brain, leucocytes, and cultured fibroblasts.

Variants of this disorder are known with later onset and slower progression. No effective therapy is available.

Gaucher's disease

This disorder is characterized by an abnormal accumulation of glucocerebrosides in involved tissues due to a lack of the enzyme glycosylceramide beta-glucosidase. Another characteristic feature is the presence in the bone marrow of peculiar large cells with a foamy cytoplasm, the so-called Gaucher cells.

In the *infantile* form of Gaucher's disease neurological symptoms dominate the clinical picture. The affected infant appears normal for the first few months. From 4–6 months of age development stagnates and the infant loses interest in his surroundings. He keeps his head thrown backwards and becomes stiff with increased muscle reflexes. A characteristic feature is a change in the voice, which becomes hoarse and crowing – usually much hoarser than in the benign condition laryngomalacia, for which it may be mistaken. Swallowing difficulties are common. Moderate hepatosplenomegaly is the rule. Anaemia, leucopenia, and thrombocytopenia may be present. The disease is progressive with death occurring during the first or second year. No therapy is available.

In the *juvenile* form hepatosplenomegaly and pancytopenia are the early dominating symptoms. If neurological symptoms occur, they usually start 6 months to 2 years after the onset of the general symptoms, and are milder but otherwise similar to those described for the infantile type. A greatly enlarged spleen may occasionally necessitate splenectomy. From a neurological point of view this is undesirable, as neurological symptoms and signs may progress more rapidly after splenectomy.

Niemann–Pick disease

This disorder is characterized by the abnormal storage of sphingomyelin in affected tissue, due to a deficiency of the enzyme sphingomyelinase. Several variants of the disorder exist, including at least one that does not involve the nervous system. The most common of the variants has its onset in early infancy with hepatosplenomegaly, jaundice, and a haemorrhagic diathesis. Psychomotor development stagnates and deteriorates. A cherry-red spot in the fundi is a common finding. Gaucher cells (*see above*) are found in the bone marrow. An increased incidence of vacuolized lymphocytes (*see* page 299 and *Figure 13.3*) is a common finding on a blood smear. Symptoms are progressive and death usually occurs during the first 2 years.

Rarer variants of this disorder show a later onset and slower progression; non-neurological symptoms and signs may dominate the clinical picture.

Some of the conditions described above, particularly generalized gangliosidosis, show clinical and metabolic features of abnormal lipid storage and mucopolysaccharidosis. At least four other types of *mucolipidosis* have been identified, characterized by physical features similar to those seen in mucopolysaccharidosis (*see* pages 135–137) and progressive mental and neurological symptoms and signs due to abnormal lipid storage in the central nervous system. In the mucolipidoses a number of hydrolytic enzymes appear displaced and are found extracellularly instead of in the lysosomes; in this way enzyme and substrate do not meet, resulting in the abnormal storage of unmetabolized products.

Wolman's disease

Under the heading generalized xanthomatosis with calcified adrenals, or Wolman's disease, a condition has been reported in which the clinical symptoms and signs and the clinical course are indistinguishable from those found in the acute form of Niemann–Pick disease. Calcification of the adrenals, which in Wolman's disease may be demonstrated radiologically, is not seen in Niemann–Pick disease. In most reported cases of Wolman's disease the diagnosis has been established on biochemical investigation of liver and brain tissue obtained at autopsy. The typical finding is an abnormal accumulation of cholesterol and triglycerides; the enzymatic defect (possibly multiple defects) is not known.

Neuronal ceroid lipofuscinosis

Most of the conditions included under this heading were previously termed late-infantile, juvenile, and adult amaurotic idiocy. They are all progressive disorders, characterized by the accumulation of lipopigments, consisting of ceroid and lipofuscin in the central nervous system, retina, and possibly other tissues. This pigment is the same as that which accumulates in ageing neurones. The localization of the abnormal pigment explains why the main symptoms are visual and cerebral. An abnormal peroxidation of fatty acids seems to be an important feature but details of this metabolic defect are not known. All types of neuronal ceroid lipofuscinosis are inherited as an autosomal recessive trait.

INFANTILE NEURONAL CEROID LIPOFUSCINOSIS (SANTAVOURI–HALTIA, FINNISH TYPE)

This disease, apparently amassed in families of Finnish origin, produces its first symptoms at the end of the first or the beginning of the second year of life. The previously normal development stagnates, the child becomes less interested in his surroundings, and is particularly uninterested in visual stimuli. Fits may start. At this stage abnormal findings may be difficult to detect, the retina may show some signs of degeneration, and motor development may be slightly delayed. Symptoms progress steadily, the patient becomes blind, spasticity with contractures develops, feeding difficulties may appear as a sign of bulbar involvement, and fits continue and may be hard to control. The patient eventually loses all contact with his surroundings and as a rule dies during the first decade, usually from a complicating respiratory tract infection. The diagnosis is difficult to establish on clinical grounds alone. The ceroid lipofuscin is also stored in the neurones of the intestinal tract and can be demonstrated on a rectal biopsy or in the appendix.

LATE-INFANTILE NEURONAL CEROID LIPOFUSCINOSIS (BIELSCHOWSKY–JANSKY)

This syndrome usually has its onset during the second year of life. The symptoms consist of ataxia and loss of interest in visual stimuli. Mental stagnation is soon apparent and all symptoms progress rapidly; the child may live for some years in a vegetative state without contact with his surroundings.

JUVENILE NEURONAL CEROID LIPOFUSCINOSIS (BATTEN–SPIELMEYER–VOGT–SJÖGREN)

This disorder usually has its onset at around 5 years of age, when impaired and deteriorating vision is detected. The eye findings, i.e. dystrophy of the macular region and pigment degeneration of the retina (see Figure 13.2, between pp. 100–101), are as a rule nonspecific. Bilateral optic atrophy appears later; a cherry-red spot is not seen. The eye abnormalities are progressive, and the child eventually becomes blind.

Neurological and mental symptoms may rarely precede the visual symptoms; they usually appear within 2 years after the detection of impaired vision. The two most common neurological symptoms are grand mal seizures and ataxia; spasticity, rigidity and other neurological symptoms may eventually appear. The mental deterioration is first apparent as irritability and difficulties at school. All symptoms are progressive. The patients usually have to be transferred from an ordinary school to a school for mentally retarded blind children, and from there to an institution. Their general condition deteriorates, and as a rule they die during their second decade. Treatment with vitamin E and selenium seems to have some beneficial effect, as this therapy is known to have stopped or at least delayed further progress in a few cases. The influence of this therapy on already established symptoms and signs is insignificant. Seizures are treated in the same way as fits of other origin.

The constellation of progressive ophthalmological, neurological, and mental symptoms and signs usually makes it possible to establish a diagnosis on clinical grounds. Examination of a blood smear for vacuolized lymphocytes is a most helpful and simple diagnostic procedure. Although about 1 per cent vacuolized lymphocytes may be found in other neurological diseases, the incidence of about 20 per cent vacuolized lymphocytes (*Figure 13.3*) found in juvenile neuronal ceroid

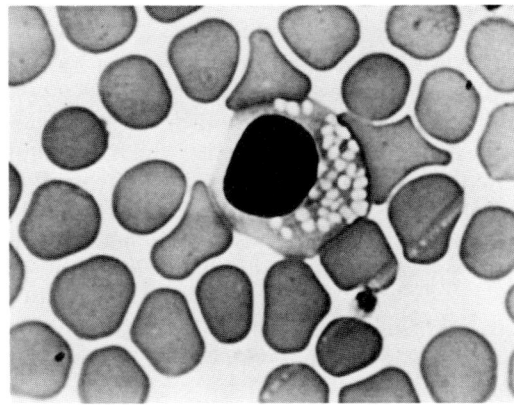

Figure 13.3. A blood smear from a case of juvenile neuronal ceroid lipofuscinosis (Batten-Spielmeyer–Vogt-Sjögren disease). Note the vacuolized lymphocyte in the centre of the picture

lipofuscinosis appears almost pathognomonic for this condition. Also, healthy heterozygotes can usually be identified by this method, as their smears contain about 1 per cent vacuolized lymphocytes. No other laboratory tests are of diagnostic help. The storage of fluorescent PAS-positive lipids is found in the neurones of the brain and the rectal wall and in the glia cells.

Poliodystrophy

Poliodystrophy (synonyms: diffuse cerebral degeneration in infancy, Alpers' disease) is a clinical condition characterized by the onset of convulsions and progressive dementia in infants between approximately 2 months and 2 years of age. Various neurological symptoms – ataxia, choreoathetosis, blindness, and spasticity – may be seen. All the symptoms are steadily progressive, and the patients die within a few years of onset. No treatment is available. The aetiology is unknown and presumably heterogeneous. The disorder has been reported in sibs; inheritance due to an autosomal recessive trait is likely in some cases.

The EEG is grossly abnormal but the changes are nonspecific. No laboratory test is of diagnostic help. At autopsy a diffuse degeneration of the grey matter in many parts of the brain is found, with widespread loss of neurones, microglial proliferation, and astrocytic gliosis. The histological findings are similar to those produced by anoxia, but the clinical picture and the progressive course do not fit such an interpretation. Pathological changes in the liver, which are more severe than could reasonably be attributed solely to malnutrition during the final stage of the illness, have been reported in some cases; it is uncertain whether or not these cases constitute a special group.

Myoclonic epilepsy

Myoclonic epilepsy comprises at least two separate conditions. Characteristic of one of them is a histological abnormality – the Lafora bodies. These consist of amorphous material which is PAS-positive and does not stain as a lipid. They are widely distributed throughout the body, occurring in the central nervous system, in the axons of peripheral nerves, and in liver, heart, and skeletal muscles; they are found both intracellularly and extracellularly. The group of patients with Lafora bodies probably represent a homogeneous disease, possibly caused by an unknown metabolic defect. The onset of this condition is in late childhood or adolescence. Patients then start to have myoclonic fits and grand mal seizures which respond poorly to antiepileptic treatment. Dementia develops. Progressive neurological symptoms – dysarthria, spasticity, and impaired vision with normal fundi – appear. The patients become increasingly handicapped and finally bedridden, and die within a decade after the onset of symptoms. Only symptomatic therapy is available.

The condition has been reported in sibs; inheritance due to an autosomal recessive trait appears likely. The EEG is grossly abnormal with continual, diffuse, high-voltage slow wave and spike-wave dysrhythmia. No laboratory methods are of diagnostic help. Histological examination of a muscle and/or a liver biopsy specimen is the best way to establish a diagnosis.

Patients with myoclonic epilepsy without Lafora bodies represent a different, probably heterogeneous condition, which is usually inherited as an autosomal recessive trait. The onset of grand mal epilepsy and of myoclonic jerks is usually in childhood. Eventually neurological symptoms and signs, such as ataxia and spasticity, appear and progress. The prognosis varies. Many patients have a mild or moderate handicap, whereas others may become severely handicapped. Their fits are often hard to control. The mental development of the patients is usually normal, even when their physical handicap is severe. The expected life-span is longer and the mortality lower than for patients with Lafora body disease.

In all types of myoclonic epilepsy the EEG is grossly abnormal with continual, diffuse, high-voltage slow wave and spike–wave dysrhythmia, sometimes reminiscent of hypsarrhythmia. The treatment is symptomatic (*see* pages 114–117). For a discussion of other aspects of myoclonic fits *see* pages 88 and 271.

Conditions with early main manifestations caused by white matter dysfunction

The leucodystrophies

The leucodystrophies can be distinguished as a special group because of the finding, common to all of them, of an increased level of total protein in the spinal fluid and a relative increase of albumin and alpha globulin. The same abnormality of the spinal fluid is found in Guillain–Barré syndrome during its early phase; the findings change during the course of that syndrome but remain essentially the same throughout the course of any of the leucodystrophies.

GLOBOID CELL TYPE

The globoid cell type of leucodystrophy (Krabbe's disease) is inherited as an autosomal recessive trait. The onset is in infancy, usually between 3 and 6 months of age. The previously normally developing child becomes irritable, hypersensitive, and stiff and has unexplained episodes of high fever. Feeding difficulties are common. The child's condition deteriorates rapidly. Within a few weeks the patient has severely increased muscle tone with legs stretched, arms bent, and the head thrown backwards; muscle reflexes are increased (*Figure 13.4*). The child loses all

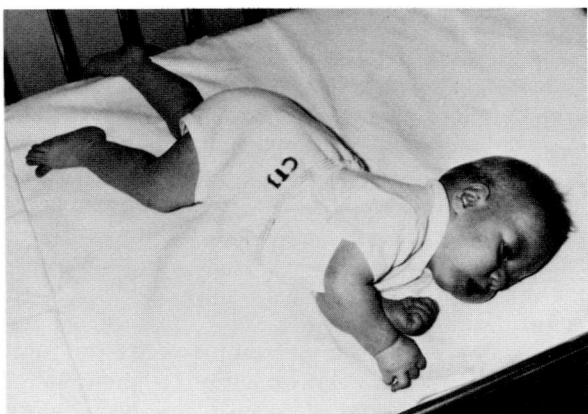

Figure 13.4. A 6-month-old girl with globoid cell type of leucodystrophy (Krabbe's disease). Note in her posture the increased muscle tone with the head thrown backwards and the hands clenched

interest in his surroundings; optic atrophy becomes apparent, and the pupils react sluggishly to light. A series of tonic fits start. Peripheral nerves are involved at an early stage. This probably partly explains the patient's irritability, which increases when he is touched and handled. Involvement of the peripheral nerves also tends to decrease the muscle tone; the increased muscle tone, which is typical of the early stage of the disease, is eventually replaced by hypotonia and weak or absent muscle reflexes. After a few months the child reaches a stage when he appears decerebrated and completely out of contact with his surroundings. With excellent nursing care he may survive for several years in this stage. No therapy is known.

The diagnosis can be suspected on clinical grounds. Repeated examination of the spinal fluid is useful in establishing a diagnosis. Throughout the course of the disease it reveals the pattern typical of leucodystrophy. The course and the lack of increased sulphatide excretion in the urine distinguishes Krabbe's disease from the other leucodystrophies.

The EEG is usually abnormal at some stage of the disease, but the abnormalities are nonspecific and not diagnostic. Involvement of the peripheral nerves is demonstrable as an abnormally low conduction velocity which decreases with time, at a period of life when it is normal for it to increase on both the motor and the sensory side.

The biochemical defect is an abnormal synthesis of sphingolipids with the accumulation of galactosylcerebrosides in globoid cells. The enzymatic defect is a lack of the enzyme beta-galactosidase which can be demonstrated in white blood cells and cultured fibroblasts. Gene carriers have an enzyme level approximately half-way between patients and normal individuals and can thus be identified. A low enzyme level is also found in the amniotic fluid of an affected fetus; prenatal diagnosis is thus possible.

At autopsy, extensive and severe demyelination is found. Within the demyelinized area there are many large multinuclear cells, the so-called globoid cells, containing a large amount of PAS-positive substance.

LATE-INFANTILE METACHROMATIC TYPE

Late-infantile metachromatic leucodystrophy (Greenfield's disease) is inherited as an autosomal recessive trait. The patients usually appear healthy and develop normally up to the age of 10–20 months, when symptoms usually start with disturbed locomotion. As a rule the first symptom is weakness of the legs, either with increased muscle tone and increased muscle reflexes which indicate damage to the corticospinal tract, or, perhaps more commonly, with flaccidity and diminished muscle reflexes which indicate damage to the ventral roots and the peripheral nerves. Eventually both the upper and lower motor neurones become involved, and the nature of the resulting weakness depends on which of them is most severely affected at the time. The general rule seems to be that findings which suggest dysfunction of the lower motor neurones dominate in the early phase and in the final stage of the disease, whereas evidence of an upper motor neurone lesion dominates in the intervening period; there are, however, exceptions to this general rule. Ataxia is practically always part of the clinical picture; it may be an early symptom or appear later during the course. After a few months the neurological symptoms have progressed considerably, and mental stagnation also becomes apparent. Attacks of tonic fits are common at this stage. Further neurological symptoms occur – rigidity, swallowing difficulties, and optic atrophy with blindness. At some stage of the disease the patients are miserable and seem to have severe pains in their arms and legs, probably due to involvement of the posterior roots. Within a year after the onset of symptoms, a stage is usually reached in which the patient appears blind and deaf, totally helpless, and with no contact with his surroundings. With good nursing care he may survive for several years in this stage. Death usually occurs between 3 and 10 years of age.

The constellation of the typical neurological symptoms and signs and the course are usually sufficiently characteristic for the correct diagnosis to be suspected on clinical grounds alone, particularly if the significance of the mixture of upper and lower motor neurone lesions is appreciated. Repeated examination of the cerebrospinal fluid shows the pattern typical of leucodystrophy (*see* page 301). The conduction velocity of the peripheral nerves is low also in cases in which the clinical findings suggest a dominating upper motor neurone lesion. The EEG is usually abnormal at some stage of the disease, but the abnormalities are nonspecific and of no diagnostic help.

The biochemical defect is an abnormal storage of sulphatide (sulphuric acid ester of galactosylceramide) in the central and peripheral nervous system, liver, kidneys, lungs, and gallbladder wall. This abnormal storage is due to a lack of the degradative lysosomal enzyme arylsulphatase A, which normally cleaves sulphatides. Arylsulphatase A is lacking in the white blood cells of the patients and abnormally low in gene carriers, making them identifiable. The demonstration of a low level of arylsulphatase A in white blood cells and urine is the best biochemical test to establish the diagnosis. However, at least one family is known with the characteristic clinical picture but normal levels of arylsulphatase A. A low enzyme level is found in the amniotic fluid of an affected fetus; prenatal diagnosis is thus possible.

A diet deficient in vitamin A would theoretically be expected to have a positive influence on patients with metachromatic leucodystrophy. It has been tried in a few patients with improvement of the laboratory findings but with insignificant influence on the clinical picture. At present no effective therapy is known.

The findings at autopsy consist of demyelination and metachromatic deposits in the central and peripheral nervous systems. Deposits are also found outside the nervous system.

Variants of metachromatic leucodystrophy are known with later (juvenile or adult) onset and slower progression.

CHRONIC TYPE

Chronic leucodystrophy (Pelizaeus–Merzbacher disease) is probably not a homogeneous disease. It is usually inherited as a sex-linked recessive trait, but clinically identical cases with evidence of autosomal recessive inheritance are also on record. The first symptom is usually nystagmus which may be observed when the patient is a few months old. It may persist for some months and then disappear. There is often a symptom-free interval of a year or two before the onset of other neurological symptoms and signs – ataxia, spasticity, and optic atrophy. The onset is so insidious and the progression so slow that it is often difficult to date when the symptoms started. By school-age the children are as a rule definitely handicapped, and they become confined to a wheelchair in adolescence or early adulthood. Difficulties at school eventually become apparent and increase slowly. Most patients die during early adulthood.

These patients are often misdiagnosed as having cerebral palsy, until the significance of the optic atrophy and the progression of symptoms and signs are appreciated. Repeated examination of the cerebrospinal fluid reveals the pattern typical of leucodystrophies (*see* page 301). The course and the lack of findings characteristic of late-infantile metachromatic leucodystrophy distinguish it from the other types of leucodystrophy.

No treatment is available. At autopsy the brain is found to be shrunken with extensive and severe demyelination and sclerosis of all the white matter. The biochemical defect is not known.

Diffuse brain sclerosis

SUDANOPHILIC TYPE WITHOUT ENDOCRINE FINDINGS

Diffuse brain sclerosis of the sudanophilic type is a poorly delineated group of disorders with an unknown and possibly heterogeneous aetiology. The onset of symptoms is fairly acute and occurs during childhood, although seldom in children below a few years of age. The most common early symptoms are cortical blindness and ataxia, followed later by spasticity and optic atrophy. Tonic fits may occur. Within a few months to a year the previously healthy child has turned into a blind, apparently decerebrated individual with no definite contact with his surroundings. With good nursing care he can live for several years in this stage.

The diagnosis can only be established on a brain biopsy, as there are no specific diagnostic laboratory tests available (*see below*, sudanophilic type with Addison's disease). The cerebrospinal fluid protein is normal.

No treatment is available. At autopsy severe demyelination and sclerosis are found. The histological picture is often described as similar to that seen in fresh plaques in cases of multiple sclerosis. Some authors have interpreted the diffuse brain sclerosis as the childhood manifestation of acute multiple sclerosis.

SUDANOPHILIC TYPE WITH ADDISON'S DISEASE

One variant of diffuse brain sclerosis occurs in association with Addison's disease; it appears to be a more homogeneous entity. It is inherited as a sex-linked recessive trait and thus occurs only in boys. It has its onset in childhood either with symptoms of Addison's disease, i.e. fatigue, irritability, brown pigmentation of the skin, attacks of vomiting with rapid dehydration, and a drop in blood pressure, or with the neurological symptoms described as sudanophilic type without endocrine findings (*see above*). Both types of symptoms may start simultaneously. Laboratory tests confirm the diagnosis of Addison's disease, i.e. elevated serum potassium, decreased serum sodium, and low plasma cortisol level which does not increase on stimulation with ACTH. The Addisonian part of the syndrome can be treated with hormone substitution, but the neurological symptoms progress steadily in spite of this treatment, and the patients die within a few years after the onset of symptoms. Autopsy findings are the same as described for the sudanophilic type without endocrine findings, plus atrophy of the adrenal cortex. The connection between the endocrine and the neurological findings is not known.

Canavan's spongy degeneration

This condition is inherited as an autosomal recessive trait; it is particularly prevalent in Jewish families. The onset of symptoms is in infancy with failure to thrive and an abnormal increase in head size (*see* page 239). Spasticity, optic atrophy, and stagnation of mental development occur. As a rule the course is fairly acute and death occurs within a few months to a couple of years; a few reported patients have survived until middle childhood. Computerized tomography of the skull may reveal the low density of the white matter and possibly the cyst formation. There are no specific diagnostic tests, and no therapy. A spongy degeneration of the white matter of the brain is found at autopsy. The existence of this syndrome as a disease entity has been doubted, as the same type of spongy degeneration may be found in known metabolic disorders, e.g. maple syrup disease.

Cockayne's syndrome

This is a rare condition, inherited as an autosomal recessive trait. Children with this syndrome appear normal during infancy. Progressive symptoms then start with a retardation of physical growth, including head circumference, hearing defect, retinitis pigmentosa, and polyneuropathy. Impairment of intellectual development is also likely but hard to evaluate in a child with severe disturbances of both vision and hearing.

Fabry's disease (ceramide trihexosidosis, angiokeratoma corporis diffusum)

This condition is inherited as a sex-linked recessive trait. Symptoms usually start at around 10 years of age and consist of bloody papules over the penis, scrotum, and umbilicus and tortuous veins in the conjunctiva. The boys complain of pains in the arms and legs, particularly after physical effort and changes of temperature. The pains are due to involvement of the peripheral nerves and may be severe; as the objective findings are small, there is a risk that the complaints may be misinterpreted as being caused by psychogenic factors. Slowly progressive kidney disease is also present and may lead to uraemia and death. The biochemical defect is a lack of the enzyme alpha-galactosidase A, leading to an accumulation of ceramide trihexoside; this accumulation can be demonstrated in cultured fibroblasts. Female gene-carriers may show mild symptoms with later onset than is seen in affected boys.

'Kinky hair' disease (Menkes' syndrome)

This disease, inherited as a sex-linked recessive trait, has its onset in early infancy with stagnation of psychomotor development and the appearance of fits. The infant loses interest in visual stimuli, develops feeding difficulties and has trouble maintaining his body temperature, which has a tendency to decrease. On examination pale discs and spasticity are found. The hair is peculiar, i.e. curly and brittle, and its shaft shows periodic narrowing, twisting, and fragmentation. The serum levels of copper and of ceruloplasmin are low, probably due to impaired copper absorption from the gut. Copper administration seems to improve the hair but has no influence on the neurological symptoms and signs. The infant deteriorates and usually dies within the first year of life. At autopsy, a serious lack of myelination is found.

Multiple sclerosis

Multiple sclerosis is rare in childhood. Early symptoms are as a rule attacks of impaired vision, ataxia, or regional paraesthesia (*see* page 260).

Other conditions

Cerebrohepatorenal syndrome

This rare syndrome, described by Zellweger and co-workers and known under his name, is inherited as an autosomal recessive trait. At birth the patient has a low birth-weight and peculiar facial features with hypertelorism, epicanthal folds, and a prominent forehead. A profound muscular hypotonia is present at birth together with areflexia and absent Moro reflex. Failure to thrive, jaundice, and convulsions are typical features. Most patients die before 6 months of age. An abnormally high level of serum ion and high iron-binding capacity may be seen and may be of diagnostic help. Its connection, if any, with the clinical picture is unknown. No treatment is available.

At autopsy the liver and kidneys are found to be abnormal: the liver is yellow and hard with micronodular cirrhosis, and multiple cysts are scattered throughout the kidneys. In the brain the white matter is greatly reduced in amount and sclerotic with severe demyelination; the histological picture is described as similar to that seen in cerebral sclerosis of the sudanophilic type.

Necrotizing encephalomyelopathy

This condition, also known as Leigh's syndrome, is inherited as an autosomal recessive trait. Two types seem to exist – one has an acute course with onset in infancy, rapid progress, and death within a few months or years, and the other has a chronic course with more insidious onset during childhood, slow progress, and survival for a decade or more.

The neurological symptoms and signs most often noted are disturbed eye movements, sluggish pupillary reactions, impaired vision and hearing, ataxia, swallowing difficulties, spasticity, and flaccid weakness due to polyneuropathy (*Figures 13.5* and *13.6*). Impaired mental development is the rule, and convulsions have been observed in a few patients.

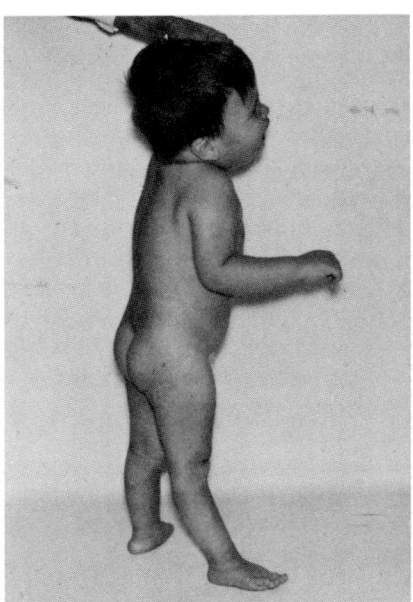

Figure 13.5. A 2-year-old boy with severe muscle hypotonia due to polyneuropathy. His clinical picture started as pure polyneuropathy, but later developed into Leigh's syndrome (*see Figure 13.6*)

The lesion found at autopsy is always bilateral and usually of a strikingly symmetrical appearance. It involves particularly the area around the third ventricle and the aqueduct (*Figure 13.7*) but extends also to the medulla oblongata, the cerebellum, the spinal cord, and the peripheral nerves; the mammillary bodies are often spared. Microscopically the picture is dominated by severe demyelination and

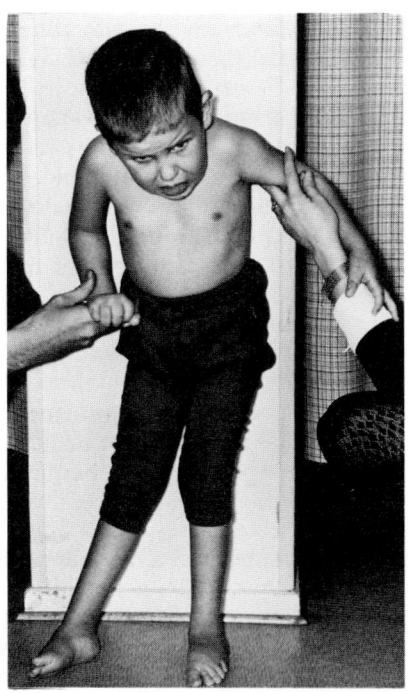

Figure 13.6. The same boy as shown in *Figure 13.5* at 6 years of age, with necrotizing encephalomyelopathy (Leigh's syndrome). Besides the polyneuropathy the boy now has ataxia, signs of involvement of the corticospinal tract, dysarthria, swallowing difficulties, and drooling

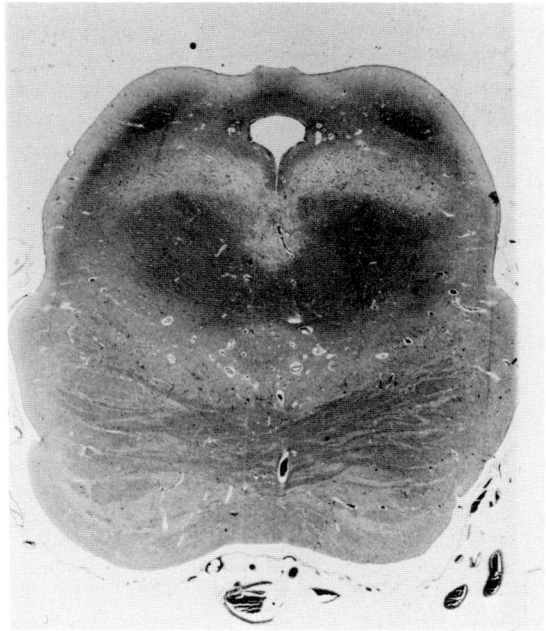

Figure 13.7. A section from the upper part of the pons of an 8-month-old boy with necrotizing encephalomyelopathy (Leigh's syndrome). Myelin staining according to Mahon; preserved myelin appears dark. Note the butterfly-shaped light area under the aqueduct, where there is degeneration with scarring and a breaking down of myelin into sudanophilic fat in macrophages

loss of neurones together with a proliferation of small blood vessels. The clinical findings are explained by the localization of the lesion, and their variability by its different extent in different patients.

The conduction velocity of peripheral nerves is low in patients with this syndrome who also have involvement of the peripheral nerves. This is, however, a nonspecific finding, noted in various disorders of the peripheral nerves. No neurophysiological measurements or laboratory tests are useful in establishing a diagnosis of necrotizing encephalomyelopathy; most reported cases have been diagnosed at autopsy. Computerized tomography of the skull is of diagnostic help in excluding other possible causes of the child's symptoms, and in revealing oedema of the brain stem, which is present at some stage but not during the whole course of the disease. This method can only give support to the diagnosis; it can neither prove nor exclude it. It is difficult to establish an antemortem diagnosis, unless the diagnosis has been proved at autopsy in a sib who during life showed a similar clinical picture.

A-betalipoproteinaemia

Abetalipoproteinaemia (Bassen–Kornzweig syndrome) is inherited as an autosomal recessive trait. The first symptoms usually occur in infancy or early childhood and consist of diarrhoea and impaired growth, suggesting malabsorption. The next symptom, which becomes apparent a few years later, is usually impaired vision and night-blindness due to atypical retinitis pigmentosa. In later childhood slowly progressive neurological symptoms and signs appear – ataxia, spasticity, and evidence of polyneuropathy.

Blood smears reveal a peculiar abnormality of the red blood cells usually described as acanthocytosis. The red blood cells are crenated and often of bizarre shape. This abnormality may be found years before the neurological symptoms appear. The cholesterol level of the blood serum is low. Analysis of lipoprotein distribution in the serum reveals a lack of beta-lipoprotein. The symptoms progress slowly and steadily. Treatment with large doses of vitamin E seems to improve the condition.

A-alphalipoproteinaemia or normal serum lipids

A-alphalipoproteinaemia seems to produce a similar clinical picture to that seen in a-betalipoproteinaemia; biochemically there is a difference as alpha-lipoprotein is absent instead of beta-lipoprotein. The same clinical picture may possibly be found in patients with normal serum lipids.

Conditions dominated by ataxia

The neurological symptoms of Refsum's disease are similar to those seen in Bassen–Kornzweig syndrome; the clinical picture is usually dominated by ataxia (*see* page 263).

Friedreich's ataxia produces slowly progressive mental and neurological symptoms and signs; the clinical picture is usually dominated by ataxia (*see* page 261).

In ataxia telangiectasia, progressive mental symptoms may appear late in the disease; the clinical picture is dominated by ataxia (*see* page 262).

Wilson's disease

Hepatolenticular degeneration (Wilson's disease) is inherited as an autosomal recessive trait. Onset is usually in childhood or adolescence. As a rule the first symptoms are caused by the liver disease; the patients show hepatosplenomegaly and laboratory tests reveal signs of liver cirrhosis, occasionally with episodes of jaundice.

Neurological symptoms usually start in adolescence or early adulthood. The characteristic findings are a Parkinson-like picture with rigidity, a mask-like facies, a coarse tremor, dysarthria, drooling, and choreoathetosis. Emotional instability is an early feature, whereas true intellectual impairment occurs late in the disease. A Kayser–Fleischer ring (a greenish-brown discoloration of the outer part of the cornea) with no visual impairment is seen only in Wilson's disease and is detectable by slit-lamp examination in practically all cases of this disease.

The diagnosis can thus usually be established on clinical examination. The biochemical defect consists of a toxic accumulation of copper within the body. This is associated with a deficiency of ceruloplasmin, the protein that is responsible for the transport of most of the serum copper. In addition there is an increased rate of absorption of copper from the intestine. Copper is deposited in various tissues, particularly the liver, brain, and cornea, and this toxic deposition explains all the clinical findings. Urinary copper is increased but not enough to prevent the accumulation of copper in the body. Laboratory tests thus reveal a decreased serum level of ceruloplasmin, a decreased level of total serum copper, increased copper excretion in the urine, and an increased content of copper in the liver, demonstrable on chemical analysis of a liver biopsy specimen. All these biochemical abnormalities, particularly the increased copper content of the liver, which may be demonstrated in a case of Wilson's disease before clinical symptoms have appeared, confirm the diagnosis.

In an untreated case, the symptoms progress and the patient becomes severely handicapped. The best treatment is a diet low in copper and administration of the chelating agent, penicillamine, which causes an increase in urinary copper and depletion of the copper stores in the body. The dose of penicillamine, which in most children and adolescents is between 1 and 3 g a day, must be determined individually. The treatment is effective in early cases but less so when symptoms have been present for a long time and irreversible tissue damage is likely. Treatment should probably be started before clinical symptoms appear in children (i.e. sibs of known patients) in whom the biochemical defect, particularly an increased amount of copper in the liver, has been demonstrated. Such early treatment has prevented the development of clinical symptoms in some individuals.

Familial idiopathic cerebral calcifications in childhood

This condition has been described in a few patients and appears to be inherited as an autosomal recessive trait. Symptoms start in early childhood with delayed mental and physical development, followed later by mental deterioration, microcephaly, spasticity and flexion contractures of the lower extremities, athetoid movements, and tremor. Skull X-ray shows calcifications of the brain, which are particularly dense in the basal ganglia, cerebral cortex, and cerebellum. Laboratory studies give normal results, and other causes of intracranial calcifications can thus be excluded.

The symptoms are progressive and the children soon become severely handicapped. There is no known treatment. At autopsy compact calcifications and tissue necrosis are found in the basal ganglia, cerebral cortex, and cerebellum. Calcified granules may be seen along the capillaries.

Hallervorden–Spatz syndrome

This is a rare, possibly heterogeneous, syndrome which has been described in sibs and seems to be inherited as an autosomal recessive trait. The symptoms usually reported consist of rigidity, involuntary movements, and dementia; they may start in childhood and are slowly progressive. Laboratory studies and neurophysiological examinations are of no diagnostic help, and it is almost impossible to establish the diagnosis during the patient's life-time.

At autopsy the globus pallidus and the substantia nigra have a rust-brown discoloration due to an iron-containing lipoid pigment located within neurones and glial cells, particularly around large blood vessels. The most striking abnormality is the thickening and fragmentation of the axons. Neuronal degeneration may also involve the cerebral cortex and the cerebellum. No treatment is known.

Familial dysautonomia

Familial dysautonomia (Riley–Day syndrome) is inherited as an autosomal recessive trait, and seems to occur mainly in Jewish families. The clinical picture is extremely variable. Symptoms from the autonomic system may start in infancy with abnormal changes in skin colour, fluctuations in blood pressure, poor temperature control, hyperhidrosis, diminished or absent lacrimation, and disturbances of the gastrointestinal tract with episodes of severe vomiting. The peripheral nervous system may also be involved with insensitivity to pain, muscular atrophy, and diminished or absent muscle reflexes. Any coincident symptoms from the central nervous system vary in extent and severity.

Abnormal catecholamine metabolism can be demonstrated as an increased urinary excretion of homovanillic acid (derived from dopamine, a pressor amine precursor); this finding in a clinically suspected case is good support for a diagnosis of familial dysautonomia. Only symptomatic treatment is available. At autopsy extensive lesions of the autonomic, peripheral, and central nervous systems may be found.

Alexander's disease

This is a rare disorder with onset in infancy, characterized by failure to thrive, stagnation of mental development, convulsions, and an abnormally rapid increase in head size with normal or slightly enlarged ventricles. There are no typical clinical or laboratory findings that can be used to establish a diagnosis during life. The characteristic features at autopsy are eosinophilic hyaline bodies deposited in a subpial and perivascular band and distributed randomly throughout the white matter. The cause is unknown.

Kearns–Sayre syndrome

This syndrome, also called 'ophthalmoplegia plus' is a diffusely delineated syndrome of unknown aetiology. Symptoms usually start during middle or late childhood. The main component is a slowly progressive ophthalmoplegia, including ptosis. Among other symptoms and signs are seizures, ataxia, retinitis pigmentosa, impaired cardiac function, particularly heart block, and often also other findings. Ragged-red fibres are often found on histological examination of muscle tissue. Only symptomatic treatment is available for the various components of the syndrome.

Rett's syndrome

This syndrome occurs only in girls. It has been reported in sisters; the number of boys in these sibships appears decreased, suggesting a sex-linked dominant inheritance of a gene which is lethal even during fetal life in the male sex. At birth the girls appear normal as does their early development. Towards the end of the first year a slowing of their development is noted. They lose interest in the purposeful use of their hands which they wring together in a stereotyped way. They are also uninterested in social contact, avoid eye contact, and do not use language, i.e. they show autistic behaviour. During childhood they show severe mental retardation, probably with some progression, and they may develop ataxia and spasticity, possibly with contractures. They may have occasional grand mal fits, but epilepsy is not a major problem. Their stereotyped hand movements make them appear to be constantly washing their hands. They need help with all activities of daily life. Although there is a tendency for the autistic behaviour to improve, they never learn to use language. The diagnosis is based entirely on the clinical picture. No radiological, physiological, or laboratory studies have revealed any characteristic features. No treatment is known.

Slow-virus encephalitis

Infections of the brain with slow virus are described here rather than in the chapter on infections because their clinical picture and course suggest a progressive degenerative disorder, whereas none of the symptoms or signs point to an infection.

SUBACUTE SCLEROSING PANENCEPHALITIS (SSPE)

The onset of SSPE is in childhood or adolescence. The first symptoms are usually mental with increasing difficulties at school and odd behaviour. Symptoms progress rapidly and involve all psychic functions, usually with an element of aphasia, agnosia and apraxia, before severe dementia renders an analysis of these problems impossible. Convulsions occur sooner or later; a series of severe fits may be the first symptom. All kinds of neurological symptoms may appear, and the order of their appearance varies. The patients may thus have spastic hemiparesis, tetraparesis, ataxia, rigidity, and disturbed eye movements. The convulsive episodes are typically associated with complex dyskinesias and hyperkinesias of various kinds, such as clonic discharges, choreic movements, myoclonic jerks, tonic fits with opisthotonos, and short and sudden lapses of tone. Unexplained periods of fever occur in many patients.

Symptoms progress rapidly and usually without remission until within a few months the child is in a stage characterized by decerebrate rigidity, complete dementia, and no apparent contact with his surroundings. Death usually occurs within a few years. No treatment has proved successful.

The cerebrospinal fluid contains few or no cells, and a normal or slightly elevated total protein with a marked elevation of gamma globulin, particularly IgG. This reaction is sufficiently characteristic to be of diagnostic help. The active production of antibodies, usually against measles, within the central nervous system is another characteristic feature. The EEG abnormalities, which are typical of the disease, consist of rhythmic complexes starting with one or a few slow spike discharges, followed by high-voltage slow waves (*Figure 13.8*). The complexes appear simultaneously in all leads. The rhythm is strikingly regular, at least during the same tracing; the frequency varies from 2 to about 18 per minute. Simultaneously with the abnormal EEG complexes, myoclonic jerks or sudden lapses of tone can usually be observed. The EEG findings may vary from day to day in the same patient, and the typical rhythmical discharges may not be present in all the tracings. However, if recordings are repeatedly performed, the characteristic abnormalities will be found in almost all patients with subacute sclerosing panencephalitis.

SSPE is caused by an early viral infection of the brain. After several inactive years the virus starts a progressive inflammatory disorder, leading to cortical necrosis. Measles virus is the usual cause of SSPE. A history, taken carefully with particular attention to this point, reveals that practically all patients with SSPE have had measles at an unusually early age, and almost always before 15 months of age.

The same clinical picture may be caused by rubella virus. Mass vaccination against these two viral diseases is the best way to reduce their incidence and their complications.

At autopsy a fibrillary gliosis is found accompanied by a subacute inflammatory reaction, evident from the accumulation of lymphocytes and plasma cells, particularly as cuffs round the blood vessels. This reaction extends diffusely throughout the white matter of the central nervous system and is occasionally also found in spinal roots and rarely in the peripheral nerves. The inflammatory reaction is noted also in the cerebral cortex, basal ganglia, and thalamus, where a severe loss of neurones is observed. Inclusion bodies may be found in the glia cells.

Other chronic viral infections of the brain

The possibility of chronic viral encephalitis must be considered in all children with signs of a progressive cerebral disease for which no other explanation is found. Even if two sibs show the same clinical picture, it might be due to a chronic viral infection. Both children may have an impaired resistance to viral infections; the inherited trait may be a congenital defect in the immunosystem.

MULTIFOCAL LEUCOENCEPHALOPATHY

A multifocal leucoencephalopathy has been described complicating Hodgkin's disease, sarcoidosis, and chronic lymphatic leukaemia in adulthood. It has also been reported in a child with generalized histiocytic reticuloendotheliosis; conceivably it may complicate other malignant diseases in childhood. Central pontine myelinolysis has been reported in a few children with malignant disease, who are receiving immunosuppressive therapy for their disease. There is good evidence that multifocal leucoencephalopathy and pontine myelinolysis are due to activation of a dormant virus in a patient who is immuno-incompetent due to a malignant disease or to the treatment for such a disease.

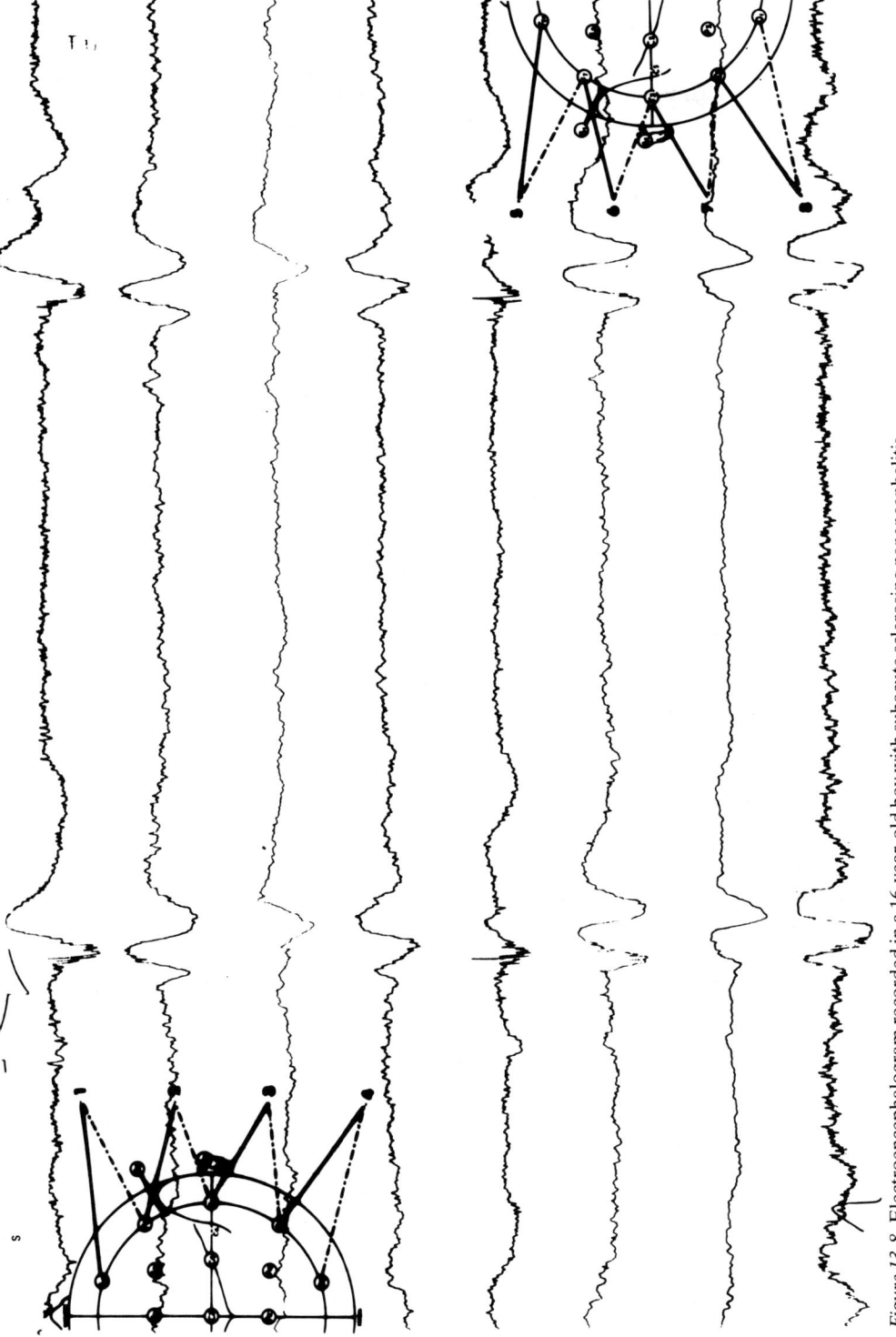

313

Figure 13.8. Electroencephalogram recorded in a 16-year-old boy with subacute sclerosing panencephalitis

The management of a child showing progressive mental and neurological symptoms and signs

The first step is a careful general paediatric examination, which may reveal, for example, hepatosplenomegaly and lymphadenopathy in disorders that also involve the reticuloendothelial system. One single neurological examination is of little specific diagnostic help, as it can only demonstrate the type and extent of the lesion at a given moment, and the findings may be the same in several different conditions. Repeated examinations, together with a careful history about the first symptoms and their further development, provide information which may make it possible to classify the condition as predominantly affecting the grey matter or the white matter. It may also suggest a localized growing process, such as a tumour.

A complete ophthalmological examination must always be performed, as abnormalities of the cornea, the retina, the macula, and the optic discs may give useful and occasionally specific diagnostic information.

Computerized tomography of the skull is performed for a wide range of indications. It may reveal, for example, a neurosurgically accessible condition in a patient previously thought to have an untreatable degenerative disorder. It can also demonstrate areas of demyelination and oedema and thus give diagnostic information.

The EEG is abnormal in practically all the conditions described in this chapter. Only in subacute sclerosing panencephalitis (*see* page 312) are the findings specific, at least on repeated examinations, and can thus be used to establish a diagnosis.

The recording of evoked potentials from the brain after visual, auditory, or tactile stimulation may reveal abnormally slow conduction within the central nervous system. Particularly useful is the recording of visually evoked potentials, the conduction of which is impaired in disorders characterized by demyelination, e.g. multiple sclerosis.

Measurement of the conduction velocity of the peripheral nerves is an easy procedure which can reveal involvement of the peripheral nervous system. Of the diseases described in this chapter, such an involvement has been demonstrated in the globoid cell type of leucodystrophy (*see* page 301), in late-infantile metachromatic leucodystrophy (*see* page 302), and in necrotizing encephalomyelopathy (*see* page 306).

The examination of an ordinary blood smear may give useful diagnostic information. An abnormality of the lymphocytes is found in juvenile neuronal ceroid lipofuscinosis, and occasionally in Tay–Sachs and Niemann–Pick diseases (*see* pages 299, 295 and 297); an abnormality of the red cells is found in a-betalipoproteinaemia and a-alphaproteinaemia (*see* page 308). If crenated red cells are found, the serum cholesterol level should be determined, and if this is low the serum lipoproteins should be analysed.

The cerebrospinal fluid must be examined in all patients with progressive mental and neurological symptoms and signs. Good diagnostic help can be obtained from the cell count, the sugar level, and the protein content, particularly the electrophoretic distribution of the different protein fractions; on the basis of these findings the leucodystrophies (*see* page 301) can be distinguished.

Histological examination of biopsy specimens may be helpful in some conditions. The bone marrow should be studied if neurovisceral gangliosidosis, or Gaucher's, Niemann–Pick, or Wolman's diseases (*see* pages 297–298) are suspected. Histological examination of muscle tissue or liver tissue may conceivably reveal

Lafora bodies (*see* page 300); a liver biopsy specimen may show evidence of cirrhosis in a case of Wilson's disease (*see* page 309). A peripheral nerve biopsy, preferably from the sural nerve, may be of value if the peripheral nervous system is also involved. Ganglion cells showing the same abnormalities as those in the brain, e.g. lipid storage in Tay–Sachs disease, can be obtained from a rectal biopsy specimen. A brain biopsy is justified in carefully selected cases.

Special laboratory tests should be performed in selected cases: investigation of Addison's disease (*see* page 304), of copper metabolism (Wilson's disease, page 309; Menkes' kinky hair disease, page 305), of the serum level of iron (*see* page 306), of the serum level of acid phosphatase (*see* page 297), of the activity of various enzymes in the white blood cells, of amino acid metabolism and the urinary excretion of organic acids and acid mucopolysaccharides (*see* Chapter 5), of serum proteins (*see* Chapter 10), and of the uric acid level in serum (*see* Chapter 5).

The possibility of a space-occupying lesion must always be kept in mind. Computerized tomography of the skull must be performed for a wide range of indications in children who show progressive mental and neurological symptoms and signs.

The first aim is always to identify the cases for which specific therapy is available. As a rule no therapy is possible, but even so a correct diagnosis is important to the whole family, as it is the basis of correct genetic counselling. A specific diagnosis is always desirable, as it allows the physician to give the family substantial information about the disease and to predict its further course.

References

ARIMA, M., KOMIYA, K., KAMOSHITA, S. and MUKAI, N. (1963) Clinical and pathological characteristics in Wilson's disease in cases under 10 years of age. Paediatria Universitatis Tokyo No 9, pp. 17–22

BAUMANN, R. J. and MARKESBERY, W. R. (1978) Juvenile amaurotic idiocy (neuronal ceroid lipofuscinosis) and lymphocyte fingerprint profiles. *Annals of Neurology*, **4**, 531–536

BERENBERG, R. A., PELLOCK, J. M., DIMAURO, S., SCHOTLAND, L., BONILLA, E., EASTWOOD, A. *et al.* (1977) Lumping or splitting? 'Ophthalmoplegia-plus' or Kearns–Sayre syndrome? *Annals of Neurology*, **1**, 37–54

BOWEN, P., LEE, C. S. N., ZELLWEGER, H. and LINDENBERG, R. (1964) A familial syndrome of multiple congenital defects. *Bulletin of the Johns Hopkins Hospital*, **114**, 402–414

CHOPPIN, P. W. (1981) Measles virus and chronic neurological diseases. *Annals of Neurology*, **9**, 17–20

COYLE, P. K. and WOLINSKY, J. S. (1981) Characterization of immune complexes in progressive rubella panencephalitis. *Annals of Neurology*, **9**, 557–562

CHRISTENSEN LOU, H. O. (1972) Angiokeratoma corporis diffusum (Fabry's sygdom). Polyteknisk Forlag, Lyngby

DOOLING, E. C., SCHOENE, W. C. and RICHARDSON JR, E. P. (1974) Halleworden–Spatz syndrome. *Archives of Neurology*, **30**, 70–83

DORFMAN, L. J., PELEY, T. A., THARP, B. R. and SCHEITHAUER, B. W. (1978) Juvenile neuroaxonal dystrophy: clinical, electrophysiological and neuropathological features. *Annals of Neurology*, **3**, 419–428

DUNN, H. G., LAKE, S. D., DOLMAN, C. L. and WILSON, J. (1969) The neuropathy of Krabbe's infantile cerebral sclerosis (globoid cells leukodystrophy). *Brain*, **92**, 329–344

DURANT, R. H., DYKEN, P. R. and SWIFT, A. W. (1982) The influence of inosiplex treatment on the neurological disability of patients with subacute sclerosing panencephalitis. *Journal of Pediatrics*, **101**, 288–293

DYKEN, P. and KRAWIECKI, N. (1983) Neurodegenerative diseases of infancy and childhood. *Annals of Neurology*, **13**, 351–364

FEIGIN, I., PENA, C. E. and BUDZILOVICH, G. (1968) The infantile spongy degenerations. *Neurology* (Minneapolis), **18**, 153–166

FULLERTON, P. (1964) Peripheral nerve conduction in metachromatic leucodystrophy (sulphatide lipoidosis). *Journal of Neurology, Neurosurgery and Psychiatry*, **27**, 100–105

GAMSTORP, I. (1968) Polyneuropathy in childhood. *Acta Paediatrica Scandinavica*, **57**, 230–238

HAGBERG, B., AICARDI, J., DIAS, K. and RAMOS, O. (1983) A progressive syndrome of autism, dementia, ataxia and loss of purposeful hand use in girls: Rett's syndrome: report of 35 cases. *Annals of Neurology,* **14,** 471–479

HAGBERG, B., HALTIA, M., SOURANDER, P., SVENNERHOLM, L. and EEG-OLOFSSON, O. (1974) Polyunsaturated fatty acid lipidosis. Infantile form of so-called neuronal ceroid lipofuscinosis. *Acta Paediatrica Scandinavica,* **63,** 753–763

HOEFNAGEL, D., BRUN, A., INGBAR, S. H. and GOLDMAN, H. (1967) Addison's disease and diffuse cerebral sclerosis. *Journal of Neurology, Neurosurgery and Psychiatry,* **30,** 56–60

HOMMES, F. A., POLMAN, H. A. and REERINK, J. D. (1968) Leigh's encephalomyelopathy: an inborn error of gluconeogenesis. *Archives of Diseases in Childhood,* **43,** 423–426

KOLODNY, E. H. and CABLE, W. J. L. (1982) Inborn errors of metabolism. *Annals of Neurology,* **11,** 221–232

LAKKE, J. P., EBELS, E. J. and TEN THYE, O. J. (1967) Infantile necrotizing encephalomyelopathy (Leigh). *Archives of Neurology* (Chicago), **16,** 227–231

LEON, G. A. DE, GROVER, W. D., HUFF, D. S., MORINIGO–MESTRE, G., PUNNETT, H. H. and KISTENMACHER, M. L. (1977) Globoid cells, glial nodules, and peculiar fibrillary changes in the cerebro-hepato-renal syndrome of Zellweger. *Annals of Neurology,* **2,** 473–484

MARTIN, J. J. and MARTIN, L. (1974) Infantile form of Hallerworden–Spatz disease. *Clinical Neurology and Neurosurgery,* **1,** 26–37

MELCHIOR, J. C. and CLAUSEN, J. (1968) Metachromatic leucodystrophy in early childhood. Treatment with a diet deficient in vitamin A. *Acta Paediatrica Scandinavica,* **57,** 2–8

MOSER, H. W., MOSER, A. B., KAWAMURA, N., MURPHY, J., SUZUKI, K., SCHAUMBERG, H. *et al.* (1980) Adrenoleukodystrophy: elevated C26 fatty acid in cultured skins fibroblasts. *Annals of Neurology,* **7,** 542–549

MULLER, D. P. R., LLOYD, J. K. and BIRD, A. C. (1977) Long-term management of abetalipoproteinaemia. Possible role for vitamin E. *Archives of Diseases in Childhood,* **52,** 209–214

PATTON, R. G., CHRISTIE, D. L., SMITH, D. W. and BECKWITH, J. B. (1972) Cerebro-hepato-renal syndrome of Zellweger. *American Journal of Diseases in Children,* **124,** 840–844

RAYNER, S. (1962) Juvenile amaurotic idiocy in Sweden. With particular reference to the vacuoles in the lymphocytes of the homo- and hetero-zygotes. Dissertation Medical Faculty, Uppsala

SANTAVUORI, P., HALTIA, M. and RAPOLA, J. (1974) Infantile type of so-called neuronal ceroid-lipofuscinosis. *Developmental Medicine and Child Neurology,* **16,** 644–653

SCHOCHET, S. S. JR, LAMPERT, P. W. and EARLE, K. M. (1968) Alexander's disease. A case report with electron microscopic observations. *Neurology* (Minneapolis), **18,** 543–549

SOFFER, D., GROTSKY, H. W., RAPIN, I. and SUZUKI, K. (1979) Cockayne syndrome: unusual neuropathological findings and review of the literature. *Annals of Neurology,* **6,** 340–348

TÖNNESEN, T., BRO, P. V., BRÖNDUM NIELSEN, K. and LYKKELUND, C. (1983) Metachromatic leucodystrophy and pseudoarylsulfatase A deficiency in a Danish family. *Acta Paediatrica Scandinavica,* **72,** 175–178

WEFRING, K. W and LAMVIK, J. O. (1967) Familial progressive poliodystrophy with cirrhosis of the liver. *Acta Paediatrica Scandinavica,* **56,** 295–300

14

Headache

Headache is a common symptom in childhood. The different causes are reviewed according to the history.

Headache with acute onset and short duration

Fever

In all ages fever is the most common cause of acute headache. It is the fever as such which causes the headache, regardless of the type of infection that produces the fever. This situation is well known to lay people and usually recognized by the patient's mother, thus differential diagnostic problems seldom arise.

Acute meningitis

In acute meningitis (*see* page 343) the acute onset is accompanied by fever, headache, backache, and vomiting. The history can usually be counted in hours when the patient first consults the doctor.

Chronic meningitis

In chronic meningitis due to tuberculosis, syphilis, or fungal infection, for example, the history is longer and may be counted in days or a few weeks. The neck is stiff, signs of increased intracranial pressure are usually present, and examination of the optic fundi may reveal pathognomonic abnormalities (*see* pages 345–348).

Leukaemic infiltration of the meninges

Infiltration of the meninges is such a common complication of acute leukaemia that routine treatment of acute leukaemia in childhood includes regular prophylactic measures to prevent its occurrence. If it occurs in spite of these measures, the onset is abrupt with headache and vomiting. On examination the child is found to have a stiff neck and papilloedema, and occasionally also sixth nerve palsy. The cerebrospinal fluid is under increased pressure and usually contains several hundred cells per cubic millimetre (many of which can be identified as blast cells), an increased protein level, and a very low sugar level. The treatment of meningeal leukaemic infiltration is part of the total antileukaemic therapy.

Subarachnoidal bleeding

Subarachnoidal bleeding often has a peracute onset, occasionally to such a degree that the patient can give not only the hour but even the minute when symptoms started. The headache is severe, and vomiting is the rule. As the blood irritates and causes an aseptic meningitis, the signs are the same as seen in meningeal infection (*see* page 343). Many patients with subarachnoidal bleeding lose consciousness within hours after the onset of symptoms. Retinal and preretinal haemorrhages may be found on eye examination, whereas papilloedema usually takes at least a couple of days to develop. The cerebrospinal fluid is bloody. Focal neurological signs may also arise, particularly if the bleeding is due to a ruptured arteriovenous aneurysm.

   Increased intracranial pressure may best be reduced with the help of steroids, e.g. dexamethasone 0.5–2 mg four time a day initially, followed by gradually decreasing doses. Computerized tomography of the skull is urgently indicated. It reveals blood in the subarachnoid space, confirming the diagnosis; the bleeding aneurysm, if large enough; and the presence of complications, such as a haematoma in the parenchyma or bleeding in the ventricles. As a rule an arteriogram is necessary to localize the bleeding aneurysm; however, this method may fail if the aneurysm is too small or if the bleeding has caused spasm of the blood vessels intense enough to obscure the picture. It is desirable to localize the aneurysm as soon as possible and to operate on it to prevent rebleeding, which may otherwise happen and worsen the prognosis. Hydrocephalus may develop as a late sequela after subarachnoidal bleeding; the management of this situation is discussed in Chapter 9.

Head trauma

During the period immediately following a head trauma, headache, usually combined with nausea and vomiting, is the rule. In a child with an uncomplicated concussion this period lasts for only a couple of hours or days. If complications, such as an intracranial bleeding, oedema due to contusion of the brain, or reactivation of a previously arrested hydrocephalus, occur, the patient's level of consciousness falls, respiration and circulation become impaired, and neurological signs may appear. A head trauma may, although seldom in childhood, be followed by more persistent headache (*see* pages 255 and 320).

Viral infection

Many viral infections are accompanied by headache, which persists after the disappearance of the fever. If the patient has a stiff neck and an increased cell count in the cerebrospinal fluid, the headache is obviously due to viral meningitis or meningoencephalitis. The same clinical picture may appear in patients without a stiff neck and with insignificant or no increase in the cell count. It is debated whether this condition should be ascribed to encephalitis without meningitis. An abnormal electroencephalogram (EEG), particularly if the abnormalities change and disappear within a few months, supports a diagnosis of encephalitis. This condition is usually benign and is only seldom followed by more persistent headache (*see* page 320) and other neurological and mental symptoms.

Sudden elevation of intracranial pressure

An acute elevation of intracranial pressure may be seen in acute meningitis (*see* page 343) and in subarachnoidal bleeding (*see* page 318). A tumour or an abscess usually produces more prolonged headache with a less abrupt onset. However, bleeding in a tumour or an abscess or a sudden blockage of the outflow of cerebrospinal fluid may cause acute symptoms. A small stalked tumour, which previously has given no symptoms, may suddenly block the aqueduct and cause increased intracranial pressure of peracute onset. This situation may also occur intermittently (*see* page 364) and with changes in the position of the head.

BENIGN INTRACRANIAL HYPERTENSION

In the condition termed benign intracranial hypertension, or pseudotumour cerebri, the raised intracranial pressure is due neither to an inflammation of the meninges nor to a space-occupying lesion. Headache and vomiting develop over a couple of days; on examination papilloedema is found, and occasionally also bilateral sixth nerve palsy and ataxia. In childhood this condition may arise as a complication of otitis media, particularly if it is inadequately treated; the term otitic hydrocephalus is occasionally used. A cerebellar abscess (*see* page 361) produces a similar clinical picture; a differential diagnosis between these two conditions is urgent (*see below*). Benign intracranial hypertension may also be seen after a viral meningitis, e.g. polio. It is a rare but characteristic complication of steroid treatment in childhood; it is particularly common when long-term therapy (several months or more) is suddenly interrupted. Exceptionally, benign intracranial hypertension occurs for no apparent reason.

A diagnosis of benign intracranial hypertension is difficult to establish on clinical grounds alone. When this diagnosis is suspected, it is advisable to perform computerized tomography of the skull to exclude a space-occupying lesion or an active hydrocephalus with increased width of the lateral ventricles. For a diagnosis of benign intracranial hypertension there must be no evidence of a space-occupying lesion and the ventricular system must be of normal or small size.

If a cause, such as otitis media, can be identified it is treated. The elevated intracranial pressure must be reduced, otherwise there is a high risk of secondary optic atrophy with permanent visual impairment. Treatment with steroids in a high dose is virtually effective but it may be very difficult to wean the patient from it without causing a relapse of symptoms. Repeated lumbar punctures may lower the intracranial pressure, but the effect is short-lasting. If these measures fail, a ventriculoperitoneal shunt (*see* page 252) or a subtemporal decompression may be considered.

Sinusitis

In sinusitis symptoms usually develop over a few days, but the onset may be acute. The headache is usually frontal, increases towards the afternoon, and is combined with signs of a common cold, low-grade fever, and an increased sedimentation rate; X-ray examination of the sinus reveals the cause.

Persistent headache of more insidious onset

Anaemia

Anaemia of various causes, including uraemia, produces fatigue and persistent headache. The symptoms may increase slightly towards the evening but the variation during the day is small.

Elevated blood pressure

Elevated blood pressure exists also in childhood and can produce headache, which may increase slightly towards the afternoon but is as a rule fairly even during the day. Blood pressure measurement is too often neglected in the examination of children; it should preferably be part of the general examination of children as well as of adults, and particularly so in a child with headache. Hypertension in childhood is usually caused by renal disease, coarctation of the aorta, or an endocrine disorder.

Refractive error

A refractive error may be one part of a complex cause of persistent headache which increases if the child has to concentrate on work at a short distance. A mild degree of hypermetropia is physiological in childhood and is easily compensated by accommodation. If the hypermetropia is more pronounced, the constant effort to accommodate may be a strain to the child and thus cause headache. Myopia and astigmatism may cause the child difficulty in seeing the blackboard, for example, and thus impair his ability to follow the teaching; tension headache (*see* page 322) may be produced in this way. Correction of a refractory error may thus be part of the treatment of headache in childhood.

Postconcussion syndrome

Postconcussion complaints may occur but are rare in childhood. The headache produced increases in warm noisy surroundings, particularly if the patient has to concentrate on work at the same time; it is combined with fatigue and irritability. The patient improves if he is allowed to work at his own speed, with nobody hurrying him, in coolish and quiet surroundings, but in reality it is often difficult to provide him with such an environment. A period of rest followed by slowly increasing demands usually improves the symptoms. Drug therapy is seldom of value; sedatives, particularly barbiturates, may worsen the condition. If EEG abnormalities are present, antiepileptic drugs (*see* page 112) may be of value. Some patients improve on a drug from the chlorpromazine or diazepam group or on an antidepressant drug, e.g. imipramine 10–25 mg two to three times a day. The prognosis is generally good. Almost all patients become symptom-free within several months to a few years. If the patient is examined within a couple of months after the trauma, it is essential to exclude a complication such as subdural haematoma. This complication of a head trauma is rare in childhood, but it does exist.

Other cerebral lesions

A similar clinical picture may arise after other types of cerebral lesion, e.g. encephalitis or operation for a brain tumour. The patient's complaints, the management, and the prognosis are the same as described for postconcussion syndrome (*see* page 320).

Space-occupying lesions

Headache due to increased intracranial pressure often, although not invariably, shows a typical variation during the day. It is worst during the early morning hours, when it may even wake the patient. It improves towards afternoon, and the patient may feel fairly well in the evening. The headache is often combined with vomiting which occurs mainly in the early morning hours before breakfast. On examination, possible findings due to the increased intracranial pressure *per se* are elevated blood pressure, decreased pulse rate, stiff neck, papilloedema, bilateral sixth nerve palsy, stretched sutures, and decalcification of the back wall of the sella turcica; however, all of these signs are not usually present in every patient. The most common cause of such findings in childhood is a tumour of the posterior fossa (*see* page 364); other types of space-occupying lesions, e.g. an abscess, and other localizations are also possible. A clinical suspicion of a space-occupying lesion is an indication for computerized tomography of the skull.

Intermittent headache

Besides acute headache due to fever, intermittent headache is the most common type of headache in childhood. Periods of hours or days with headache alternate with symptom-free intervals lasting for days, weeks, or months. The symptoms have usually persisted for months or years before the child is brought to the doctor.

Costen's syndrome

Costen's syndrome is due to malocclusion of the teeth, causing an arthrosis of the jaw-joint. The significance of this syndrome as a cause of headache is debated; it is probably small in childhood. If the dentist finds an indication of this dental anomaly, it does no harm to correct it.

Vascular malformation

A malformation of an intracranial blood vessel may cause intermittent headache. In childhood an arteriovenous malformation is more common than an arterial aneurysm. Both may cause attacks of headache because of their size or because of small haemorrhages from them. The arteriovenous aneurysm also often produces convulsions and focal neurological signs, as the brain may suffer from localized anoxia due to the direct shunting of the blood from the arterial to the venous side. An intracranial bruit may be heard over an arteriovenous aneurysm. If the arteriovenous malformation is large, it may produce hydrocephalus (*see* page 252), engorged veins on the skull, enlargement of the heart, and cardiac failure. Both arterial and arteriovenous malformations may cause subarachnoidal bleeding as their most serious complication. In many cases these malformations can be treated neurosurgically; a correct diagnosis as early as possible is therefore desirable. An arteriovenous aneurysm may definitely be suspected on clinical grounds; the local brain damage may also often cause EEG abnormalities. An arterial or arteriovenous aneurysm may, if large enough, be diagnosed on computerized tomography of the skull, but an arteriogram is usually also necessary. Treatment is surgical.

Intermittent elevation of intracranial pressure

A stalked tumour of the third ventricle may intermittently block the passage through the aqueduct and cause an acute and intermittent elevation of intracranial pressure; peracute attacks of severe headache thus occur, often combined with vomiting, and occasionally with an impaired level of consciousness. The attacks may be provoked if the head is kept in a certain position and may be relieved if this position is changed. This is a rare cause of intermittent headache, which is difficult to diagnose and easily mistaken for migraine. Examination during an attack may reveal increased blood pressure and decreased pulse rate as evidence of the elevated intracranial pressure; papilloedema is seldom present. Examination between attacks usually reveals no abnormalities. Computerized tomography of the skull is the best way to demonstrate the tumour. Lumbar puncture is dangerous and must not be done.

A steadily growing tumour of the posterior fossa may also cause intermittent symptoms (*see* page 364).

Tension headache

In childhood, as in adulthood, tension headache is probably the most common kind of headache. The headache is intermittent, intensifying during periods of increasing stress and subsiding during vacations and other periods of diminishing stress. It is seldom present in the morning, appears during school hours, and disappears again in the evening when the child has had time for food, rest, and play. Nausea and vomiting are not part of the clinical picture. The most common cause of the stress is a discrepancy between the child's academic ability and his own or his parents' ambition for his career at school. Hereditary factors probably play a great role in the patients' disposition to develop tension headache.

On examination, tense muscles may be found in the neck and at the temples. Complete general and neurological examination reveals no other abnormalities, neither does an EEG. A refractory error may be found on eye examination, which is normal in all other respects.

The best treatment is to explain the condition to the patient and to try to get him to adjust realistically to his situation. A reassuring description of the benign nature of the condition, given both to the patient and to the parents, is of great therapeutic value. The headache may diminish if the patient is trained to relax his tense muscles by a physiotherapist. This training is important as the headache may recur, perhaps together with other symptoms of tension, when the patient is subjected to unavoidable stress. The type of reaction and the sensitivity to stress is individual and lifelong; it is of great help to the patient to know how to cope on his own with his stress-induced, benign but unpleasant symptoms. Relaxation may be more effective if it is combined with a short introductory period of treatment with diazepam. On the whole, however, drugs have no place in the management of this condition and should be avoided, particularly in children.

Migraine

Migraine is another common cause of headache in childhood. In older children the clinical picture is the same as in adults with headache as the chief complaint, but symptoms and signs are different in small children. One type of symptom may follow another in the same patient; if an older child with headache is suspected to have migraine, the mother should be asked specifically about typical manifestations of migraine in earlier childhood. Migraine is inherited, probably as an autosomal dominant trait. Thus, if a child has migraine, one of the parents and other members of the family usually also have it. Because of the high incidence of migraine in the general population, however, the fact that migraine runs in the family does not prove this diagnosis in a child with headache.

MANIFESTATIONS OF MIGRAINE DURING THE FIRST TWO YEARS OF LIFE

A child of this age cannot describe his symptoms. The earliest sign to suggest an attack of migraine is ophthalmoplegia. Attacks of ophthalmoplegia due to migraine may occur in infants less than a year old. In practically all cases of ophthalmoplegic migraine the first attack has occurred during infancy or early childhood. The attack of ophthalmoplegia, which usually comes on suddenly and involves the muscles innervated by the third nerve on one side, may last from a few hours to a few weeks, usually several days. It is accompanied by obvious discomfort, pallor, nausea, vomiting, and possibly bellyache and/or headache.

MANIFESTATIONS OF MIGRAINE IN TODDLERS AND PRESCHOOL CHILDREN

These are usually attacks of bellyache and vomiting. The attacks come on for no apparent reason, and the child is obviously uncomfortable, pale, and nauseated. The vomiting may be persistent and cause ketoacidosis. The attack may last from an hour to a couple of days, usually a few hours, and end with several hours of deep sleep, after which the child awakes recovered. Ophthalmoplegic attacks may also be seen in this age-group, either as the first evidence of migraine or in a child who previously has had ophthalmoplegic attacks or attacks of bellyache. A child of 5–6 years of age may start to complain of headache, but abdominal pain and vomiting usually dominate the clinical picture.

MANIFESTATIONS OF MIGRAINE IN SCHOOLCHILDREN

In the age-group 7–10 years the clinical picture slowly changes from predominant abdominal discomfort to predominant headache. The headache comes on suddenly for no apparent reason, is not usually strictly one-sided, and is practically always accompanied by nausea and vomiting. Other vegetative symptoms may also be noted such as perspiration, pallor, and diarrhoea. Teenagers may describe visual aura as flickering spots or lines or scotomata, but younger children seldom report such an experience, even when they are carefully questioned. The attack may be accompanied by other neurological symptoms, e.g. hemianopsia (often described by the child as impaired vision in one eye), localized paraesthesia, hemiplegia, and aphasia. Ophthalmoplegic attacks may also occur in this age-group (*Figure 14.1*). The whole attack usually lasts for several hours. During the attack the patient wants to be left alone in a coolish, darkened, and quiet room. After he has vomited

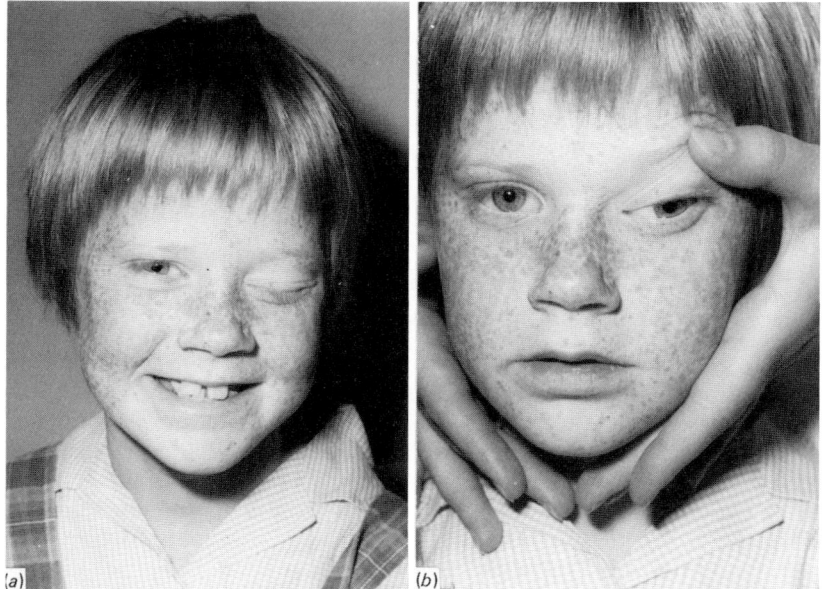

Figure 14.1a and *b*. A 10-year-old girl during her third attack of left-sided ophthalmoplegic migraine

a few times, he usually falls asleep and awakes recovered after several hours. The attacks may occur almost daily or at intervals of weeks or months. The patient usually has periods of frequent attacks alternating with periods, perhaps lasting several months, when he has only a few attacks.

Examination in an attack-free interval reveals nothing abnormal. Negative neurological and ophthalmological findings are necessary for the diagnosis, which is based on the typical history alone; this must therefore be taken very carefully. The EEG gives no specific diagnostic help. It is often normal but may be abnormal in about a third of the patients; temporal abnormalities provoked by sleep are often seen.

The most important differential diagnosis is between migraine and malformation of an intracranial blood vessel. This possibility, though rare compared with migraine, must be considered in all children with migraine-like headache. The suspicion increases if the patient has ophthalmoplegic attacks, particularly if they recur on the same side, or attacks accompanied by other neurological signs such as hemiplegia. In this situation computerized tomography of the skull is indicated. It may reveal an arteriovenous aneurysm, if large enough, and the brain atrophy surrounding such a lesion. An aneurysm is better demonstrated on an arteriogram, but this examination carries a certain risk and the indication for it must be more definite.

The rare possibility of a stalked tumour suddenly blocking the aqueduct and thus causing acute attacks of severe headache and vomiting must also be considered (*see* page 319).

An acute migraine attack in childhood can usually be treated simply and effectively with salicylate 0.25–1 g, possibly combined with caffeine 50 mg. The effect is better if the medication is given as soon as the attack starts. The patient should therefore be provided with a few tablets, which he knows he can take immediately wherever he may be, including school. The child's very knowledge that he carries with him something that may help often has a beneficial influence on the attacks. In older children salicylates alone are usually not enough, and a specific antimigraine preparation, e.g. a combination of ergotamine, an antiemetic drug (often an antihistamine), and caffeine, has to be given. This preparation must be given in a fairly large dose at the very onset of the attack to have the best effect; the dose must be determined individually and in most teenagers is half to two-thirds of the adult dose. Because of the great tendency to vomiting, a suppository is often the best way to administer the drug, but difficult for the child to handle on his own.

Many children with migraine respond to long-term treatment with antiepileptic drugs, particularly phenytoin and carbamazepine. They must be given in the same dose and for the same length of time as for epilepsy. It is possible that children with EEG abnormalities respond better than those without, but children with a normal EEG may also improve with this treatment. Another drug recommended for the prophylaxis of migraine attacks is propranolol in a dose of 20–40 mg three to four times a day. It has a direct effect on the blood vessels, which makes it particularly useful in children with migraine attacks accompanied by neurological symptoms and signs. Its unpleasant, but not dangerous, side effect is sleep disturbance and nightmares. A serotonin antagonist may also be tried. Cyproheptadine in a dose of 2–4 mg two to four times a day for a 3-month period is suggested as the drug of choice. It may cause drowsiness but only rarely has more serious side effects. This side effect has a tendency to disappear in spite of continued therapy and should not provoke the immediate interruption of treatment. Methysergide may be more effective, but its side effect, retroperitoneal fibrosis, is too serious to justify its use in childhood except in a rare and extremely severe case. If this dangerous drug is used, the duration of treatment must not exceed 3 months, and must be followed by a period of at least 3 months during which the patient is kept free of medication.

The evaluation of long-term therapy for migraine is always difficult as the disease fluctuates spontaneously and the patients show a high incidence of placebo response. In controlled double-blind studies, both carbamazepine and propranolol have proved more effective than placebo in reducing the number and severity of migraine attacks. Most children do not need long-term treatment for migraine; the disease is so benign that there is almost no justification for using any of these drugs if side effects occur. It is important that children with migraine live a fairly regular life with enough sleep, regular meals, and not too much stress. If the attacks steal much time from school and play, a trial period of drug treatment for a few months is justified; its effect should then be evaluated and the treatment stopped if it is ineffective or if side effects are more unpleasant than the attacks.

The long-term prognosis is fairly good, as at least 50% of children with migraine who have been restudied 15–20 years after the original diagnosis appear well or considerably improved.

Overuse of salicylates

The overuse of salicylates in all forms may *cause* headache. The patient then enters a vicious circle: he takes salicylate for his headache but the drug causes more headache. Careful questioning on this point is important, as the patient may not be aware of the mechanism and may not regard salicylate as a medication. Measurement of the serum level of salicylate is useful in establishing the diagnosis. Treatment consists of explaining to the patient the nature of the vicious circle he is in, and convincing him that he must reduce, and preferably stop, the use of the drug.

Horton's vascular headache or cluster headache

This usually starts in young adulthood and is more common in males than in females. It may, however, also be seen in childhood, particularly in youngsters at or around puberty; its appearance in young childhood is known down to the age of 4 years, but it is rare in such a low age. The headache usually starts during the small hours of the night and wakes the patient up. It is localized to the temple and around the eye and is usually so severe that the patient yells out loudly. It continues for 10–20 minutes and then subsides, only to recur 10–30 minutes later. After 4–8 attacks they subside and the patient is free of pains but tired for the rest of the day. Next morning the attacks recur in the same way. During an attack the patient usually has ample secretion from the mucous membrane of the nose on the same side as the headache and the eye on that side is red, running, and injected. The period of daily attacks usually lasts for 1–4 weeks; towards the end of this period the patient may have pains only every second morning. The patient may have only one series of attacks in his life, or they may recur from 6 months to several years later; the number of attacks during a patient's life-time is quite unpredictable.

The diagnosis is established from the history, if possible supplemented by clinical observation during the attack; no special studies are helpful. It is also important that the paediatric neurologist knows of the existence of the disorder, as many unnecessary studies may otherwise be performed in a case of Horton's headache. The condition is extremely uncomfortable but is not in itself dangerous. The treatment is symptomatic, and includes analgesics and all drugs used in the treatment of migraine (*see* page 325).

Management of the child with headache

The general clinical and neurological examination should also include measurement of blood pressure, eye examination, and simple laboratory tests to exclude anaemia and chronic renal disease. Lumbar puncture must be performed in all cases in whom there is a suspicion of meningitis (due to bacterial, viral, or fungal infection, or to blood or leukaemic infiltrations); lumbar puncture must not be done if there is a suspicion of increased intracranial pressure. The indications for performing an EEG are wide. Computerized tomography of the skull should be performed in selected cases and an arteriogram on strict indications. Salicylates are usually adequate as symptomatic treatment in childhood, but the physician must also warn against overuse. In older children with migraine, specific drugs, of the same composition as used in adults, are often necessary. Long-term treatment with phenytoin, carbamazepine, propranolol, or a serotonin antagonist may reduce the suffering in children with migraine.

References

BILLE, B. (1962) Migraine in school-children. *Acta Paediatrica* (Uppsala), suppl. 136

BILLE, B. (1982) Migraine in childhood. *Panminerva Medica Europa Medica,* **24,** 57–62

BILLE, B., LUDVIGSSON, J. and SANNER, G. (1977) Prophylaxis of migraine in children. *Headache Journal,* **17,** 61–63

CONGON, F. J. and FORSYTHE, W. I. (1979) Migraine in childhood; a study of 300 children. *Developmental Medicine and Child Neurology,* **21,** 209–216

EGGER, J., CARTER, C. M., WILSON, J., TURNER, M. V. and SOOTHILL, J. F. (1983) Is migraine food allergy? A double-blind controlled trial of oligo-antigenic diet treatment. *Lancet,* **ii,** 865–869

HJERN, B. and NYLANDER, I. (1964) Acute head injuries in children. Traumatology, therapy and prognosis. *Acta Paediatrica* (Uppsala), suppl. 152

KOCH, C. and MELCHIOR, J. C. (1969) Headache in childhood. A five year material from a pediatric university clinic. *Danish Medical Bulletin,* **16,** 109–114

MILLICHAP, C. G. (1959) Benign intracranial hypertension and otitic hydrocephalus. *Pediatrics,* **23,** 257–259

15

Malformations of the nervous and the muscular systems

Congenital malformations play a great role in producing neurological symptoms and signs, which are occasionally progressive, in infancy and childhood.

Malformations of the brain and the cranium

ANENCEPHALY

Anencephaly (acrania or exencephaly) is a severe malformation of the brain and the skull, which is immediately apparent at birth. Its incidence, which varies in different parts of the world, is higher in the West than in the East and is higher in a cold than in a warm climate. Some authors have postulated an infectious aetiology, among other factors, because of a seasonal variation, with an increased incidence of anencephaly among 'summer conceptions' (in the northern hemisphere); others have denied such a variation. A genetic factor seems to have some influence, as the risk of having an anencephalic child increases from about 0.5–5:1000 up to about 1:30 if the sibship already contains affected children. The aetiology and pathogenesis of this malformation are probably not the same in all cases.

The child is born with a defective convexity of the skull, and a severely malformed brain is exposed or covered only by a thin membrane (*Figure 15.1*). The cerebral tissue is badly disorganized; the brain stem and the basal ganglia are usually better preserved than the hemispheres. The neurohypophysis is usually absent; the adenohypophysis may be developed, although it is often abnormally situated.

The neck is usually short, the tongue sticks out of a narrow oral cavity with a high palate arch, and the eyes protrude (*Figure 15.2*). Other malformations of the central nervous system may be present. Adrenal abnormalities are the rule and malformations of other organs, e.g. hypoplasia of the lungs, are often seen.

Because of the fairly well-preserved basal structures these infants may survive for up to a couple of weeks, although most of them die within a few days. No therapy is possible.

ENCEPHALOCELE AND CRANIUM BIFIDUM

A defective closure in the midline of the skull is called cranium bifidum. If the dura is strong enough to prevent herniation through the skeletal defect, and if no

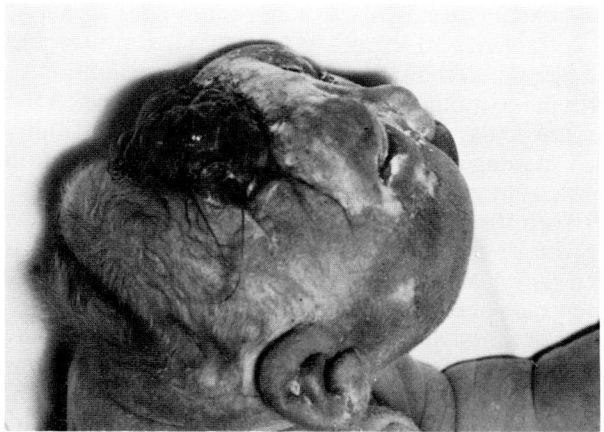

Figure 15.1. A newborn infant with a large cranial defect and an exposed malformed brain

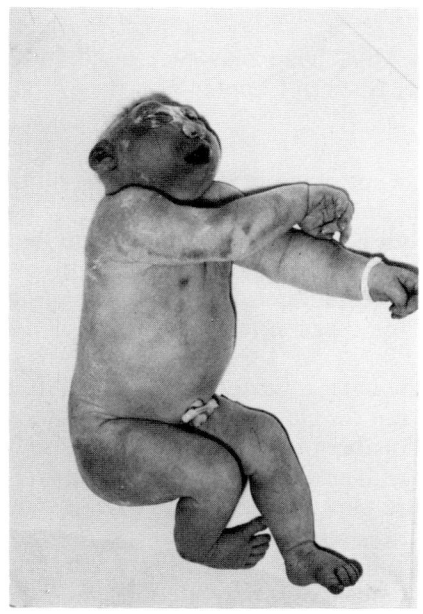

Figure 15.2. A newborn infant with a large cranial defect. Note the protruding eyes and the small size of the cranium, contrasting with the otherwise fairly well-developed face, limbs, and body

connection exists between the skin and the meninges (*see* page 330), the skeletal defect *per se* has no clinical significance. A hernia may occur, containing only meninges (a meningocele) or meninges and cerebral tissue (an encephalomeningocele). These hernias may be found anywhere in the midline; their most common localization is in the occipital area and thereafter in the frontal region or at the root of the nose.

An encephalomeningocele may vary in size from very small, producing no symptoms except the cosmetic effect, to large, perhaps larger than the skull. A small encephalomeningocele may be mistaken for a lipoma or an atheroma; a large one causes no diagnostic difficulties. If the hernia is large and contains brain tissue, the whole of the brain is usually malformed.

All meningoceles and encephalomeningoceles, particularly large ones localized in the occipital region, carry a certain risk of exposure to trauma, rupture, and infection. They should therefore be operated on as soon as the child's condition so allows. All operations on a growth in the midline of the skull or face, even when the primary diagnosis is a lipoma or atheroma, must be performed with the possibility of a meningocele in mind. Small meningoceles have a good prognosis. Children with a large encephalomeningocele seldom develop normally.

An incomplete separation between the skin and the intracranial structures may be associated with defective closure of the skull, and a thin string or channel, a *dermal sinus,* may thus connect the skin with the dura. A dermal sinus easily becomes infected and may be the cause of repeated attacks of purulent meningitis. Its opening, which is usually in the occipital area, may be difficult to detect; it may be necessary to examine the area, after it has been shaved, with a magnifying lens to find the opening. A dermal sinus should be operated on during a period when it is not infected in order to prevent further attacks of purulent meningitis. The opening may also be in the midline of the back (*see* page 337).

ABNORMAL GROWTH OF THE HEAD

Both an abnormally small and an abnormally large head may be caused by a primary malformation. These conditions are described in Chapter 9.

HYDRANENCEPHALY

Hydranencephaly is a severe malformation of the entire brain, which is turned into a large cyst, lined with ependyma and with only a small amount of or no disorganized cerebral tissue in the wall; the skull is intact. It is debated whether hydranencephaly should be considered a primary malformation or the result of a destruction, e.g. by the sudden impairment of circulation during fetal life, of an originally normally developed brain; it is possible that the mechanism is not the same in all cases.

The infants appear normal at birth and the neonatal reflexes are present. After some weeks it becomes apparent that they are not developing normally, and they are not starting to fix or follow with their eyes. An abnormal increase in head size is the rule, as hydranencephaly is often associated with elevated intracranial pressure. Transillumination (*see* pages 7–8) shows a diffuse glowing of the whole head. The electroencephalogram (EEG) may be isoelectric or reveal small areas of brain activity. Computerized tomography of the skull outlines the severe cerebral malformation. No therapy is possible. Most patients die during infancy.

PORENCEPHALIC CYST

A porancephalic cyst may be a primary malformation or caused by localized brain destruction due to prenatal or perinatal impairment of the cerebral circulation. Symptoms may not be evident until during the child's second half-year, when signs of hemiparesis and, occasionally, hemianopsia appear. The child may also have seizures and be slightly retarded in his development. If the fluid within the cyst is under pressure, the skull may become asymmetrical (*see Figure 9.3,* between pp. 100–101). The symptoms produced by a porencephalic cyst depend on its size and localization.

If the cyst reaches the cerebral surface it can be demonstrated on transillumination, which then reveals a localized zone of abnormal illumination.

Focal abnormalities are often found on the EEG. Computerized tomography of the skull reveals the defect.

The treatment is symptomatic (*see* page 234). The prognosis depends on the extent of the brain destruction.

AGENESIS OF THE CORPUS CALLOSUM

Agenesis of the corpus callosum may occur as an isolated malformation or together with other malformations within the central nervous system, e.g. hydrocephalus or malformation of the cerebellum, or outside the central nervous system, e.g. cleft lip and palate; it may also be part of a syndrome due to a chromosomal aberration, e.g. trisomy 13–15 or 17–18. It is also an obligate part of Aicardi syndrome (*see below*).

The diagnosis is established through ultrasound examination or computerized tomography of the skull, which shows the absence of the septum pellucidum and an upward dislocation of the third ventricle between the lateral ventricles, which are more widely separated than in normal individuals. The clinical symptoms that lead to the diagnostic procedures are usually convulsions, abnormal growth of the head, and mental retardation. Agenesis of the corpus callosum has been found at autopsy in individuals who during life have had no known symptoms from the central nervous system.

Symptomatic treatment should be given (*see* Chapter 4, 5, and 9); the malformation *per se* cannot be treated. The prognosis probably depends more on the complicating abnormalities than on the agenesis of the corpus callosum.

AICARDI SYNDROME

This syndrome affects only girls and may occur in sisters. The likely explanation is inheritance due to a sex-linked dominant gene which is lethal during fetal life in the male. Symptoms start with infantile spasms (*see* pages 88–92) when the girl is 3–9 months of age. Slow psychomotor development is usually apparent, even before the start of the fits, and mental retardation becomes more obvious as the child grows older. Eye abnormalities, mainly choreoretinopathy with depigmented zones in the epithelium, but also coloboma, iris synechiae, and micro-ophthalmia, together with agenesis of the corpus callosum and vertebral malformations are the typical features of the syndrome. The fits are treated as outlined in Chapter 4 (*see* page 117). The prognosis is poor and mortality is high during early childhood.

CYST OF THE SEPTUM PELLUCIDUM

A cyst of the septum pellucidum is an anomaly of no practical significance, occasionally found on computerized tomography of the skull. No treatment is necessary.

ABNORMAL DEVELOPMENT OF THE CEREBRAL GYRI

A reduction in the number of cerebral gyri (pachygyria) down to a completely smooth cortical surface (lissencephaly or agyria, *Figure 15.3*) is seen only rarely. This malformation, if severe, causes mental retardation and convulsions. An increased number of abnormally small gyri (micropolygyria, *Figures 15.4* and *15.5*)

332

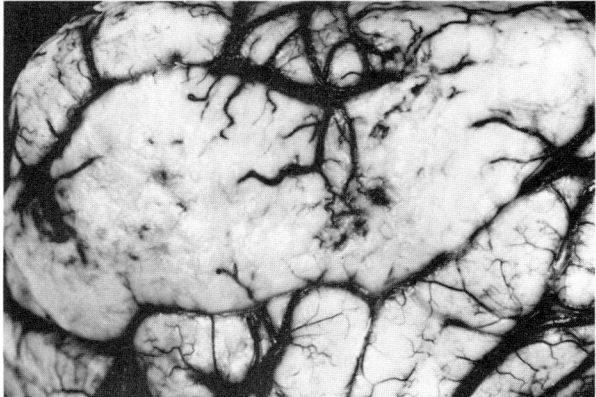

Figure 15.3. Agyria. Note the complete lack of convolutions in the central part of the picture, contrasting with the normal gyri in the lower third of the picture

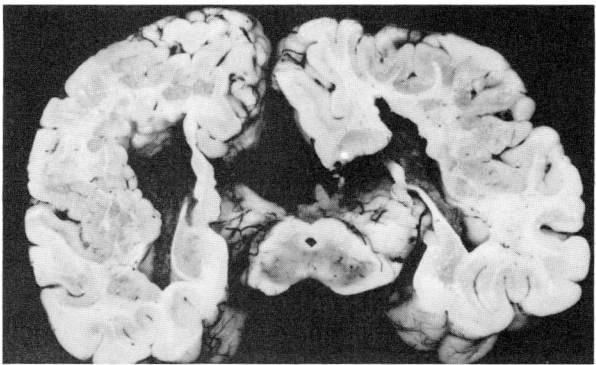

Figure 15.4. Micropolygyria (section through the parietal lobes). In the upper part of the picture note the small close-set, abnormal convolutions, and in the white matter the abnormally placed grey areas which reach into the ventricular system as polypoid formations; compare with the essentially normal gyri in the basal parts of the temporal lobes, in the lowest part of the picture

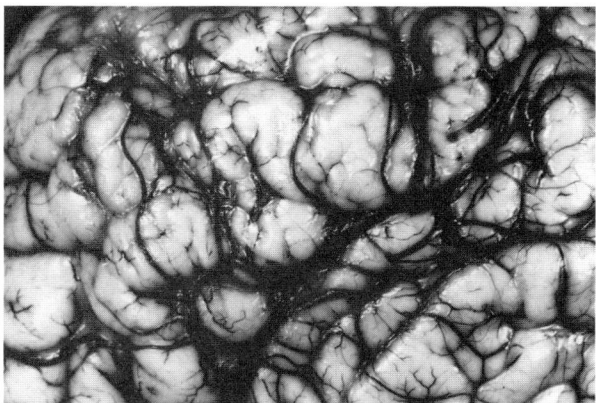

Figure 15.5. Micropolygyria. Note the frontal operculum with small, close-set, irregular convolutions in the central part of the picture; compare with the essentially normal gyri of the temporal lobe in the lower right corner of the illustration

is a more common malformation. It may cause seizures and mental retardation. Computerized tomography of the skull may reveal some nonspecific cortical abnormalities, but is often normal. An exact diagnosis can only be established at operation or autopsy. The treatment is symptomatic.

CEREBELLAR HYPOPLASIA

Cerebellar hypoplasia is a fairly common malformation. It may cause either no symptoms or ataxia that is present from an early age. It is part of the Dandy–Walker syndrome (*see* pages 250–251).

VASCULAR MALFORMATIONS

Malformations of intracranial blood vessels may cause convulsions (*see* page 98), abnormal growth of the head (*see* page 252), and headache and subarachnoidal bleeding (*see* page 318).

Malformations of the spine, spinal cord, and nerve roots

The most common and clinically most important type of malformation is incomplete separation and closure of the posterior structures; it occurs most commonly in the lumbosacral region and thereafter in the cervical region. The term spinal dysraphism covers all of these disorders. The severity of this defect of separation and closure varies.

SPINA BIFIDA OCCULTA

Spina bifida occulta means an incomplete closure of one or more vertebral arcs with no herniation of meninges or nervous tissue and intact skin covering the defect. Such a cleft in the first sacral vertebra alone is a common finding of no clinical significance. Under a differently localized or more extensive spina bifida occulta there may be a dysplasia of the cord and the nerve roots, and this may cause neurological symptoms, which may be progressive (*see* pages 337–338). If the neural tissue is malformed there is often, though not invariably, an abnormality of the skin, e.g. a tuft of hair (*Figure 15.6*), a haemangioma, or a deep indentation (not a shallow dimple, which is a common finding and unrelated to malformation of the nervous system). The most common localization of such abnormalities is the lumbosacral area.

Spina bifida occulta with myelodysplasia in the cervical region is an unusual malformation which may cause symptoms from the arms and hands, such as weakness and impaired sensation of varying severity, depending on the extent of the cord lesion. Similar symptoms are often present in cases of syringomyelia, a condition which might be classified as a malformation of the spinal cord (*see* page 393). In myelodysplasia the crossing of the cortisospinal tracts is often affected, causing incoordination of movements of the hands, e.g. mirror movements – one hand involuntarily makes the same movement as that performed intentionally by the patient with the other; mirror movements cause difficulties for the patient e.g. at the table or climbing a ladder. Severe mirror movements are a serious handicap,

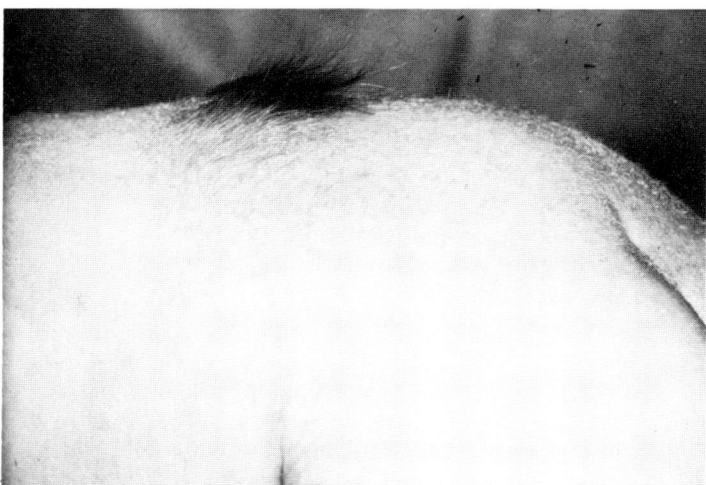

Figure 15.6. A tuft of hair in the lumbar area of a newborn girl. This girl had a diastematomyelia for which she was operated on at the age of 7 months

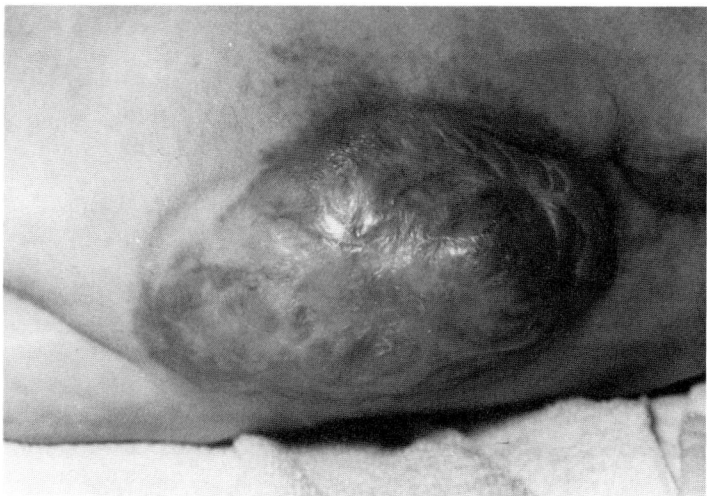

Figure 15.7. An unoperated myelomeningocele in an infant a few months old

impairing all activities that require the use of the two hands together. For further discussion of spina bifida occulta in the lumbosacral region with malformation of the nervous tissue *see* pages 337–339.

SPINA BIFIDA CYSTICA

Spina bifida cystica means a herniation of meninges and neural tissue through the skeletal defect (*see Figure 3.15,* page 56). The hernia may contain only meninges, a meningocele, or both meninges and neural tissue (a myelomeningocele; *Figure 15.7*). A meningocele may be covered by skin, whereas a myelomeningocele is at birth almost always covered only by a thin membrane which may rupture and provide a route of entry for infection. Spina bifida cystica is always apparent at birth on inspection of the child.

The incidence of spina bifida cystica is usually estimated to be 1–4:1000 newborns. The incidence appears to be particularly high in the western part of the United Kingdom and low in Japan. As in anencephaly, a genetic factor probably plays a role, since the risk of a child being born with spina bifida cystica increases if a previous child in the family has already been born with this defect.

Meningocele

A simple meningocele, which is a rare condition, usually causes no neurological signs, at least not in the newborn period. However, there is usually some dysplasia of the neural tissue, even when the hernia contains only meninges, and neurological symptoms may eventually develop. The most common localization of a meningocele is the sacral region and thereafter the cervical region. If the localization is sacral, incontinence and difficulty in emptying the bladder completely can be expected; if the localization is cervical, symptoms may appear from the arms and hands (*see* page 333).

Myelomeningocele

A myelomeningocele is a severe malformation of nervous tissue, and neurological signs below a certain cord level are already apparent in the newborn period. The most common localization is the lumbosacral region, and the neurological signs usually extend up to the L2–L3 level. This means a flaccid paralysis of all leg muscles except the hip flexors (iliopsoas), loss of sensation in the legs, and impaired innervation of the sphincters with urinary and faecal incontinence and usually an inability to empty the bladder completely. The pelvic floor is lowered and the anus is displaced anteriorly and gaping. Occasionally the myelomeningocele is in the thoracolumbar region, in which case all the hip muscles and the lower abdominal muscles are also involved. If the localization of the lesion is at a lower level there is better preservation of the function of hip muscles and knee extensors. If the localization of the lesion is even further down, only the function of the sphincters and some foot and lower leg muscles may be affected. Symptoms are bilateral but seldom strictly symmetrical.

If the lesion is left unoperated the thin membrane will usually rupture, leading to meningitis and the death of the child. A few children survive and in them the lesion may become covered by skin; nevertheless, neurological symptoms usually progress and more function is lost in the legs. This is due to drying and infection of the sac with further damage to the neural elements. An early operation thus not only gives the child a better chance of survival but also the chance of survival with less neurological deficit. Spina bifida cystica should therefore be operated on within the child's first 2 days of life. No antibiotic therapy is then necessary, which is another advantage of an early operation.

Figure 15.8 shows the skin-covered lesion in an unoperated child with weakness and atrophy of the hip, pelvic, and leg muscles and malposition of the left foot.

The first complication occurring in a child with an operated myelomeningocele is usually hydrocephalus. Approximately 80 per cent of all children with a lumbar or lumbosacral myelomeningocele develop signs of hydrocephalus, and most of them do so within the first few weeks of life. The usual cause of hydrocephalus in these cases is an Arnold–Chiari malformation (*see* page 252), which may, although

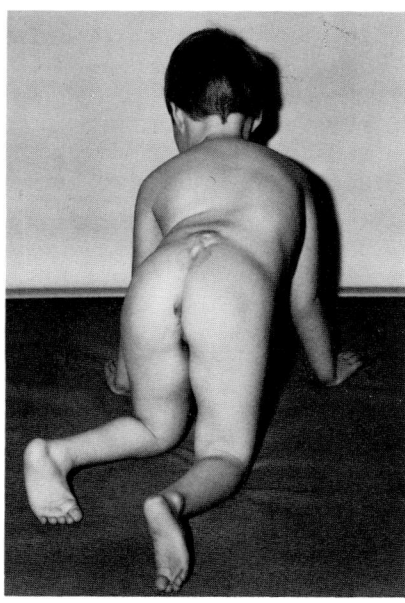

Figure 15.8. A 6-year-old girl with an unoperated myelomeningocele. Note the weakness and atrophy of the buttocks and legs and the abnormal posture of the left foot

rarely, be seen in patients without a myelomeningocele. The management of hydrocephalus is discussed in Chapter 9 (pages 252–255).

The second postoperative problem is paralysis and deformities of the legs. Physiotherapy should be started early. The children are stimulated to perform as much active movement as they can with their legs, and passive movements are used to prevent the deterioration of present contractures and the development of new ones. The more severely paralysed are the legs, the more important it becomes to train the shoulder and arm muscles also, as the children's ability to walk with the help of technical aids depends on the strength of these muscles. The physiotherapist must be aware of the child's lack of sensation in the feet. The child must also be taught as early as possible to be careful with his feet and to avoid ulcerations.

Orthopaedic measures are important in helping the patient to learn to walk and should be combined with physiotherapy. Attempts must never be made to correct these paralytic deformities by forcible splints, traction, or serial plasters, as such measures are ineffective and can cause damage, e.g. pressure sores and fractures. Surgical correction of the deformities by division of soft tissue, followed by appropriate tendon transplantation, is the primary need. When the deformities have been corrected, night splints to maintain the corrected position and calipers and irons to support flail or weak joints are used after individual testing. With the best possible care and training about 80 per cent of children with myelomeningocele learn to walk.

The third problem arising in children with myelomeningocele involves the urinary tract. About a quarter of these children have a primary malformation of the urinary tract. Practically all other affected children have impaired innervation of the urinary bladder, causing incontinence and difficulty in emptying the bladder completely. Incontinence is a severe social handicap. Some children may be trained to reasonably good bladder control through manual emptying of the bladder at regular intervals during the daytime. If this method fails, the child and/or his parents are taught to empty the bladder with the help of a clean unsterile catheter at regular intervals. Many children learn to master this technique which is a great help to them. Stagnation of the urine always leads to urinary tract infection and often to the formation of stones, dilatation of the urinary tract, and eventually impaired renal function. Children born with a myelomeningocele must be watched for urinary tract infection, and urological operations may become necessary.

Incontinentia alvi may also be a problem. This social handicap can often be diminished by teaching the child to evacuate his bowel once or twice a day by manual pressure on the lower abdomen. As both diarrhoea and obstipation increase the patient's difficulties in controlling the bowel, the diet must be properly balanced and laxatives used with judgement and caution.

A diet sufficiently low in calories must be started as early as possible to prevent the patient becoming obese. Because of his paralysed legs and lack of activity, a child with a myelomeningocele needs less calories than a healthy child of the same age, and a heavy child is more difficult to mobilize.

The prognosis for most children born with spina bifida cystica must be judged as serious. Without therapy most of them die during childhood from meningitis, hydrocephalus, or renal failure. Early treatment will prevent the described complications and, in combination with continuous medical attention and technical help, diminish the child's problems, but no child born with a myelomeningocele will grow up entirely free of a handicap. In Scandinavia few of these children have a mental handicap. The severity of the physical handicap varies, depending mainly on the extent and level of the malformation; roughly 80 per cent of Scandinavian children (the majority of whom have a lumbosacral myelomeningocele) learn to walk independently with or without aids, but only few walk and run normally.

Prenatal diagnosis is possible in most cases of myelomeningocele and hydrocephalus. A myelomeningocele usually gives an abnormally high level of alpha-fetoprotein in the amniotic fluid. Hydrocephalus may be demonstrated on ultrasound examination of the pregnant uterus; this method may in some cases also reveal a malformation of the back.

DERMAL SINUS

A dermal sinus may have its opening in the midline of the back, most commonly in the sacral region and occasionally in the cervical area. Its aetiology, symptoms, complications, and treatment are the same as when its localization is the cranium (*see* page 330).

LIPOMENINGOCELE

A lipomeningocele is a rare condition which, in the newborn infant, resembles a soft skin-covered meningocele (*Figure 15.9*). Neurological signs are absent or insignificant in the young infant. However, the lipoma grows, and the intermingled nervous tissue becomes stretched when the lower end of the cord moves upwards in relation to the spine during the growth of the infant. Slowly progressive symptoms therefore appear from the legs and the urinary bladder (*see* page 338). This malformation should be operated on early, preferably around 6 months of age, to prevent the development of progressive symptoms. The operation is difficult because the nervous tissue is so intermingled with the lipomatous tissue that removal of the latter without causing damage to the neural structures can only be achieved through very careful dissection.

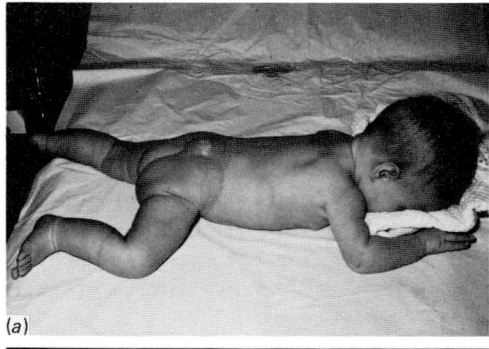

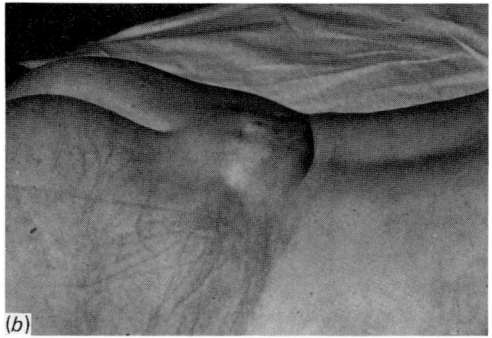

Figure 15.9a and *b*. A 6-month-old girl with a lipomeningocele. Note the skin-covered dimpled protuberance in the lumbosacral area

AGENESIS OF THE SACRUM

Agenesis of the sacrum implies a severe disturbance of the function of the sacral roots, which are often entirely absent. This defect causes incontinence and often also an inability of the patient to empty the bladder completely. The diagnosis can be established on X-ray examination of the lower back. The malformation *per se* cannot be treated; the complications from the urinary tract require the same management as myelomeningocele (*see* page 336).

OTHER MALFORMATIONS OF THE LOWER CORD AND CAUDA EQUINA

Diplomyelia, diastematomyelia, and tight filum terminale are all malformations of the lower part of the cord and the cauda equina, which are often, though not invariably, connected with spina bifida occulta and a tuft of hair over the lumbosacral region. A lipoma or a haemangioma may be present over the neural malformation. In diplomyelia the lower part of the spinal cord is doubled; in diastematomyelia it is divided into two portions by a bony or fibrocartilaginous spicule that arises from the vertebral body and transfixes the cord; the tight filum terminale attaches the lower end of the cord to skeletal structures. The symptoms produced are due to the hindrance of the normal cranial migration of the cord in relation to the spine during the growth of the infant, leading to impaired blood circulation and pulling on the nerve roots with impairment of their function.

Neurological signs are absent or insignificant at birth but usually develop during early childhood. They consist of flaccid weakness of certain muscle groups in the feet and legs, variable sensory disturbances, which occasionally include pains in the legs, and impaired control of the urinary bladder. The muscle imbalance causes deformities of the feet; pes equinovarus, pes calcaneus, and pes cavus are most commonly seen. The symptoms that bring the patient to the doctor are usually gait disturbances, commonly difficulties in learning to walk, with or without deformities of the feet. Medical advice is most commonly sought when the patients are a few years of age. The findings are usually bilateral, although not symmetrical. Other early symptoms, caused by impaired innervation of the urinary bladder, are recurrent urinary tract infection and incontinence. A child presenting with any of these symptoms, and particularly with a combination of them, should have his back carefully examined both clinically and radiologically (*see* page 56). If there is a reasonable suspicion of a malformation in this area, computerized tomography of the back or a myelogram must be performed.

The treatment of these conditions is neurosurgical. All adhesions are removed, and a bony or fibrocartilaginous spicule, when present, is excised. Little or no improvement can be expected after the operation, but the further progression of symptoms is prevented. A correct diagnosis is therefore desirable as early as possible.

SPINA BIFIDA ANTERIOR

Spina bifida anterior is a rare malformation. A defect is present in the vertebral bodies, through which meninges and neural structures can herniate forwards. In the sacral region the hernia consists of a meningocele, which often produces no symptoms, unless it is so large that it causes mechanical difficulties at delivery. In other regions there is, as a rule, severe malformation of the spinal cord which causes various neurological symptoms. Other malformations, e.g. rib deformities or malformations of the lungs or the gastrointestinal tract, may also be present. Treatment is only seldom possible.

Malformations of the peripheral nerves

An anomaly of the course of a peripheral nerve or of connections between peripheral nerves is a rather common occurrence of no clinical significance. Only when a peripheral nerve is damaged (e.g. by trauma) does an abnormal course of the nerve or a connection between nerves become important for the interpretation of neurological findings and neurophysiological measurements.

Malformations of muscles

The absence of extraocular and facial muscles, Möbius' syndrome, is described in Chapter 8, page 222.

Congenital absence of the abdominal muscles, known as the prune belly syndrome, may occur as an isolated phenomenon, causing a bulging abdomen and some impairment of respiration; it is often combined with malformation of the lower urinary tract. Such abnormalities should be looked for in a patient with congenital absence of the abdominal muscles.

A congenital defect of the diaphragm may cause a displacement of abdominal content into the thoracic cavity. The usual symptom in the newborn is respiratory distress. The diagnosis can be established on a chest X-ray; urgent surgical treatment is needed.

Congenital absence of one or more skeletal muscles, most commonly the major pectoral muscle, may occur. This produces mild cosmetic problems (*Figure 15.10*) but only exceptionally causes any significant difficulties. The condition is benign and nonprogressive and needs no treatment.

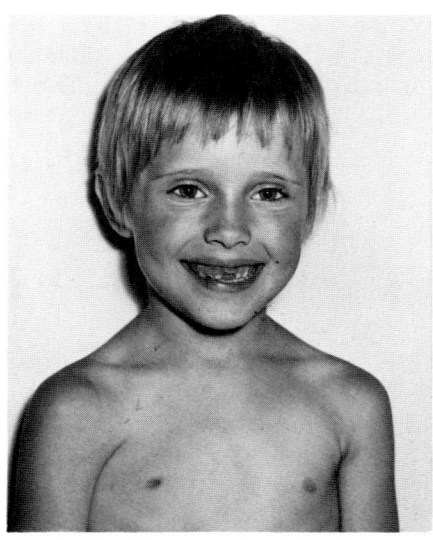

Figure 15.10. A 7-year-old girl with congenital aplasia of the right major pectoral muscle

Arthrogryposis multiplex congenita is a clinical syndrome characterized by deformities of several joints (*Figure 15.11*), already present in the newborn infant. The condition can be regarded as prenatally arising contractures of a few or many joints, due to the impaired ability of the fetus to move normally, e.g. paralysis of one or several muscle groups. Dislocation of the hips, as well as foot deformities, are often seen; any joint may be involved, and the severity of the joint involvement varies. The localization of the primary cause also varies. The condition may be due to an extensive lesion of the upper motor neurones, the lower motor neurones, the peripheral nerves, the muscles, or the joints; the onset is prenatal in all cases.

The cause should be localized as far as possible with the help of clinical neurological examination, X-ray examination of the joints and of the soft tissue of the limbs, examination of the spinal fluid, measurement of the conduction velocity of the peripheral nerves, electromyography, and histological examination of a muscle biopsy specimen (*see* pages 165–169). The treatment consists mainly of physiotherapy and orthopaedic measures. The prognosis depends on the extent of the lesion and its aetiology.

Management of the situation around a newborn infant in whom a malformation is apparent immediately after birth

The diagnosis of a malformation in a newborn infant creates more problems than those related to the medical management of the infant. The parents must be informed, and this information starts in them a series of emotional reactions, which basically consist of grief for the loss of the expected healthy infant and a struggle to receive the infant with a malformation, which they did not expect. In the medical staff around the family the situation arouses feelings of agony, panic, and compassion, mixed with a wish to be free from the duty to inform the parents. It is important that the physician is aware of his own feelings and learns to handle them in such a way that he can be of help to the parents.

The way the first information is given is important for the family's future ability to manage the situation. If the infant needs resuscitation, this need must of course be attended to first. As soon as possible the infant must be brought to his parents,

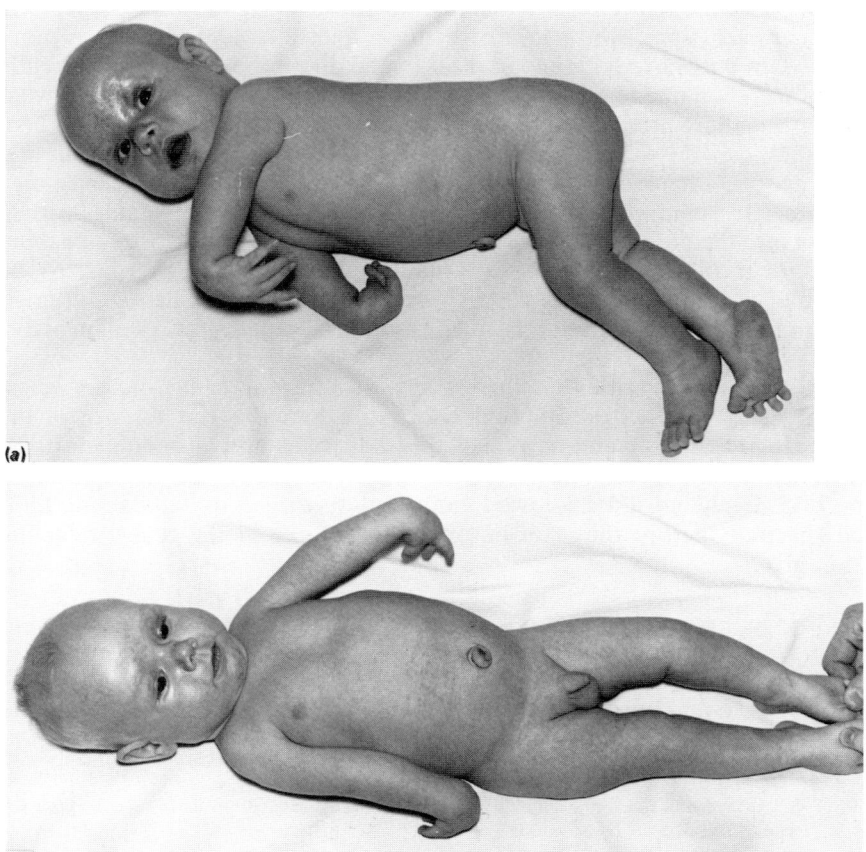

Figure 15.11a and b. A boy with arthrogryposis multiplex congenita and involvement mainly of the arms and hands

who are told without delay about the malformation. The term 'a malformed infant' should never be used as it may to lay-people imply 'a monster'. Instead the term 'a malformation of . . .' is used, indicating a *localized* abnormality of an *otherwise entirely normal child*. Both parents must be present and preferably also the infant. This very first information, given within minutes after delivery, must be short and practical, as the parents at this point are unable to take in much information and unable to think too far into the future. They must be allowed to show their feelings openly. The physician, midwife, and nurse must in their attitude and words show that they find it natural for the parents to see and to handle their infant, even if the infant's malformation is as serious as acrania; if necessary, the parents should be encouraged to have this contact. Reality is never as frightening as the picture imagination may create when one does not know. Reality is also a good starting point for a normal grief process. Photographs should be taken and made available if the parents wish to have them. This is particularly important if the infant is born dead or dies very early. Parents should be encouraged to give their infant a name, even if it is stillborn or dies too early for any name-giving ceremony to take place. A name makes the infant a real person.

The parents must then have daily regular contact with a physician, preferably the same physician each time, who can answer their questions and give them more information when they have had time to react to and digest the information already given. All information must be honest and realistic. The physician must stress what optimistic aspects there are and support the parent's own resources, showing them how much they can do themselves, and not trying to take over their parental responsibility for their child. Both parents must take an active part in the exchange of information. It is impossible for the physician to change the child with a malformation into the parent's expected healthy child, but it is his duty to give them support and help in their grief. The situation requires the physician to be knowledgeable, not only about the child's medical condition but also about crisis reactions, and to have an insight into his own emotions, empathy, and skill in active listening.

The parents of children with a malformation that is insignificant from a medical point of view need some extra attention also. An example is the absence of the pectoral muscle. The physician knows that this defect has only insignificant or no influence on the child's further life, but to the parents a part is missing from their newborn child. They must be allowed time and the right to talk about their emotional reaction, before they can be expected to take in the realistic factual information given.

References

BROCKLEHURST, G., FORREST, D., SHARRARD, W. J. W. and STARK, G. (1976) Spina bifida for the clinician. Clinics of Developmental Medicine No. 57. London: William Heinemann Medical Books

CLARREN, S. K. and HALL, J. C. (1983) Neuropathological findings in the spinal cord of 10 infants with arthrogryposis. *Journal of Neurological Science,* **58,** 89–102

DODGE, P. R. (1961) Congenital neuromuscular disorders. *Research Publications of the Association for Research in Nervous and Mental Disease,* **38,** 479–527

HAGEMAN, G. and WILLEMSE, J. (1983) Arthrogryposis multiplex congenita. *Neuropaediatrics,* **14,** 6–11

JAMES, M. C. C. and LASSMAN, L. P. (1972) Spinal dysraphism. Spina bifida occulta. London: Butterworth & Co

KOLIN, I. S., SCHERZER, A. L., NEW, B. and GARFIELD, M. (1971) Studies of the school-age child with meningomyelocele: Social and emotional adaption. *Journal of Pediatrics,* **78,** 1013–1019

LAGERGREN, J. (1981) Children with motor handicaps. Epidemiological, medical and socio-paediatric aspects of motor handicapped children in a Swedish county. *Acta Paediatrica Scandinavica,* suppl. 289

LAURENCE, K. M. and TEW, D. J. (1971) Natural history of spina bifida cystica and cranium bifidum cysticum. Major central nervous system malformations in South Wales IV. *Archives of Diseases in Childhood,* **46,** 127–138

NAGLO, A. S. and HELLSTRÖM, B. (1976) Results of treatment in myelomeningocele. *Acta Paediatrica Scandinavica,* **65,** 565–569

RECORD, R. G. and MCKEOWN, T. (1949) Congenital malformations of the central nervous system. I. A survey of 930 cases. *British Journal of Social Medicine,* **3,** 183–219

ROBIN, O. and GORCE, F. (1972) Arhinencephalie. Etude clinique, anatomique et etiologique de 13 cas. *Archives Franchaises Pédiatrie,* **29,** 861–879

16

Infectious diseases and immunization

Acute purulent meningitis

Acute purulent meningitis is an acute bacterial invasion of the meninges, usually from the bloodstream and occasionally from a focus near the meninges, e.g. sinusitis, otitis, or spondylitis.

CASES OUTSIDE THE NEWBORN PERIOD

The vast majority of cases occurring in children outside the newborn period are caused by one of three types of bacteria: pneumococci, meningococci, and *Haemophilus influenzae*. Purulent meningitis in children above 6–8 years of age is rarely due to infection with *H. influenzae*, which is the dominating infection in young children, whereas the other two organisms may cause meningitis in all age-groups.

The onset of purulent meningitis is abrupt with high fever, headache, backache, and vomiting; convulsions may occur. The previously healthy child appears seriously ill within a few hours to a day. Examination reveals an acutely ill child with a high fever, often an impaired level of consciousness, a stiff neck, and positive Lasègue's, Kernig's, and Brudzinski's signs (*see Figure 2.15*, page 16); an infant will have a bulging fontanelle, provided he is not dehydrated. Slightly swollen discs may be found on examination of the fundi, but severe papilloedema has seldom had time to develop. If this is present, the diagnosis of uncomplicated meningitis must be doubted and a space-occupying lesion suspected.

A characteristic finding in septicaemia due to meningococci, with or without meningitis, is petechiae and ecchymoses in the skin. Meningitis complicating otitis is often due to *H. influenzae*. An aseptic meningitis, e.g. due to subarachnoidal bleeding or leukaemic infiltration of the meninges (*see* page 317), causes a clinical picture indistinguishable from that of purulent meningitis. A diagnosis of bacterial meningitis or of the type of infecting organism can never be proved on clinical examination alone.

Lumbar puncture must be performed immediately to establish the diagnosis and to get fluid for bacteriological culture. The cerebrospinal fluid, which is under increased pressure and cloudy, contains many cells, most of which are polynuclear; the protein level is elevated and the sugar level is low. In many cases the organism can be identified correctly on a smear, or within several hours by the demonstration of fluorescent antibodies. Specimens must always be taken not only from the spinal fluid but also from the blood and from the nose and throat. The cerebrospinal fluid must be kept warm and be added to the culture medium as rapidly as possible after the lumbar puncture to enhance the chances of obtaining a positive answer; meningococci are particularly sensitive and do not grow out if the spinal fluid is allowed to cool. Treatment with antibiotics, even a single dose, before the lumbar puncture may prevent the bacteria growing out. A false negative culture is found in 5–30 per cent of all cases of purulent meningitis; a negative culture thus never excludes bacterial invasion of the meninges.

As soon as lumbar puncture has been performed and cultures taken, treatment is started without waiting for the results of the bacteriological examinations. Antimicrobial therapy must therefore cover the three likely possibilities and their likely resistance pattern. This may vary with time and between different geographical areas. As soon as the resistance pattern is known, the therapy is adjusted to provide maximum specificity for the infecting organism. Antimicrobial treatment is given for at least 2 weeks and the spinal fluid checked before and after stopping therapy. Intrathecal administration of antibiotics is rarely needed and is permissible only under special circumstances, e.g. when ventriculitis complicates the picture.

Other bacteria, e.g. streptococci, staphylococci, pseudomonas, and salmonella, may be the cause of acute purulent meningitis.

Dehydration must be corrected and water and electrolyte balance maintained. If electrolyte-free solutions are infused, the risk of producing water intoxication and brain oedema is particularly great in cases of acute meningitis. A blood transfusion may be effective, particularly in children with meningococcal septicaemia, haemorrhages, and shock. If the intracranial pressure appears to be dangerously increased, corticosteroids, e.g. dexamethasone 0.5–2 mg four times a day, may be of value. The risk of convulsions is high, and intravenous anticonvulsant therapy (see pages 109–111) must be started at the slightest sign of a fit.

Almost all untreated patients with purulent meningitis succumb. In the early phase of the disease the cause of death is either septic shock or increased intracranial pressure with herniation of the brain stem; it is therefore necessary to prevent and neutralize these factors in the period before antibiotics have had time to influence the situation. If vigorous treatment is started soon after the onset of symptoms the prognosis is fair, as at least 80–90 per cent of the patients survive and only few have permanent sequelae. If treatment is delayed, the risk of a permanent handicap, e.g. cerebral palsy, convulsions, deafness, or impaired mental development, increases considerably. Tiredness and irritation are often observed for several weeks to a few months after a purulent meningitis.

A subdural hygroma (see page 240) may occur within a few days to a few weeks after the onset of a purulent meningitis; it should be suspected in a child who does not recover completely after the infection or has signs of increased intracranial pressure, neurological findings (e.g. hemiplegia), or a persistently abnormal cerebrospinal fluid, particularly an increased level of protein. The diagnosis and therapy of subdural hygroma are discussed in Chapter 9.

CASES IN THE NEWBORN PERIOD

In newborn infants the most common invading organism is a Gram-negative rod, usually belonging to the coli-group. Other organisms seen are beta-haemolytic streptocci group B and *Listeria monocytogenes*; both are acquired from an infection of the mother, who usually has no symptoms. The symptoms of purulent meningitis are vague in the newborn period – impaired general condition with poor, greyish colour, jaundice, feeding difficulties, vomiting, and sometimes fever. The fontanelle is often bulging, and Brudzinski's sign is positive. The clinical diagnosis is difficult, and a lumbar puncture must therefore be performed for a wide range of indications. The findings in the spinal fluid are the same as those in purulent meningitis in other age-groups (*see* page 343).

Treatment must be started immediately and consists of broad-spectrum antibiotics to cover the common organisms and their likely resistance pattern in this age-group. This may vary with time and between different geographical areas. When the invading organism and its resistance pattern are known, the treatment is adjusted to provide maximum specificity for that organism. The newborn infant's ability to metabolize drugs, which differs from that of older children, must be taken into account when the type and dose of antibiotic are chosen. The dose should preferably be monitored by measurement of the drug level in the serum and occasionally in the spinal fluid. Therapy must be continued for at least 2 weeks, and sometimes longer.

Meningitis in the newborn period, although usually followed by complete recovery, carries a higher risk of mortality and permanent sequelae than does purulent meningitis occurring in later childhood. The common sequelae are cerebral palsy, hydrocephalus, subdural hygroma, impaired mental development, and epilepsy. Hydrocephalus and subdural hygromas can be treated neurosurgically (*see* Chapter 9) and epilepsy can be treated medically (*see* Chapter 4).

RECURRENT PURULENT MENINGITIS

If the same child has several attacks of purulent meningitis, a predisposing factor must be suspected. This factor may be general or local. Children with a generally impaired resistance to infection due to a disease of the immunosystem or to immunosuppressive therapy of leukaemia, for example, may contract repeated attacks of purulent meningitis. Possible local factors to be considered are a focus of osteitis, e.g. in a processus mastoideus which has not healed completely during antibiotic treatment; an infected dermal sinus (*see* pages 330 and 337); and a traumatic lesion of the dura with a connection between the subarachnoid space and, for example, the nasal sinus. It is essential to look for such predisposing factors and to treat them in every child who has more than one attack of purulent meningitis or who has an attack which does not respond in the usual way to prompt treatment (*see also* pages 347 and 361–362).

If a child has a history of repeated attacks of meningitis, not proven by characteristic findings in the cerebrospinal fluid, the possibility of repeated subarachnoidal bleeding must be kept in mind (*see* page 318).

Chronic meningitis and meningoencephalitis

TUBERCULOUS MENINGITIS

Tuberculous meningitis is rare in countries with a high social standard for the whole population, rigid control of all individuals infected with tuberculosis, and a programme for BCG vaccination of all infants and children at risk.

The infecting organism is carried by the bloodstream from the primary focus to the meninges; tuberculous meningitis is thus a feature of miliary tuberculosis, although this phase of the disease may give no specific symptoms or signs.

The first symptoms are vague. The child becomes tired and irritable, stops playing, and does not eat. Constipation is a common early symptom. The temperature is subfebrile. After a few days vomiting starts, and the older child complains of headache. The patient starts to squint. The level of consciousness may decrease, and convulsions may occur. On examination a drowsy, irritable, subfebrile child with a stiff neck and evidence of increased intracranial pressure (cracked-pot sound, bilateral abducens paresis, and papilloedema) is found. Examination of the fundi may reveal tuberculous retinochoroiditis. Lung X-ray usually, although not invariably, reveals a primary complex and/or miliary tuberculosis. The tuberculin reaction is of little help; it may be positive, but if the child is ill enough, it is negative.

Examination of the spinal fluid reveals an increased cell count, increased protein content with a cobweb clot, and decreased level of sugar and chloride. No bacteria are found on routine bacteriological examination or culture. The tubercle bacilli may occasionally be found on direct microscopy of the cobweb clot; they can also be cultured on a specific medium. As this takes a few weeks, treatment has to be started before bacteriological diagnosis is established.

The basic of antituberculous treatment is isoniazid (INH), which in a case of tuberculous meningitis is used in a dose of 20–25 mg/kg per day. The occasionally complicating polyneuropathy is prevented by the administration of pyridoxine. All modern treatment schedules contain at least one, and often several, drugs besides INH. The classic antibiotic is streptomycin, used intramuscularly in a dose of 15–30 mg/kg per day. Rifampicin, in a dose of 9 mg/kg per day, is used either as a supplement to this regimen or as a substitute for streptomycin. Ethambutol and pyrazinamide are drugs which may increase the efficiency of the regimen but also increase its toxicity; as a rule, when these drugs are used they are given for periods of 6–8 weeks, regularly alternating with each other or with streptomycin and/or rifampicin. Corticosteroids, e.g. prednisolone 0.5 mg/kg per day, are often added to the regimen in order to diminish the risk of a complicating hydrocephalus. The total duration of therapy should never be less than 1 year.

All untreated children with tuberculous meningitis die within 3–6 weeks after the onset of symptoms. With early, intense, and prolonged treatment most children survive, and the incidence of permanent sequelae is reduced. The mortality can be reduced to below 5 per cent and the incidence of severe handicap to about 10 per cent. However, an early diagnosis is often missed, giving a poorer prognosis; in reality one can expect that of children with tuberculous meningitis one-third will die, one-third will survive with a handicap, and one-third will survive without sequelae.

A complication of tuberculous meningitis is hydrocephalus, which is treated neurosurgically (*see* page 252) after the infection has subsided. Other sequelae are impaired vision due to optic atrophy, hearing defects, cerebral palsy, convulsions, and impaired mental development.

SYPHILITIC MENINGITIS

Syphilis, which in infancy and childhood is practically always congenital, may cause meningitis. The symptoms are variable, ranging from an acute fulminant disease with vomiting, bulging fontanelle, convulsions, and an impaired level of consciousness to no clinical symptoms at all. Syphilitic symptoms and signs from other organs support the clinical diagnosis, but their absence has no diagnostic significance. The spinal fluid contains an increased number of cells, which are mainly mononuclear, and an elevated level of protein, particularly globulins. The serological reactions are positive in the mother and in the child's blood and cerebrospinal fluid. The treatment is penicillin 0.1–0.15 g/kg per day by intramuscular injection for at least 10 days, preferably 3 weeks. If treatment is started early, the prognosis is excellent. Any delay in treatment increases the risk of permanent sequelae such as mental retardation, cerebral palsy, and convulsions. Occasionally the spirochaete is resistant to penicillin; other antibiotics then have to be used, the first choice after penicillin being erythromycin.

The disease can be entirely prevented by examination of all pregnant women and treatment of all syphilitic mothers during pregnancy.

FUNGAL MENINGITIS

Fungi may infect the meninges, usually from a primary focus in the lungs or the tonsils. The symptoms usually have a less abrupt onset than in purulent meningitis, but are otherwise the same, i.e. fever, headache, vomiting, and stiff neck. Lumbar puncture reveals an increased cell count, an elevated protein level and a low sugar level. No bacteria can be identified on direct smear or on routine cultures; the fungi can, however, be cultured on specific media. The possibility of a fungal meningitis must be kept in mind if a patient who appears to have a purulent meningitis does not respond in the usual way to treatment and has no demonstrable bacteria in the spinal fluid.

Fungal meningitis is treated with amphotericin, which is given daily in a dose of 1 mg/kg in an intravenous infusion of 5 per cent glucose over a 6-hour period. Treatment must be continued for 3–6 months. Occasionally, intrathecal administration is also necessary in a daily dose of 10–20 mg; this therapy may have to be continued for up to 3 months. The drug has many side effects, and almost all patients react with headache, nausea, vomiting, and fever. If the patient does not respond or shows severe toxic reactions to amphotericin, fluocytosine may be added or given as a substitute. The standard dose is 0.1–0.2 g/kg per day, given in four divided doses at 6-hourly intervals; preparations are available both for peroral use and for intravenous infusion. The duration of treatment varies from a few weeks to several months. The mortality is still high in fungal meningitis, but treatment as outlined above reduces it from 100 per cent, which is the mortality in untreated cases.

TOXOPLASMA MENINGOENCEPHALITIS

Congenital toxoplasmosis
In congenital toxoplasmosis there is usually meningoencephalitis with an onset in fetal life (*see also* page 125). Examination of the cerebrospinal fluid reveals a moderately increased cell count, a greatly elevated protein level, and a normal or slightly decreased sugar level. Treatment with pyrimethamine 3–6 mg/day and a sulphonamide, e.g. sulfaisodimidine 0.3–0.4 g/kg per day, is recommended but seldom seems to have a great influence on the course of the disease. Another recommended treatment is a combination of trimethoprim 6 mg/kg per day and sulphamethoxazole 30 mg/kg per day (i.e. co-trimoxazole 36 mg/kg per day); the

effect of this treatment is also hard to evaluate. The sequelae are mental retardation, cerebral palsy, convulsions, impaired vision, and hydrocephalus; neurosurgical treatment of the hydrocephalus is recommended in most cases to reduce the brain damage and abnormal growth of the head (*see* page 252).

Acquired toxoplasmosis
This may also cause meningoencephalitis. The symptoms are headache, vomiting, fever, and stiff neck. As a rule the onset is fairly insidious, and the child does not appear to be seriously ill. Lumbar puncture reveals a moderately increased cell count and protein level and a normal sugar level. No organisms can be identified. Rarely the clinical picture is that of acute encephalitis with acute onset, impaired level of consciousness, and severe convulsions; stiffness of the neck and abnormalities of the spinal fluid may be absent. The diagnosis is established on positive serological reactions and the presence of manifestations of the infection, particularly in the eyes, where retinochoroiditis is found. The recommended treatment is the same as for the congenital type. The influence of treatment is debated. The prognosis is usually good, although it takes several months for the child to recover. When severe encephalitis dominates the clinical picture, neurological and mental sequelae may occur in addition to convulsions.

Viral infection of the central nervous system

ACUTE VIRAL MENINGITIS

Acute viral meningitis is a common disease in childhood. The onset is acute, although not as abrupt as in purulent meningitis. A period of fever, vomiting, and diarrhoea or symptoms of a common cold may precede the meningeal symptoms. The patients have fever, headache, vomiting, and a stiff neck; they are usually conscious, and their general condition is only mildly impaired. Convulsions may occur as in all febrile diseases in childhood (*see* page 92); they may also be caused by a complicating involvement of the brain. Examination of the spinal fluid reveals a moderately increased cell count with almost only mononuclear cells (occasionally polynuclear cells may dominate very early in the disease), a normal or slightly elevated protein level, and a normal sugar level; no organisms can be identified.

Many viruses may cause the same clinical picture: viruses belonging to the ECHO and Coxsackie groups appear to be the most common types. Poliovirus is a common cause of viral meningitis in areas where a vaccination programme has not eradicated the virus. In some areas in northern and eastern Europe the tick-transferred virus causing Russian Spring-Summer Encephalitis (RSSE) is a common cause of viral meningitis. Epidemic parotitis is often complicated by meningitis; the same virus may cause meningitis with no signs of parotitis. Poliovirus, in particular, but also Coxsackie and RSSE virus may attack the anterior horn cells and cause a flaccid weakness (*see* page 169).

An aetiologic diagnosis can seldom be established on clinical examination. A specific rise in the serum antibody titre can be demonstrated in several viral diseases during the weeks after the onset of the disease. Occasionally the virus can be cultured and identified from the nasopharynx or from a rectal swab, and very occasionally from the cerebrospinal fluid.

There is no specific treatment for any type of viral meningitis. Good general care, which includes maintenance of nutrition and of water and electrolyte balance and relief of pain, is all that is needed. The permanent sequelae of polio are well-known (*see* page 169). In other types of viral meningitis the prognosis is generally good. Many patients have a prolonged convalescence, when they are tired, irritable, difficult to manage, and have problems at school. It is important that parents and teachers understand and accept the child's difficulties and are aware of their temporary nature. Almost all patients recover completely within 6–12 months after the acute phase of the disease.

HERPES SIMPLEX ENCEPHALITIS

Herpes simplex virus may cause severe, often fatal, encephalitis. The onset is usually abrupt with convulsions, loss of consciousness, and various neurological symptoms, particularly hemiplegia. The onset may be so abrupt that intracranial bleeding is suspected, and death may occur within 24 hours after the onset of symptoms. Blisters on the skin or in the mouth, which suggest infection with herpes simplex virus, may be present or may appear during the course of the disease, but are often absent. Some patients, particularly young infants, may have signs of a disseminated disease such as hepatomegaly. Papilloedema and haemorrhages in the fundi are occasionally found. Signs of meningeal involvement, such as a stiff neck, are often mild or may be entirely absent.

The cerebrospinal fluid may be normal. There is, however, usually mild to moderate pleocytosis and an elevated protein level. In many cases the cerebrospinal fluid is bloody.

The diagnosis is difficult and cannot be proved on clinical grounds alone. A rising antibody titre in the serum is good support for the diagnosis of herpes simplex. The EEG shows severe one-sided abnormalities which are characteristic of herpes simplex encephalitis (*Figure 16.1*); in young infants the EEG abnormalities may be atypical. Computerized tomography of the skull, performed a few days after the onset of symptoms, shows severe oedema, mainly of the temporal lobe (*Figure 16.2*). Later, the oedematous areas become necrotic and eventually cysts will be formed (*Figure 16.3*). Antibodies to herpes simplex virus may be demonstrated in the spinal fluid with the fluorescent technique; the virus may also be cultivated from the spinal fluid. A rise in the serum antibody level indicates that the child has been infected with the herpes simplex virus, but this finding occurs too late to be of help in the management of the patient. Brain biopsy is a direct method of rapidly establishing the diagnosis of herpes simplex encephalitis. Histological examination of the specimen reveals a haemorrhagic necrotizing encephalitis with inclusion on bodies; it is possible to cultivate the virus from the specimen.

The prognosis is poor; mortality is high, as is the incidence of neurological and mental handicap in surviving patients. Treatment consists of an antiviral drug and corticosteroids to diminish the brain oedema, which precedes and causes the necrosis. Antiviral drugs are still experimental but experience is gathering which suggests that those belonging to the arabinose group may be of value if given early in the course. Steroids must be started on a high dose, e.g. dexamethasone 1–4 mg four times a day for several days, and thereafter continued in decreasing dosage. The incidence of fits is high and intravenous anticonvulsant therapy must start at the slightest suspicion of a seizure.

REYE'S SYNDROME

The provoking factor in this syndrome, when it occurs in young children, is an infection of several days duration. The two viruses most commonly associated with

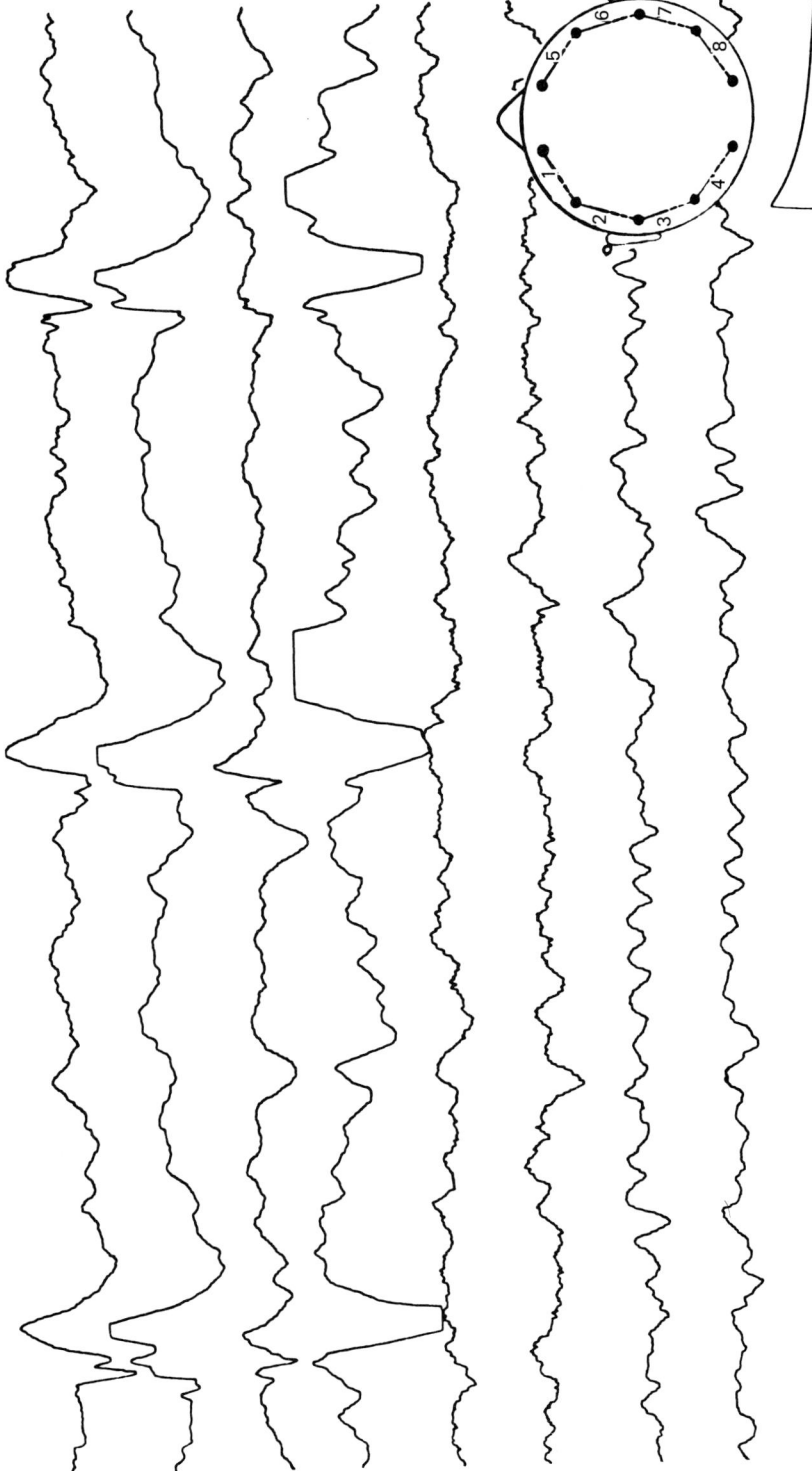

Figure 16.1. The EEG of a 7-month-old child with herpes simplex encephalitis, recorded on the third day after the onset of symptoms

Reye's syndrome are influenza B and varicella. The relationship of other environmental factors and/or genetic predisposition to this syndrome is unclear. Towards the end of the phase of acute infection, vomiting starts and becomes severe, leading to confusion which may deteriorate into delirium and coma. The liver becomes swollen. Laboratory studies show a severely disturbed homeostatis with metabolic acidosis, respiratory alkalosis, hypoglycaemia, and abnormal liver tests, including an elevated ammonia level. The EEG is grossly abnormal. The intracranial pressure is increased.

Treatment consists of intense supportive care. Mannitol infusion to decrease the intracranial pressure, glucose infusions to normalize the blood sugar, vitamin K to prevent bleeding, and assisted ventilation to maintain normal oxygenation and elimination of carbon dioxide are the main features of this regimen. Some physicians also suggest exchange transfusion to remove a postulated toxic factor, mechanical ventilation after pharmacological paralysis of the patient's own respiratory muscles, and high doses of barbiturates to protect the brain against the high intracranial pressure, brain swelling, and a postulated toxic factor. The condition is serious; the mortality in untreated patients, and in patients in whom treatment is begun when they are in deep coma, is close to 100 per cent; it may be reduced to 15–20 per cent by early and intense therapy.

Neurological complications of common infectious diseases and immunizations

Febrile convulsions (*see* pages 92–95) may occur in any infectious disease with fever.

MEASLES

Encephalopathy occurs in about 1–1.5 per 1000 cases of measles. Symptoms usually start 2–4 days after the appearance of the rash; occasionally they begin in the catarrhal stage or at any time up to several days after the disappearance of the rash. The temperature rises again, and the child becomes irritable and drowsy, and may lose consciousness. Convulsions are common and may be difficult to control. Any type of neurological symptoms and signs may occur.

The cerebrospinal fluid generally shows pleocytosis and an elevated protein level, although normal findings do not exclude measles encephalopathy. Severe diffuse EEG abnormalities are usually found (*Figure 16.4*).

The course is variable. Many patients improve within a few days and may eventually recover with no sequelae; the EEG improves (*Figure 16.4*). A few patients die in status epilepticus or from respiratory difficulties in the acute stage, and sequelae (cerebral palsy, disturbed mental development, or convulsions) are seen in some surviving patients. There is no specific treatment; the effect of gamma globulin and steroids is equivocal. The best possible care in the acute stage (intense antiepileptic therapy, the maintenance of free airways, and prompt treatment in a respirator when needed) is important for the prognosis, as some of the residual symptoms may be due to brain anoxia in addition to the measles encephalopathy.

At autopsy a disseminated demyelination is found in the brain. Perivascular cuffs of lymphocytic infiltrations are found in both the grey and the white matter.

Rare neurological complications of measles are a Guillain–Barré syndrome and myositis (*see* pages 175 and 205). Transverse myelitis, causing paralysis and

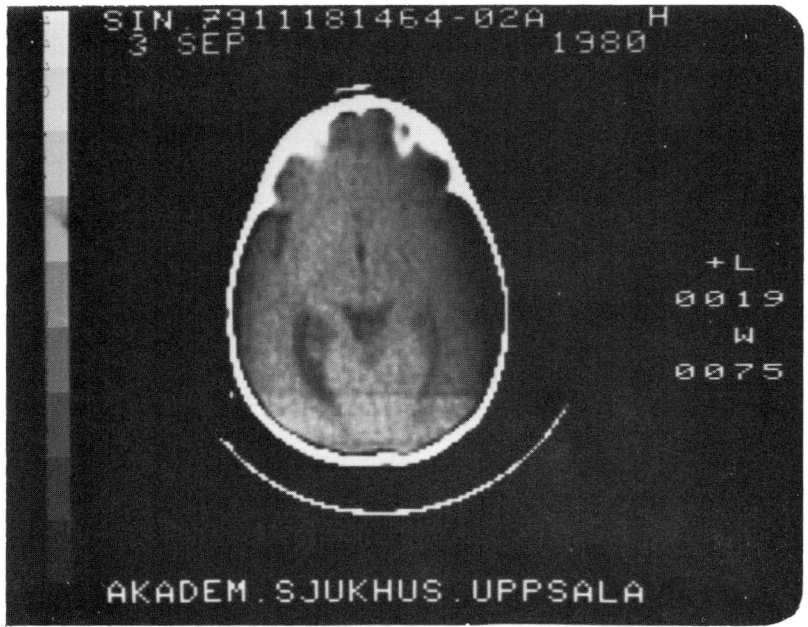

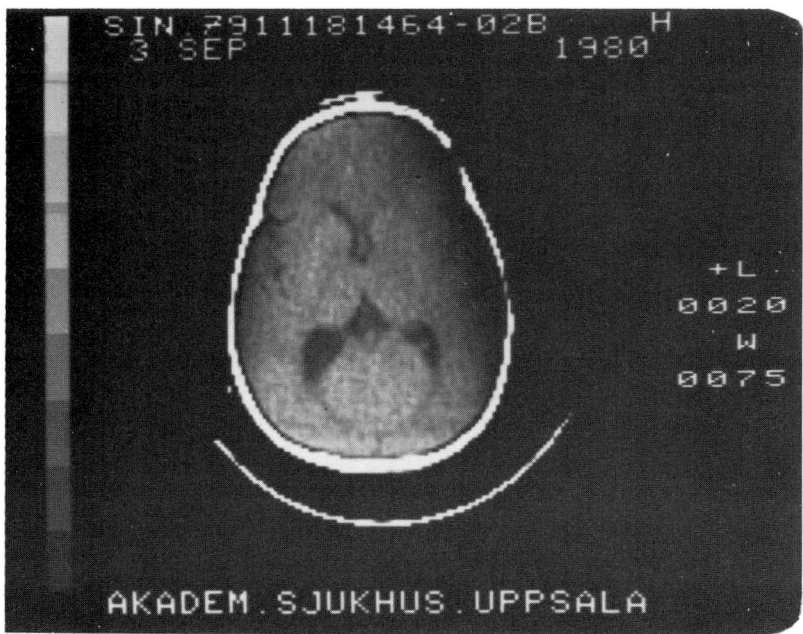

(a)

Figure 16.2. Computerized tomography of the skull of a 10-month-old child with herpes simplex encephalitis, 1 day (*a*) and 1 week (*b*) after the onset of symptoms

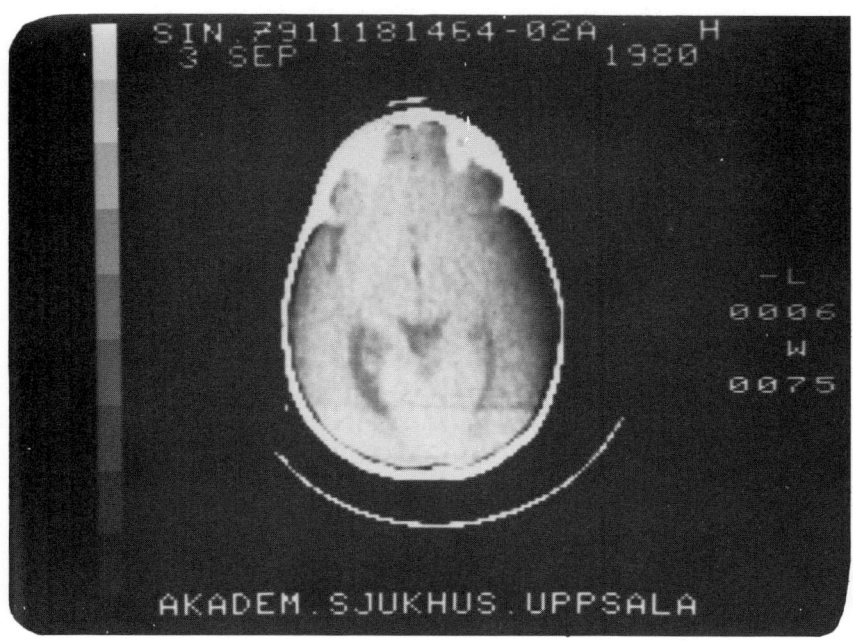

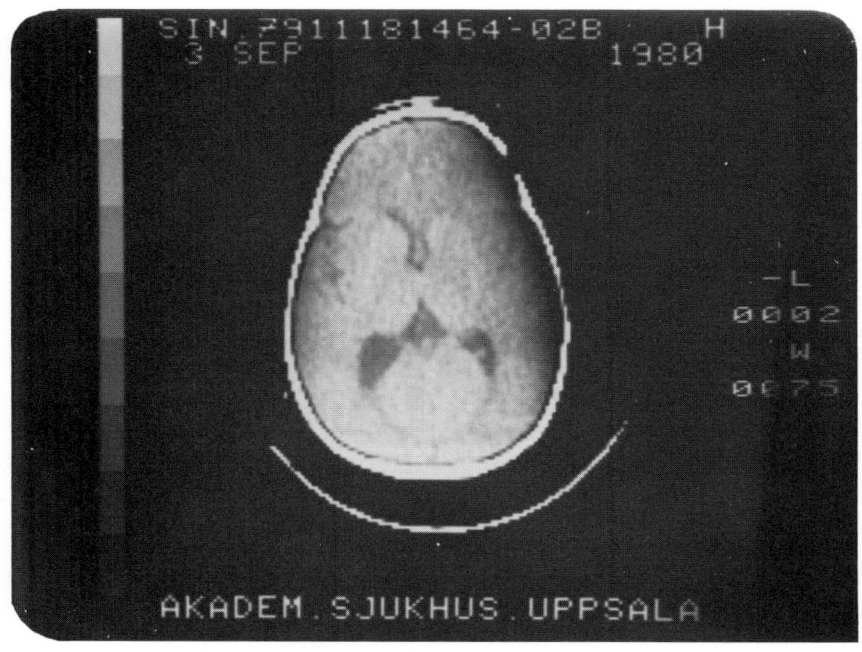

Figure 16.2a (contd)

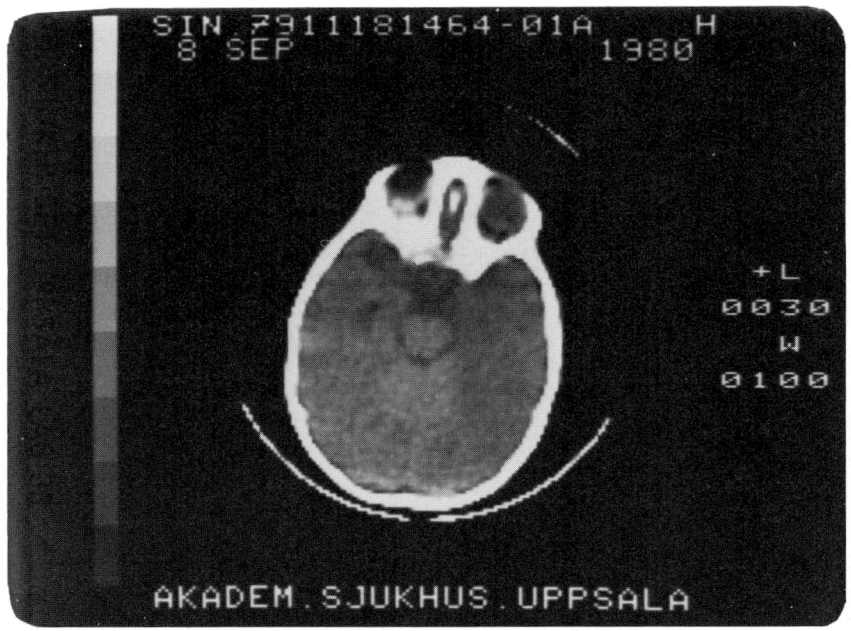

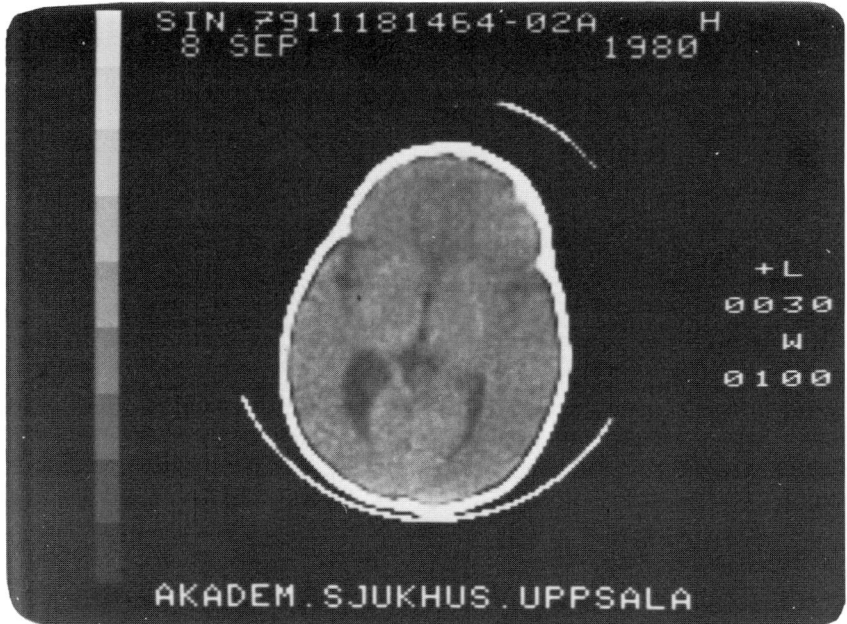

Figure 16.2b (contd)

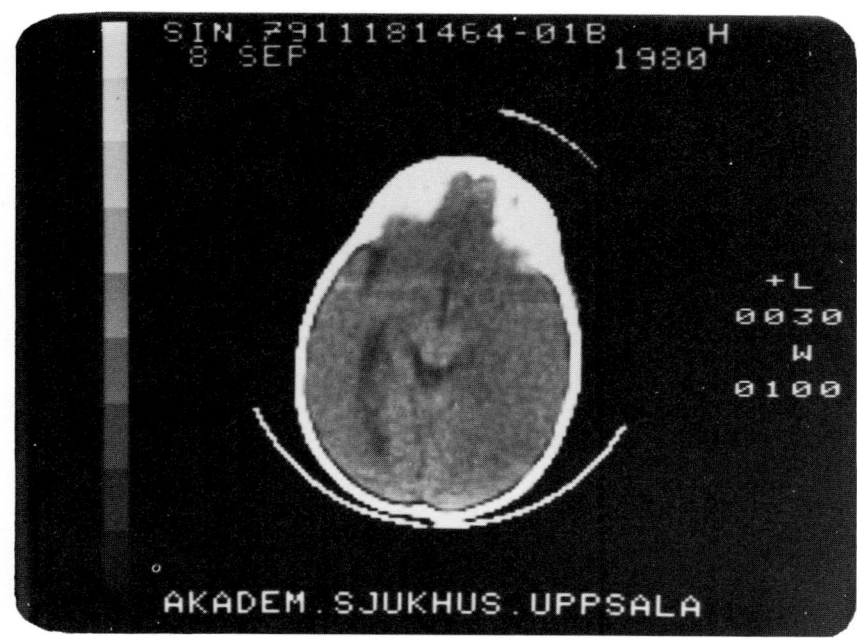

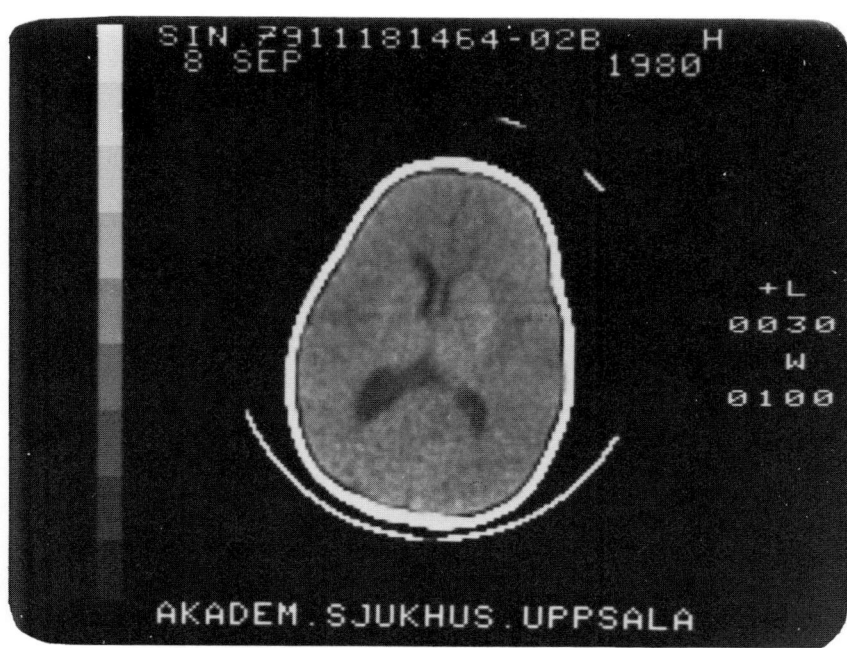

Figure 16.2b (contd)

356

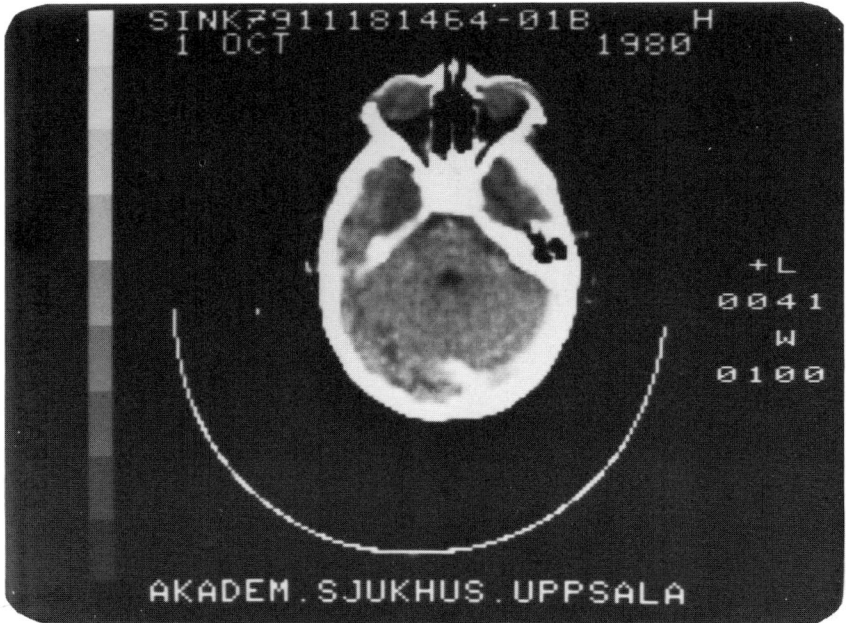

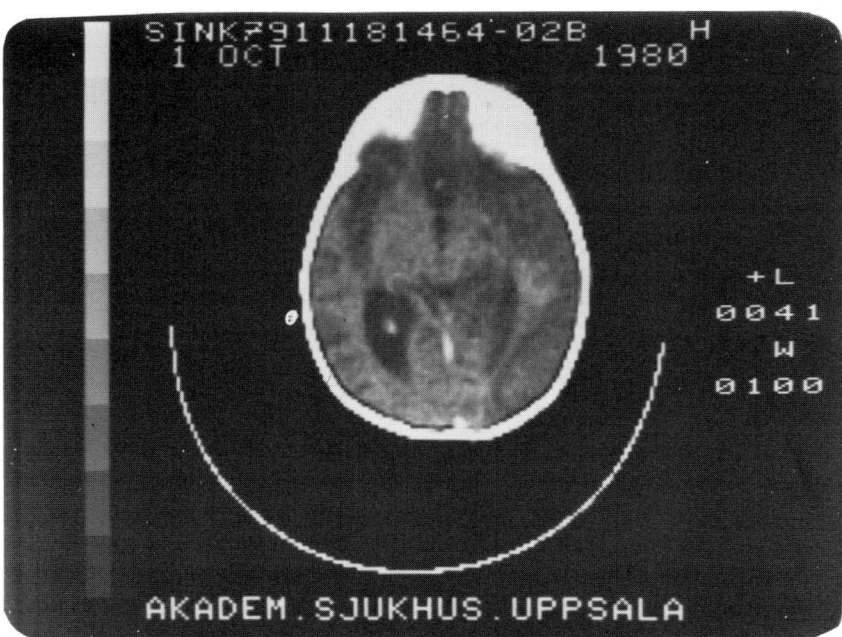

Figure 16.3. Computerized tomography of the skull of the same child as in *Figure 16.2,* approximately 1 month after the onset of symptoms

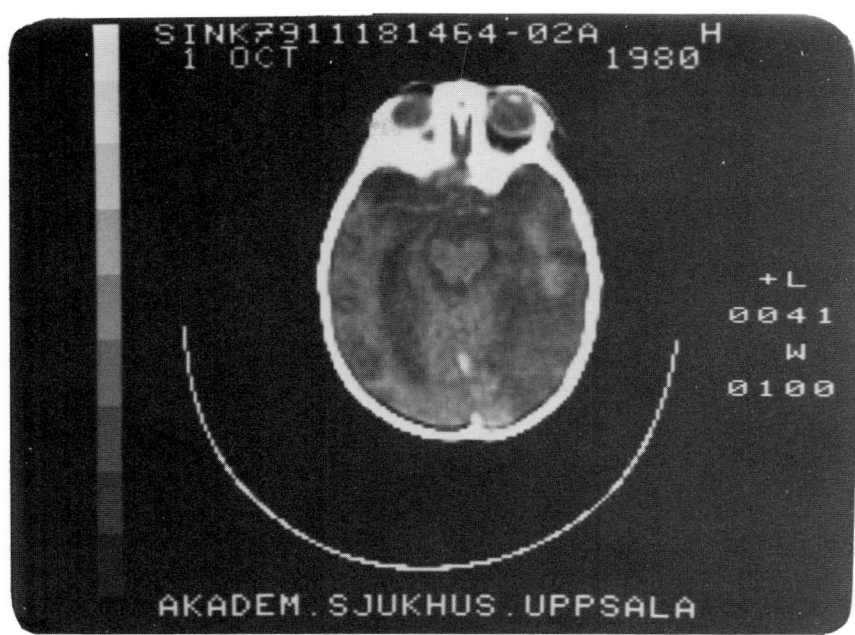

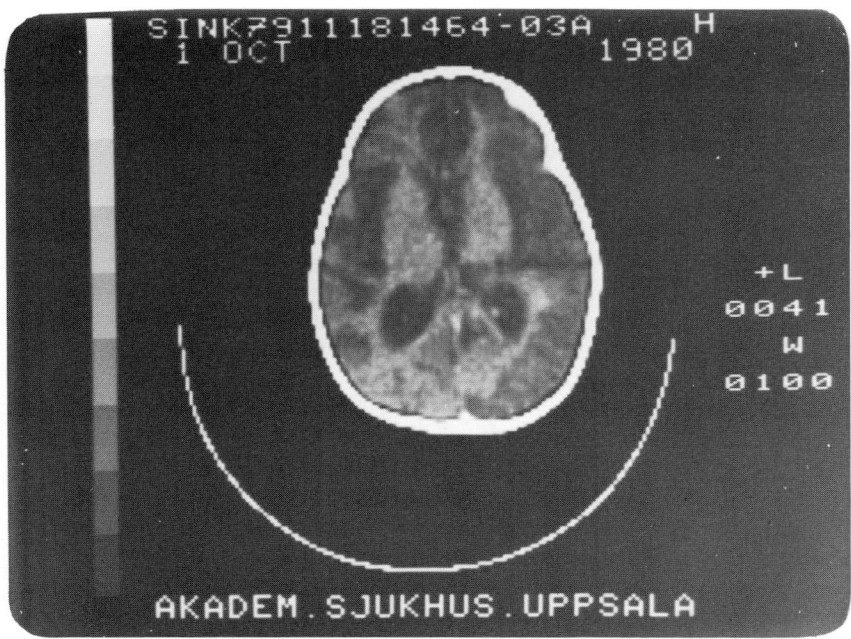

Figure 16.3 (contd)

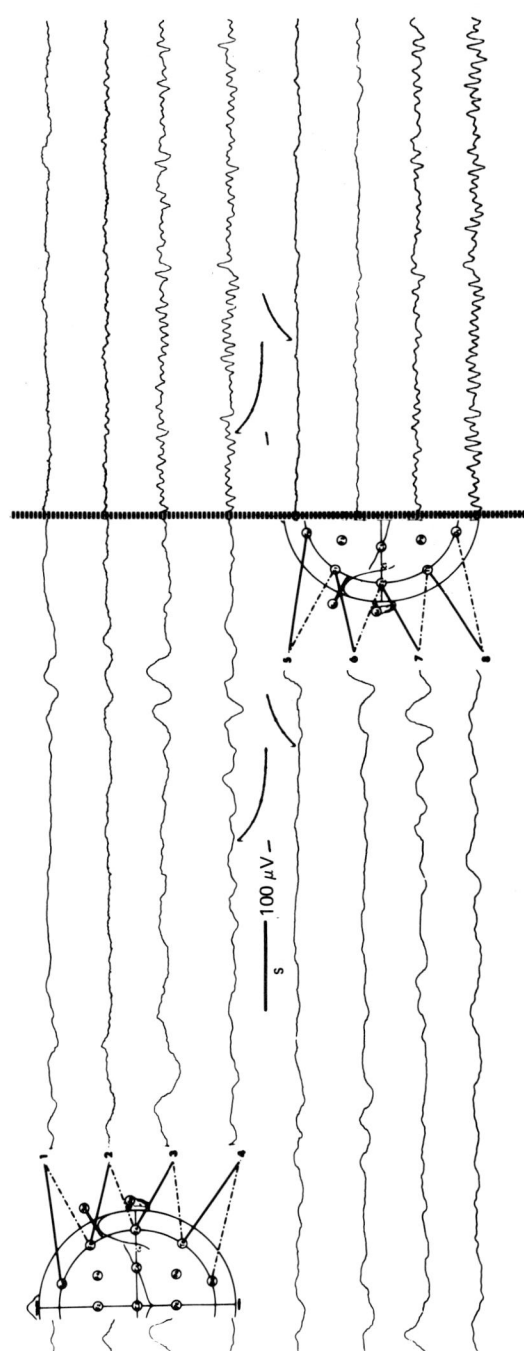

Figure 16.4. The EEG of an 8-year-old girl with measles encephalopathy; during the acute phase of the disease (left) and during convalescence (right)

anaesthesia below a certain spinal level, may also be a complication of measles. Subacute sclerosing panencephalitis is a late complication of measles (*see* page 311).

CHICKENPOX

Neurological complications of chickenpox are rare, at least in childhood. One type consists of ataxia and muscular hypotonia lasting for a couple of weeks, occasionally with convulsions. The prognosis is good, and the symptoms disappear completely. An acute hemiplegia may occur; it usually regresses completely within a couple of months, but mild signs may rarely persist. In a few patients the clinical picture is the same as described for measles encephalopathy with convulsions and coma; the prognosis is grave in this group, and the findings at autopsy are the same as in measles encephalopathy. No specific therapy is available.

RUBELLA

Neurological complications of rubella are rare. Encephalopathy, myelopathy, and peripheral neuropathy may occur. The clinical picture and the histological findings are similar to those described for measles. No specific therapy is available. Rubella may cause subacute sclerosing panencephalitis with a clinical picture indistinguishable from that seen in measles (*see* page 312). Rubella may also infect the fetus during pregnancy (*see* page 124).

MUMPS

The viral meningitis seen in mumps is so common that it should possibly be considered not a complication but an inherent part of the disease. Common complications are unilateral deafness, which may become permanent, and peripheral facial palsy. Rarely a more serious clinical picture may occur, indicating an involvement of the brain – mumps encephalitis. The signs associated with mumps encephalitis are disturbed consciousness, convulsions, confusion, psychosis, dysarthria, and ataxia. The EEG usually shows generalized slow activity. Only symptomatic treatment, e.g. anticonvulsant therapy, is available. Most of the symptoms abate slowly over many months, but sequelae such as deviant behaviour, concentration difficulties, clumsy movements, and ataxia may become permanent.

CYTOMEGALIC INCLUSION BODY DISEASE

This virus may infect the fetus during pregnancy and cause prenatal encephalitis (*see* page 125). It may also rarely cause encephalitis in an individual with impaired resistance to infection, either due to a disease of the immunosystem or to immunosuppressive therapy, e.g. for leukaemia. Symptoms and signs are similar to those of acquired toxoplasma encephalitis (*see* page 348); no effective treatment is known.

WHOOPING COUGH

Whooping cough may, particularly in children below 2 years of age, cause cerebral symptoms and signs. These usually appear during the second or third week when the whooping is most severe. The main symptoms are convulsions, although irritability, stupor, coma, and localized neurological findings, such as hemiplegia, may occasionally be seen. It is debated whether the neurological symptoms and signs are due mainly to the anoxia and bleeding tendency caused by the disease or to the infection *per se*. In children dying from this condition the findings are small haemorrhages due to asphyxia and cortical atrophy with neuronal degeneration. In surviving children, impaired mental development is a common sequela. No specific therapy is available; measures to prevent anoxia are important. Whenever possible, pertussis should be prevented in children below 3 years of age; this goal can be achieved by vaccination of infants and by the administration of gamma globulin to exposed unvaccinated children below 3 years of age within a few days after exposure.

DIPHTHERIA

The diphtheria toxin may attack the peripheral nerves causing polyneuropathy with a characteristic distribution. The first and most common symptoms consist of nasal speech and regurgitation of fluid on swallowing, due to paresis of the soft palate. These symptoms usually appear during the second week after the onset of diphtheria, whereas other neurological symptoms, if any, begin during the following week. Impaired accommodation due to paresis of the intrinsic eye muscles is another characteristic feature. Weakness of the neck muscles may be seen. Occasionally the peripheral nerves of the limbs are involved, causing the typical picture of weakness, muscular hypotonia, areflexia, and sensory disturbances (*see also* page 177). Although rare, respiratory difficulties may occur due to involvement of the diaphragm and the intercostal muscles. Symptoms usually progress for a few weeks and then slowly subside over many weeks.

Prophylaxis against diphtheritic polyneuropathy consists of the active immunization of healthy children and the administration of antitoxin during the acute phase of diphtheria. The management of patients with acute polyneuropathy is discussed in Chapter 6 (pages 175–177). The ultimate prognosis is usually good, although the course is protracted.

TRIPLE VACCINATION

Triple vaccination (pertussis, tetanus, and diphtheria) may in rare cases be followed by the clinical picture of infantile spasms (*see* pages 88–92). In almost all cases of infantile spasms the onset of symptoms occurs at the same age as that at which the three injections of triple vaccine are given, thus the causal connection between vaccination and the encephalopathy is hard to evaluate and much debated.

SPILLANE'S NEURITIS

Spillane's neuritis with weakness and atrophy of the shoulder muscles has been seen as a rare complication of serum treatment, usually as a feature of serum sickness; the same type and localization of weakness (*see* page 227) has very occasionally been observed in patients after injection of a vaccine in the upper arm; the connection between the symptoms and the injection is uncertain.

Brain abscess

A brain abscess may be a complication of meningitis; be caused by an infection
originating from a focus in the ear, nose and throat region or the skin, or spread by
the bloodstream from a more distant focus of infection, e.g. in the lungs; or it may
occur for no apparent reason. The abscess is a growing, space-occupying lesion
which causes signs of increased intracranial pressure – headache, vomiting,
drowsiness, irritability, papilloedema, cracked-pot sound and separated sutures,

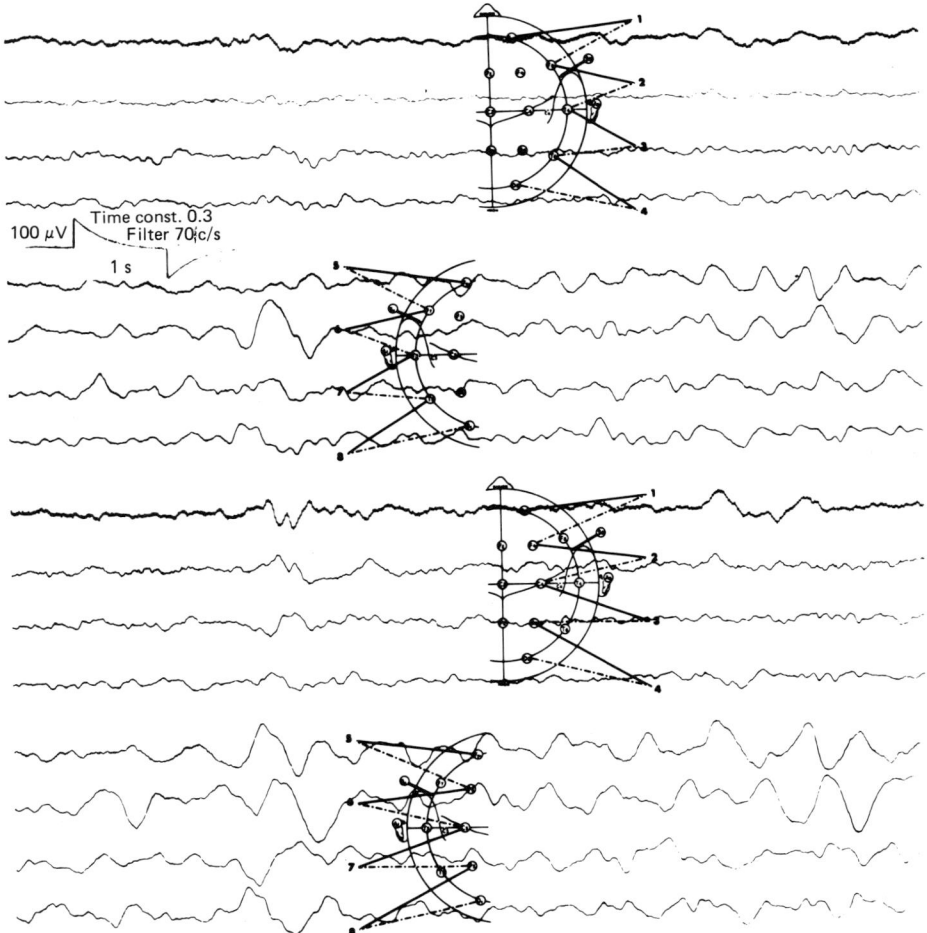

100 μV   Time const. 0.3
          Filter 70 c/s
    1 s

Figure 16.5. The EEG of a 9-year-old boy with a left-sided brain abscess

and focal neurological signs depending on its localization. Focal convulsions of the
Jacksonian type or epilepsia partialis continua (*see* pages 78 and 271) are signs of
the cortical irritation often found in a patient with a brain abscess. Some evidence
of infection is usually also found. Most patients, though not all, have a subfebrile
temperature, leucocytosis, and increased sedimentation rate.

The symptoms of a brain abscess usually develop over a period of a couple of weeks and increase steadily. As a rule, the patient's condition becomes serious within 1–2 months after the onset of symptoms.

The cerebrospinal fluid may be normal but usually shows slight pleocytosis, dominated by mononuclear cells. It is sterile, provided the brain abscess is not caused by or has caused a free meningitis. The characteristic EEG abnormality is a focal area of very slow activity and no spikes (*Figure 16.5*). This pattern is often seen in cases of brain abscess but is otherwise rare in childhood.

The diagnosis is established on computerized tomography of the skull. The treatment consists of intense antibiotic therapy (*see* page 344) combined with neurosurgery. It is advantageous to begin effective antibiotic therapy before operation, but in some cases urgent surgery may be needed.

There is a high risk of convulsions in patients who have been successfully operated on for a brain abscess. The EEG must therefore be followed-up after the operation; it is often advisable to give antiepileptics as a prophylactic measure.

Subdural abscess

A subdural abscess may be localized either intracranially or around the spinal cord. An intracranial subdural abscess causes evidence of increased intracranial pressure, focal convulsions, focal neurological signs, focal slowing on the EEG, a sterile cerebrospinal fluid with pleocytosis, fever, leucocytosis, and increased sedimentation rate. The differential diagnosis between a subdural abscess and a superficially located brain abscess is difficult. The treatment is the same as for a brain abscess – operation and intense antibiotic therapy. The risk of convulsions is high.

A subdural abscess localized around the spinal cord is, as a rule, a complication of spondylitis, which has usually caused pain and tenderness of the back and perhaps also fever, leucocytosis, and an increased sedimentation rate before the neurological symptoms start. These begin acutely with increasing pain and stiffness of the back, weakness and impaired sensation below a certain spinal level, and disturbed sphincter function. X-ray of the back reveals the spondylitis and possibly also the abscess as a mass in the soft tissue in front of the vertebrae; in other cases the abscess can be demonstrated on a myelogram. The treatment is neurosurgical evacuation of the abscess and intense antibiotic therapy. Neurosurgery is urgently required to relieve the pressure on the spinal cord and prevent permanent cord damage. Immobilization of the spine is often necessary after the operation to prevent the development of severe kyphosis.

References

GRIFFITH, J. F. and CH'IEN, L. T. (1983) Herpes simplex virus encephalitis. Diagnostic and treatment considerations. *Medical Clinics of North America*, **67**, 991–1008

IDRISS, Z. H., SINNO, A. A. and KRONFOL, N. M. (1976) Tuberculous meningitis in childhood. Forty-three cases. *American Journal of Diseases in Children*, **130**, 364–367

KAPLAN, S. L. and FEIGIN, R. D. (1983) Treatment of meningitis in children. *Pediatric Clinics of North America*, **30**, 259–269

KOSKINIEMI, M., DONNER, M. and PETTAY, O. (1983) Clinical appearance and outcome in mumps encephalitis in children. *Acta Paediatrica Scandinavica*, **72**, 603–609

KRAVITZ, G. R., DAVIES, S. F., ECKMAN, M. R. and SAROSI, G. A. (1981) Chronic blastomycotic meningitis. *American Journal of Medicine,* **71,** 501–505

LEADING ARTICLE (UNSIGNED) (1978) Treatment of tuberculous meningitis. *Journal of Antimicrobial Chemotherapy,* **4,** 1–13

MIZRAHI, E. M. and THARP, B. R. (1982) A characteristic EEG pattern in neonatal herpes simplex encephalitis. *Neurology* (NY), **32,** 1215–1220

SIEVERS, M. L. and FISHER, J. R. (1981) Coccidioidal meningitis and intrathecal corticosteroids. *Annals of Internal Medicine,* **95,** 242–243

WEINSTEIN, L. and IRVING, J. (1980) Successful treatment of cerebral cryptococcoma and meningitis with miconazole. *Annals of Internal Medicine,* **93,** 569–571

17

Tumours of the nervous system

Intracranial tumours

Intracranial tumours have an annual incidence of about 3–5 new cases per 100 000 children below 15 years of age. They represent roughly 10–15 per cent of malignant tumours of childhood. The symptoms and signs produced by an intracranial tumour can be divided into those due to increased intracranial pressure caused by blockage of the flow of cerebrospinal fluid, and those due to the direct local effect of the tumour.

Increased intracranial pressure

SYMPTOMS

The symptoms of increased intracranial pressure are headache, vomiting, slow cerebration, an impaired level of consciousness, double vision due to unilateral or bilateral sixth nerve palsy, tilting of the head, opisthotonos, tonic fits, and impaired respiration and circulation. The headache may occur at any time of the day, but is usually worst during the early morning hours, when it may waken the patient, and improves towards the afternoon. Over a longer period of time it may be intermittent and disappear for days or weeks. These periods of seeming improvement are presumably connected with a yield of the sutures. They may cause diagnostic difficulties, as steadily progressive symptoms are usually expected in a case of brain tumour, and the intermittent headache may be misinterpreted as due to migraine, for example. Vomiting may be of the projectile type, unaccompanied by nausea and occurring during the early morning hours. In infants and young children it may be less specific and occur at any time of the day. Slow cerebration means that the child answers questions only after a considerable delay, talks slowly, appears to think slowly, and responds to any stimulus in a slow fashion. The sixth nerve palsy is caused by pressure on the nerve, the intracranial course of which is longer than that of the other cranial nerves; sixth nerve palsy is thus a sign of increased intracranial pressure and is not a localizing sign. The blocking of the flow of cerebrospinal fluid may diminish when the head is kept in a certain position; this is one of the factors involved in the explanation for the head tilting often seen in children with a tumour in the posterior fossa (*see Figure 17.1,* page 366). When the increased intracranial pressure causes opisthotonos and tonic fits, the patient is usually stuporous. A patient in this stage often rubs his face, as if it were itching.

On examination a bulging fontanelle is found in the young infant and papilloedema and a cracked-pot sound in the older child. On skull X-ray stretched or widened sutures (*see Figure 3.14,* page 55) and decalcification of the back of the sella turcica may be found. Papilloedema usually takes at least several days to develop, whereas the cracked-pot sound and the changes on skull X-ray only become apparent after a few weeks of slowly increasing intracranial pressure. Thus, the absence of papilloedema, a cracked-pot sound, and abnormalities on the skull X-ray does not exclude the possibility of increased intracranial pressure.

The symptoms and signs of increased intracranial pressure are found mainly in patients with an infratentorial tumour localized in the posterior fossa. A description of them will not be repeated for each separate type of tumour.

Local effect of the tumour

The direct local effect of the tumour consists of focal neurological signs, the nature and extent of which depend on the localization of the tumour. These symptoms and signs are described for each type of tumour.

Description of the various types of tumour

INFRATENTORIAL NEOPLASMS

Cerebellar astrocytoma
Infratentorial neoplasms dominate in the age-group 2–15 years. Cerebellar astrocytoma is a slow-growing, often cystic, tumour of the cerebellum. It causes slowly increasing intracranial pressure, and consequently headache, often of the intermittent type (*see* page 364). Ataxia is a localizing sign which usually has a subacute onset and only becomes apparent after some time, as the symptoms caused by the increased intracranial pressure progress slowly. It is common for a child with a cerebellar astrocytoma to keep his head tilted in a fixed position, always to the same side (*Figure 17.1*). The child is usually unaware of this tilting and insists that he is keeping his head straight. The typical head tilting in a case of cerebellar astrocytoma is probably due to impaired proprioceptive impulses. It is an early symptom, occasionally the first, and is often present before the increased intracranial pressure has had time to develop and contribute to the head tilting. Early diagnosis is urgent, as the tumour is operable and can be removed completely with little or no sequelae. The diagnosis is established on computerized tomography of the skull.

Medulloblastoma
This is a common type of brain tumour in children. It produces evidence of increased intracranial pressure with symptoms that progress rapidly over several weeks; occasionally the progression is slower, symptoms may become intermittent (*see* page 364), and ataxia, usually of the truncal type, has time to develop. The

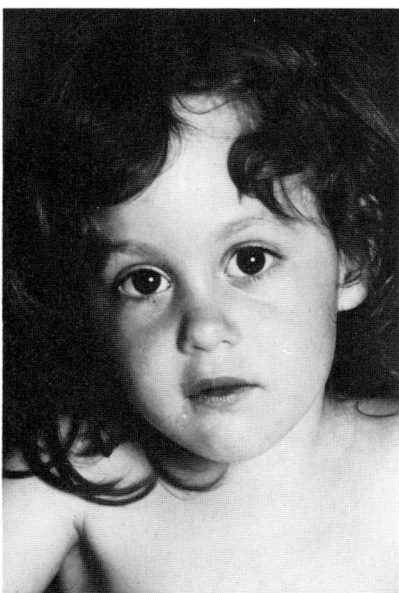

Figure 17.1. A 3-year-old girl with a cerebellar astrocytoma, keeping her head constantly tilted to one side

diagnosis is established on computerized tomography of the skull. The neurosurgeon's aim is to remove as much of the tumour as possible, preferably all of it. The border between tumour and normal tissue may, however, be difficult to distinguish, and part of the tumour may be impossible to remove. The tumour is radiosensitive and operation is followed by radiotherapy combined with courses of antimetabolite therapy. The radiotherapy is given not only over the tumour area, but also along the spinal cord. This latter area is treated because metastases along the spinal cord and in the cauda equina are common in cases of medulloblastoma and may cause symptoms due to the infiltration of tumour cells around the nerve roots. This combined therapy has improved the prognosis, with the result that 50 per cent of the patients may survive without recurrence. Some of these patients show growth retardation caused by the X-ray treatment over the spine.

Ependymoma of the fourth ventricle
This lesion produces the same symptoms and signs as does medulloblastoma, possibly with slightly slower progress. A definite differential diagnosis between these two conditions may not be possible before operation. Treatment and prognosis are the same as described for medulloblastoma.

Brain-stem glioma
The early symptoms of a brain-stem glioma are usually due to the local effect of the tumour, whereas signs of increased intracranial pressure appear late in the course. The neurological signs are caused by damage to the nuclei of the cranial nerves, localized in the brain-stem. Depending on the level at which the glioma is localized, they may consist of palsy of various extraocular muscles causing strabismus with double vision or gaze paralysis; peripheral facial weakness; weakness, atrophy, and fasciculations of the tongue; and swallowing difficulties. The long tracts passing through the brain stem may also be affected, causing hemiplegia and eventually

tetraplegia and ataxia. The findings are slowly progressive, as more and more structures of the brain stem are involved.

The diagnosis can usually be established on computerized tomography of the skull, but the brain-stem area is difficult to examine and a small tumour may be missed. Rarely, a tumour may be better demonstrated on a pneumoencephalogram. No surgical treatment is possible in this area. Radiotherapy will usually produce at least a temporary arrest of the progress. If evidence of increased intracranial pressure appears, these symptoms can be controlled temporarily by a shunt procedure. The prognosis is poor.

SUPRATENTORIAL NEOPLASMS

These are the dominating type of tumour in adulthood, but they represent less than half of the brain tumours that occur in childhood. Symptoms due to the local effect of the tumour are usually present for some time before evidence of increased intracranial pressure appears.

Glioma of the cerebral hemispheres

A slow-growing astrocytoma may infiltrate the cortex, causing focal grand mal or psychomotor attacks, possibly for several years before the appearance of neurological signs. This type of tumour, which is often difficult to diagnose, must be suspected in patients with fits that cannot be controlled, particularly if these are connected with mental changes. Even some years after the onset of fits, the tumour may be difficult to demonstrate both on computerized tomography of the skull and on a carotid arteriogram. Occasionally, when patients are operated on for severe epilepsy, supposedly caused by an epileptic cortical scar, this type of tumour is found at operation or on histological examination of the removed tissue.

A cerebral astrocytoma is operated on without delay, once the diagnosis has been established. The operation is performed as radically as possible without causing the patient further neurological symptoms. It is difficult to distinguish the border between tumour tissue and normal brain tissue; complete removal is seldom possible. Radiotherapy is given after the operation. The convulsions may become easier to control, and the patient may otherwise remain symptom-free for several years after this treatment; there is, however, always a risk of recurrence.

A rapidly growing oligodendroglioma and an undifferentiated glioma are more common tumours of the cerebral hemispheres than an astrocytoma. They cause convulsions, hemiparesis, hemianopsia, and mental disturbances; all these symptoms are progressive, and the patient is as a rule severely handicapped within several months after the onset of symptoms. The diagnosis can usually be established on computerized tomography of the skull, possibly combined with a carotid arteriogram. If the tumour is well demarcated, as much of it as possible, and always enough for a histological diagnosis, is removed. The operation is followed by radiotherapy and treatment with antimetabolites. The prognosis is poor and survival short.

Glioma of the midline structures

The dominating early findings are evidence of increased intracranial pressure and endocrine disturbances. An optic glioma (*see below*) is a common type of tumour in this region, but other types of glioma may be seen. The diagnosis can be established on computerized tomography of the skull, possibly combined with a carotid arteriogram. Radical removal is often difficult. The increased intracranial pressure is controlled by a shunt. Radiotherapy is given after the operation. The prognosis is generally poor, although survival for several years has been reported.

Optic glioma

This lesion may arise in the optic disc, where it is seen on examination of the fundi. It may be localized along the intracranial part of the optic nerves, causing impaired vision and visual field defects, or at the chiasma. When the localization is at or near the chiasma, the tumour is a glioma of the midline structures (*see above*) and endocrine disturbances such as obesity, emaciation, and growth disturbances caused by damage to the diencephalon (*see* pages 383–385) are common. Visual disturbances, abnormalities of the visual fields, and evidence of increased intracranial pressure may also be present. The spinal fluid protein is usually increased. The diagnosis can usually be established on computerized tomography of the skull; rarely, a pneumoencephalogram may also be needed. The treatment is surgical removal of as much of the tumour as possible without rendering the patient blind; a shunt is applied if the intracranial pressure is increased. Surgery is followed by radiotherapy. With this treatment the symptoms may remain stationary for many years, although there is always a risk of recurrence of the tumour and the development of new symptoms.

Diencephalic syndromes

These are growth disturbances (*see* pages 383–385) caused by a lesion of the diencephalon. The most common cause is an optic glioma (*see above*), although other types of glioma may occur in this region; a diencephalic syndrome may also be caused by other conditions, such as an atrophic lesion in the same area.

Craniopharyngioma

This is the most common type of tumour in the hypothalamic–hypophyseal region in childhood. It is localized above the sella turcica and is often cystic. Endocrine abnormalities are as a rule the first symptoms noted. These usually consist of disturbed growth and sexual development, most commonly a retardation of the child's growth and sexual maturation, and occasionally the opposite, i.e. pubertas praecox. If the posterior part of the hypophysis is involved, diabetes insipidus may also be present. The neurological findings consist mainly of visual disturbances and visual field defects; evidence of increased intracranial pressure may also be present. Optic atrophy is a common finding. Calcifications of the cystic tumour are found on skull X-ray in 80–90 per cent of patients with craniopharyngioma. The diagnosis is established and the extension of the tumour demonstrated on computerized tomography of the skull.

   The treatment is surgical. When as much of the tumour as possible has been removed and the cysts are emptied, the progression of symptoms is temporarily arrested. If the diagnosis is established early, complete removal of the tumour may be possible. It must be followed by endocrine substitution therapy. Early diagnosis and complete removal of the tumour carry a good prognosis, although the need for endocrine substitution therapy remains lifelong. If removal is incomplete the tumour may recur.

Pinealoma and teratoma in the region of the pineal

This type of lesion may cause both endocrine and neurological symptoms. The clinical picture is usually dominated by the neurological symptoms, which consist of evidence of increased intracranial pressure and abnormal eye movements, particularly a paralysis of upward gaze. The endocrine symptoms consist of diabetes insipidus and pubertas praecox. Too much emphasis has been put on pubertas praecox, which may occur but is a rare finding. Skull X-ray often reveals a large calcification of the pineal; this finding in a child must always arouse a suspicion of a pinealoma or a teratoma. The diagnosis is established on computerized tomography of the skull; occasionally it must be supplemented by a pneumoencephalogram or a vertebral arteriogram. The treatment is operation followed by radiotherapy. Complete removal may be possible in some cases, and survival for many years has been reported.

Ependymoma of the lateral ventricles
This lesion causes the same symptoms as does an oligodendroglioma or an undifferentiated glioma of the cerebral hemispheres; treatment and prognosis are the same (*see* page 367).

Plexus papilloma
This causes an increased production of cerebrospinal fluid and thus hydrocephalus, which is poorly controlled by a shunt (*see* page 250). The diagnosis is established on computerized tomography of the skull, which should be performed in most cases of hydrocephalus before a shunt is applied. The treatment is surgical, and if possible complete, removal of the tumour; a shunt may also be needed. The tumour is rare, and its prognosis is difficult to evaluate.

Meningioma
A rarity in childhood, a meningioma grows slowly and causes slowly progressive neurological symptoms and signs, such as progressive hemiparesis and hemianopsia. Evidence of increased intracranial pressure appears late in the course. The tumour may irritate the periosteum and cause a thickening of the skull above the tumour, visible on a skull X-ray. The diagnosis is established on computerized tomography of the skull. Children with this rare tumour may easily be misdiagnosed as having cerebral palsy if the slow progression of symptoms and signs is overlooked. The tumour is benign and can often be removed completely. An early diagnosis is urgent, as only limited regression of already established neurological signs can be expected.

Acoustic neurinoma
A tumour of the cerebellopontine angle, an acoustic neurinoma, is rare in childhood and occurs almost exclusively in cases of Recklinghausen's disease (*see* page 373). It causes tinnitus, a progressive impairment of hearing, dizziness, and a slowly progressive facial weakness without the abrupt onset typical of Bell's palsy (*see* pages 220–221); occasionally the fifth and sixth nerves and the cerebellar tracts are also involved. Evidence of increased intracranial pressure appears late. Examination reveals hearing defects, an irresponsive labyrinth on caloric testing, peripheral facial weakness, possibly also impaired corneal sensation, sixth nerve palsy, and ataxia. Skull X-ray may reveal destruction of the bone around the porus acusticus; the cerebrospinal fluid protein is often increased. Other signs of Recklinghausen's disease may be evident (*see* pages 373–374). The usual type of acoustic neurinoma is rarely bilateral. Bilateral occurrence is, however, often seen

in Recklinghausen's disease and thus in cases of acoustic neurinoma with the onset in childhood, although symptoms rarely start simultaneously on both sides.

The diagnosis is established on computerized tomography of the skull. The treatment is surgical removal of the tumour. If the diagnosis is established early, complete removal is usually possible. The risk of new intracranial tumours is high in Recklinghausen's disease.

RARE INTRACRANIAL TUMOURS

These tumours may be infratentorial or supratentorial.

Metastatic tumours
Metastatic tumours with an intracranial localization may occur but are extremely rare in children, except for leukaemic infiltration of the meninges and occasionally of the nervous tissue (*see* pages 317–318).

Tumours originating from the structures surrounding the brain
These may infiltrate the nervous tissue and cause neurological symptoms and signs. Examples of such tumours are sarcomas of the nasopharynx and of the skull.

Lindau's tumour
Angioma of the retina and the cerebellum, Lindau's tumour, is seldom seen in persons below 20 years of age.

Sturge–Weber angiomatosis
The angiomatosis of Sturge–Weber syndrome (*see* page 97) is more a malformation than a tumour, although a slow progression of symptoms may occasionally be seen.

Tuberous sclerosis
Angiomas, as well as all types of glioma, are common in tuberous sclerosis (*see* page 97); they are often multiple.

Brain tumours in infants

Special problems arise in the diagnosis of brain tumours occurring in infants and children below 2 years of age. Both symptoms and signs are less characteristic than in later childhood. The vomiting may occur at any time of the day and is particularly pronounced with tumours of the hypothalamic area; emaciation and growth disturbances are common with this localization of the tumour. The increased intracranial pressure causes a bulging fontanelle and an abnormal increase in the head circumference but not necessarily papilloedema. These patients may be misinterpreted as having expansive hydrocephalus; if a shunt is applied without preoperative computerized tomography, the symptoms may be controlled for some time and the correct diagnosis unnecessarily delayed. Convulsions that do not respond to antiepileptic therapy and neurological symptoms such as hemiplegia may be signs of a brain tumour; neurological symptoms starting in this age-group are easily misinterpreted as due to cerebral palsy. Several of the intracranial tumours that occur in this age-group can be removed completely, if the diagnosis is established early. The possibility of a brain tumour must therefore be kept in mind when an infant shows failure to thrive, growth disturbances, expansive hydrocephalus, uncontrolled fits, or progressive neurological signs.

Enclosed infectious processes

An enclosed infectious process may cause symptoms and signs indistinguishable from those produced by a tumour. Purulent infection, i.e. a brain abscess, is described in Chapter 16 (*see* pages 361–362). Chronic infections, e.g. a tuberculoma, a luetic gumma, or an echinococcus cyst, may be the cause of symptoms and signs interpreted as evidence of a brain tumour; they are rarely seen in countries with well-developed programmes of paediatric preventive medicine.

Tumours of the spinal cord

Tumours of the spinal cord are rare in childhood; they have an incidence of 5–10 per cent of that of intracranial neoplasms. Most of them are benign, and the symptoms they produce are reversible for a limited period; the delay in establishing a diagnosis of these rare conditions must therefore be minimized as far as possible. The most common symptoms caused by all types of spinal cord tumours are gait disturbances, impaired sphincter control, and pain in the back irradiating in an extremity or around the body. The pain increases on movements of the spine; the patient therefore keeps his back stiff. Scoliosis may develop with the concavity on the affected side. Children with alleged cerebral palsy showing symptoms and signs, particularly if they are progressive, in the lower limbs only, and children who lose sphincter control once achieved, should be strongly suspected of having a spinal cord tumour.

Extradural tumours

Extradural tumours constitute about one-quarter of spinal tumours occurring in the paediatric age-group; the majority of them are sarcomas arising from the vertebrae. Operation and radiotherapy may provide temporary relief.

The extradural space may be infiltrated by leukaemic cells, causing pain which irradiates along the infiltrated nerve roots, sensory disturbances, and weakness of muscles innervated by the affected nerve roots. As a rule these symptoms respond rapidly to local X-ray therapy. This palliative procedure is important, as the limited life-span of these patients must be made as comfortable as possible.

The tumour may arise from the autonomic nervous system and be a neuroblastoma or a ganglioneuroma. These tumours produce the common symptoms of a spinal cord neoplasm (*see above*). They grow slowly, and there is a fair chance that complete surgical removal may be successful.

Metastases along the spinal cord and the nerve roots may come from a medulloblastoma (*see* page 365). They are radiosensitive. X-ray therapy over the spinal cord is therefore given routinely as a prophylactic measure at the time of the treatment of the primary tumour. They also respond to vincristine, and combined treatment with radiotherapy and vincristine may relieve the symptoms, at least temporarily. These metastases may cause symptoms, although only rarely before the primary tumour has been diagnosed.

Metastatic carcinoma is an extremely rare condition in childhood with a poor prognosis.

An enclosed infectious process localized in the extradural space may cause symptoms and signs indistinguishable from those caused by an extradural tumour, together with general signs of infection such as fever and leucocytosis (*see* page 362).

Intradural–extramedullary tumours

These lesions constitute only about 10–15 per cent of spinal cord tumours in childhood and are extremely rare in children below the age of 10–12 years. The two types seen are meningioma and neurofibroma. Both are slow-growing benign tumours, which can be completely removed. The symptoms are those commonly seen in spinal cord tumours (*see* page 371) and are reversible for a period of time. These tumours must be suspected in teenagers who, for no apparent reason, have persistent backache with pain radiating around the body or in an extremity, possibly with a stiff back, scoliosis, progressive weakness, abnormal posture of the feet and legs, and impaired sphincter control. In childhood, neurofibromas occur almost exclusively in cases of Recklinghausen's disease (*see* page 373).

Intradural–intramedullary tumours

These tumours constitute about one-quarter of spinal cord tumours in childhood. The types seen are various kinds of gliomas and blood vessel tumours. The intramedullary tumours seldom cause back pain and stiffness of the back, but slowly progressive neurological symptoms occur from the level below the tumour. Early diagnosis of this type of tumour is less urgent as it can seldom be removed without causing further damage to the spinal cord; an operation is therefore not performed early in the disease.

Tumours extending both extradurally and intradurally

These lesions constitute the largest group of spinal cord neoplasms in childhood. They consist of lipomas, dermoids, and teratomas. They usually arise as a hamartomatous mass from a primary malformation of the lower part of the cord or the cauda equina. Some kind of local abnormality is therefore often found – a dimple, a hairy tuft (*see Figure 15.6,* page 334), or a palpable soft tumour such as a lipoma (*see Figure 15.9,* page 338). Thus, such a lesion may be diagnosed even before neurological symptoms have appeared. An abnormal posture of the feet may already be present at birth or arise later. Slowly progressive gait disturbances and impaired sphincter control are the most common symptoms in older children. These conditions should be operated on as soon as the diagnosis is established. By careful dissection, as much of the tumour tissue as possible is removed without causing damage to the normal nervous structures. The long-term prognosis is excellent if all the tumour tissue can be extirpated; if only part of the tumour can be removed the prognosis is fair, as these tumours grow slowly.

The most important procedure in the diagnosis of a spinal cord tumour is a complete X-ray of the spine. This should be performed in all children who arouse the slightest clinical suspicion of a spinal cord neoplasm. In almost all cases it reveals some kind of abnormality, e.g. destruction of a vertebra in a case of sarcoma, widening of the interpediculate distance at the level of the tumour, enlargement of intervertebral foramina (*Figure 17.2*), or malformation of the spine in congenital hamartomatous lesions (*see* page 339). The cerebrospinal fluid protein is increased if there is a partial or complete block of the subarachnoid space and the lumbar puncture is performed below this block. If the clinical suspicion is strong or if X-ray of the spine has revealed any abnormalities, a myelogram is performed. This procedure demonstrates the presence, localization, and extent of the tumour.

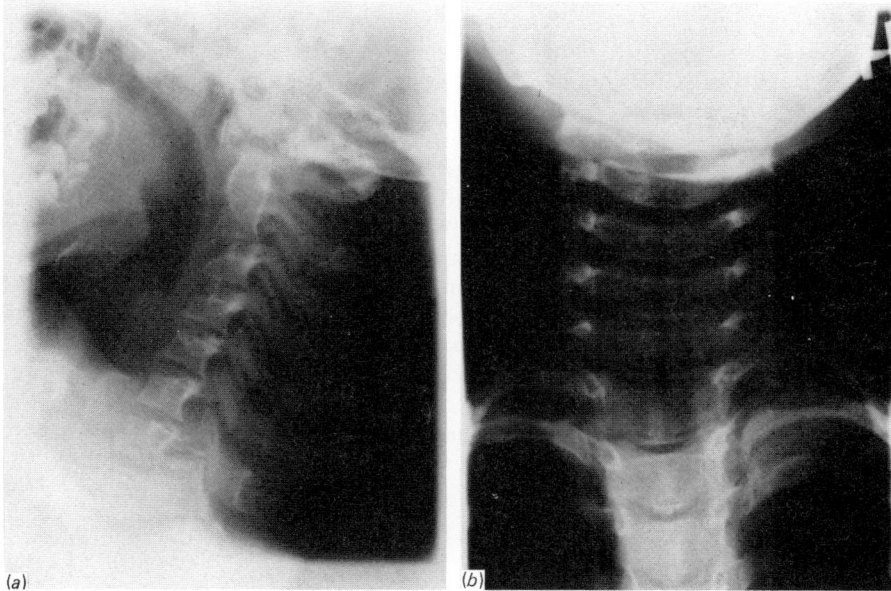

Figure 17.2. X-ray of the cervical spine of a 5-year-old boy with neurofibromatosis von Recklinghausen, showing neurofibromas of the cervical cord and nerve roots. Note the widening of the interpediculate distance (*a*) and enlargement of the intervertebral foramina (*b*)

Tumours of the peripheral nerves

Tumours of the peripheral nerves occur almost exclusively in the neurofibromatosis von Recklinghausen. This condition, inherited as an autosomal dominant trait, is characterized by abnormalities of the skin, subcutaneous tissue, bone, and the nervous system. The typical skin lesion is café-au-lait spots, which are usually large in size and number in affected individuals (*Figure 17.3*). Other types of skin lesions,

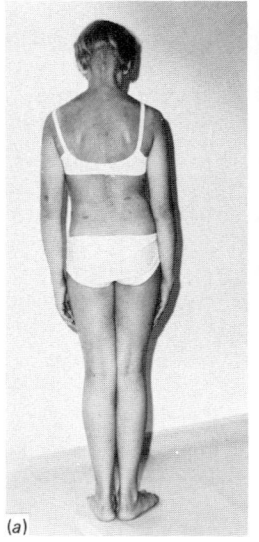

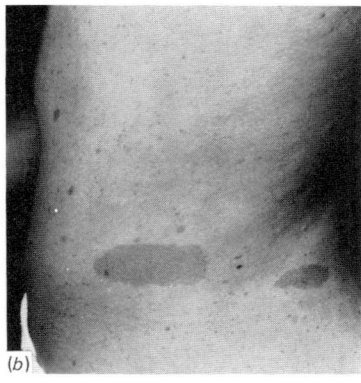

Figure 17.3a and *b*. A 15-year-old girl with Recklinghausen's disease and numerous café-au-lait spots. Note also the scar on the neck where a neurofibroma has been removed

e.g. depigmented areas and adenoma sebaceum, may also be seen. The subcutaneous tissue and the bones may show a diffuse overgrowth causing gigantism of a limb or enlargement of part of the face. Tumours of the nervous system are common. They may be intracranial (*see* page 369) or originate from the spinal cord (*see* page 373), nerve roots, nerve trunks, or peripheral nerves. Peripheral tumours may cause irradiating pains, sensory disturbances, and weakness of the muscles innervated by the affected nerve. They are often palpable along a superficially located nerve. Neurofibromas can be excised, but they recur easily in the same place or new tumours appear with a different localization. There is a definite risk of sarcomatous degeneration of these tumours, particularly if they recur several times in the same place. Operation should therefore be avoided, unless the tumour causes the patient pain or other discomfort.

The prognosis is variable. Some individuals have the café-au-lait spots as the only evidence of the disease and live an entirely normal life; others die in adolescence or early adulthood from sarcomas or intracranial tumours. No treatment is known for the disease *per se*.

References

COHEN, M. E. and DUFFNER, P. K. (1984) *Brain Tumours in Children: Principles of Diagnosis and Treatment,* (International Review of Child Neurology Series). New York: Raven Press

GUNNESSON-NORDIN, V., BLENNOW, G., GARWICZ, S., BRUN, A. E., BYNKE, H., LANDBERG, T. G. *et al.* (1982) Gliomas of the anterior visual pathway in children. Tumour behaviour and effect of treatment. *Neuropediatrics,* **13**, 82–87

KOOS, W., LAUBICHLER, W. and SORGO, G. (1973) Statistischer Untersuchungen bei spinalen Tumoren in Kindes- und Jugendalter. *Neuropädiatrie,* **4**, 273–303

SAMUELSSON, B. (1981) Neurofibromatosis (v. Recklinghausen's disease). A clinical–psychiatric and genetic study. Academical Dissertation, Medical Faculty, Göteborg

18

Physical injury to the nervous system after the neonatal period

Head trauma

Head trauma is common in childhood. Few individuals pass their childhood without experiencing several head traumata; fortunately these do not generally cause either acute problems or late sequelae.

Of children with head traumata severe enough for the parents to seek medical advice about two-thirds are boys. Among children hospitalized because of head trauma, there is an overrepresentation of children who, before the trauma, showed symptoms of mental problems and behaviour disorders and who came from home environments characterized by tension and anxiety; the likelihood of the family having psychosocial problems is particularly high if the same child needs hospitalization several times for physical injuries, including head trauma.

SYMPTOMS, SIGNS, TREATMENT, AND PROGNOSIS

Most mild head traumata cause no symptoms at all, and the parents never seek medical advice. No treatment is needed and there are no sequelae.

If the blow is a little harder, the child may become unconscious for a few minutes. On regaining consciousness he is usually pale, irritable, and perhaps confused; he is nauseated and vomits. After a while he falls asleep and sleeps for several hours; on waking the child may be recovered or still have headache and nausea. In this situation, which corresponds to *concussion of the brain,* many parents seek medical advice. Children with this history must be carefully observed for 1–2 days for evidence of intracranial bleeding or brain contusion with oedema severe enough to render neurosurgical intervention necessary. The child must be roused from his sleep at short, regular intervals to confirm that he is asleep and not unconscious; he must be watched for the appearance of focal neurological signs; and pulse, blood pressure, and respiration must be monitored. Skull X-ray is of some help in selected cases, as an impression fracture is often operated on early and a fracture across the temporal bone must alert the physician to the possibility of extradural bleeding. The presence or absence of a skull fracture has otherwise little influence on the management and prognosis of a patient with a head trauma, thus skull X-ray need not be performed routinely. Neither electroencephalography nor lumbar puncture is of help in the acute situation; the latter procedure may even be dangerous. Ultrasound examination of the skull is a safe procedure which gives reliable information about dislocation of the midline structures; when necessary it can be repeated at short intervals.

It is often advisable to hospitalize a child for this short period of intense observation. If, at the end of this time, the patient is fully awake with normal vital signs, no focal neurological findings, and no other evidence of intracranial bleeding or brain contusion with oedema, he is discharged. At discharge the parents are informed about the excellent prognosis in cases of uncomplicated head trauma in children. The child is entitled to a period of rest from school or other stressful activities, but he must not be confined to bed, and should be allowed to play and move around as much as he likes. At discharge from the hospital, patients with a head trauma may still be tired and irritable and have headache, but these symptoms disappear within a few days or weeks without any treatment. This reassuring information, given when the child is discharged, is the best prophylaxis against the postconcussion syndrome (*see* page 320). If the parents so wish the child may be checked a few weeks after the head trauma and the reassuring information repeated. From a strict medical point of view a check is not needed, provided the child feels well and behaves normally. The belief that a mild head trauma may cause serious mental or neurological sequelae and that prolonged bed-rest is necessary to avoid them has produced great and unnecessary concern and possibly caused stress headache in both child and parents; *the good prognosis of uncomplicated head trauma in childhood cannot be stressed enough,* and this information is the best prophylaxis against later problems.

COMPLICATIONS

If, during the initial observation period, the patient shows a decreasing level of consciousness, unstable vital signs, or increasing neurological findings, a complication should be suspected.

One complication that must be considered when there is a discrepancy between a mild trauma and serious symptoms which indicate increased intracranial pressure is a previously arrested hydrocephalus, now reactivated by the trauma (*see* page 255). Other serious complications are an intracranial haemorrhage or brain contusion with so much brain swelling that the intracranial pressure is increased; all these situations need immediate neurosurgical attention. Evaluation by a neurosurgeon is also necessary if the patient has an impression fracture or a fracture across the temporal bone, which crosses the course of the medial meningeal artery and carries a high risk of epidural bleeding.

Intracranial bleeding may be intracerebral, subarachnoidal, subdural, or epidural. An intracerebral haemorrhage must be removed if it is large enough, and the same is true for a severely contused part of the brain; both give rise to increased intracranial pressure which must be counteracted as effectively as possible. Subarachnoidal bleeding may eventually lead to hydrocephalus (*see* page 251).

Subdural haematoma
A subdural haematoma is usually acute in children, causing signs of increased intracranial pressure and dislocation of the midline structures, even in the acute phase. Rarely it may be of the chronic type and produce symptoms and signs of increased intracranial pressure and focal neurological signs a few weeks after the

trauma. The diagnosis is best established by computerized tomography of the skull, possibly supplemented by a carotid arteriogram. The haematoma is removed neurosurgically.

Epidural haematoma

Epidural bleeding is a serious complication of a head trauma. The trauma may be mild; in a small child it may be so mild that it is overlooked by the mother. It may cause no loss of consciousness or only a short period of unconsciousness followed by a symptom-free interval of one to a few hours. Symptoms then start with a rapidly falling level of consciousness, a dilated pupil on the side of the haematoma, and hemiparesis as a rule on the other side. Of these two localizing signs, the dilated pupil is the most reliable one, as the hemiparesis may occasionally be on the same side as the haematoma. The child soon becomes deeply unconscious, both pupils dilate, respiration stops, and finally circulation ceases. Immediate removal of the haematoma is life-saving. The severity of permanent symptoms and signs (convulsions or cerebral palsy), if any, depends on the degree of cortical damage caused by the haematoma.

Convulsions

A fit may occur in the period following a head trauma. If it is short and appears within the first few hours after the trauma, it has no serious significance (*see* page 96) and is probably due to transient oedema. Repeated or persistent convulsions usually indicate a complication that requires neuroradiological studies and neurosurgical help.

TRAUMA TO THE NECK CAUSING CEREBRAL SYMPTOMS AND SIGNS

A trauma to the neck may in rare instances cause an occlusion of the carotid artery with the appearance of hemiparesis a couple of hours to a day after the trauma. The mechanism can usually be proven on a carotid arteriogram, which shows the occlusion of the carotid artery. By this time, however, it is generally too late for surgical therapy, and treatment with anticoagulants seems to have no influence on the course. Most patients survive with permanent hemiparesis; impaired mental development is common and seizures may occur.

SUMMARY OF THE MANAGEMENT AND PROGNOSIS OF HEAD TRAUMA IN CHILDHOOD

A child who is unconscious for a short period after a closed head trauma should be observed, at home or in a hospital, for 1–2 days for evidence of increasing intracranial pressure, reappearance of a decreasing level of consciousness, and focal neurological signs. As a rule, only clinical observation is needed; in selected cases X-ray and ultrasound examination of the skull may be of value. X-ray of the cervical spine is advisable in all patients with a severe trauma, as an injury of the cervical cord is easily overlooked in an unconscious patient. If no signs of a complication have developed during this period, the child is discharged and allowed to take part in any normal activity he wants; he is entitled to some days of rest and play before going back to school. The parents should be informed that the patient may be irritable and tired for some days or weeks, but that there is no need for bed-rest or other restriction of the child's activity. Uncomplicated head traumata in childhood have an excellent prognosis; the parents must be fully informed on this point at the end of the initial observation period. Persistent headache or convulsions are exceptional complications of head traumata in childhood. Neither a single short convulsion, appearing within a couple of hours after the trauma, nor a skull fracture without impression or signs of intracranial bleeding impairs the good prognosis.

Children with an open head trauma, prolonged or reappearing unconsciousness, an impression fracture, a fracture across the temporal bone, repeated convulsions, increasing intracranial pressure, or focal neurological signs are referred for neurosurgical evaluation, as operation may rapidly become necessary. During transportation, free airways must be maintained and the increased intracranial pressure reduced (see page 319). When brain injury is substantial, sequelae such as cerebral palsy, impaired mental development, and convulsions are common but do not always occur.

Spinal cord injury

Injury to the spinal cord may be due to a direct localized trauma to one or a few vertebrae, or to a longitudinal trauma to the spine, such as may occur when a person dives into water that is too shallow or falls from a horse. Vertebral fractures are common. The spinal cord may be damaged by direct laceration, pressure from a fractured vertebra, bleeding around or into the cord, or impaired circulation.

If the lesion is severe, all of the body below the injured segment is paralysed, sensation is lost, and sphincter function is impaired. The paralysis is usually flaccid during the first few days or weeks after the trauma. Muscle tone reappears as a rule after 1–2 weeks and becomes increased; muscle reflexes return and become hyperactive with clonus, and the Babinski sign appears. Sensation improves, and the upper level of hypoaesthesia is slightly decreased.

The usual treatment is traction of the spine by different devices in order to reset the fractured vertebrae and to reduce the pressure on the spinal cord and its blood supply. Traction must continue until the fractures have healed and the spine is stable; renewed damage to the cord may otherwise occur. Active treatment to prevent bedsores and contractures must be initiated at this stage. An indwelling catheter is often inevitable in the acute stage, but training in the manual and automatic emptying of the bladder is started immediately in order to minimize the length of time for which a catheter is necessary. Very occasionally a patient may benefit from laminectomy and surgical reposition and fixation of the fractured vertebrae.

The prognosis is always serious in patients with an injury to the spinal cord. Some improvement is the rule during the weeks following the injury, but complete recovery is an exception. A trauma to the cervical cord is particularly serious, as it leaves the patient with the severe handicap of a tetraparesis. Complications involving the urinary tract need continuous attention. Intense and persistent rehabilitation is rewarding in patients with spinal cord injuries, as their cerebral function is undamaged, and they can cooperate actively and make good use of technical aids.

Injuries to the nerve roots and the peripheral nerves

This type of trauma causes denervation and impaired sensation within the area innervated by the damaged root or nerve (see also Chapter 7). The peripheral nervous system is capable of regeneration; an injured nerve may grow out and reinnervate the denervated area. In some instances a nerve suture may help the regenerating nerve to find the way to denervated structures. In childhood a nerve fibre grows at the rate of 1–3 mm/day.

References

BABCOCK, J. L. (1975) Spinal injuries in children. *Pediatric Clinics of North America*, **22**, 487–500

FRANTZEN, E., JACOBSEN, H. H. and THERKELSEN, J. (1961) Cerebral artery occlusion in children due to trauma to the head and neck. *Neurology* (Minneapolis), **11**, 695–700

HJERN, B. and NYLANDER, I. (1964) Acute head injuries in children. *Acta Paediatrica* (Uppsala), suppl. 152

KRETSCHMER, H. (1982) Prognosis of severe head injuries in childhood and adolescence. *Neuropediatrics*, **14**, 176–181

ROSMAN, N. P., HERSKOWITZ, J., CARTER, A. P. and O'CONNOR, J. F. (1979) Acute head trauma in infancy and childhood. *Pediatric Clinics of North America*, **26**, 707–736

19

Abnormal growth as a symptom of a neurological disorder

Short stature with normal body proportions

Short stature with normal body proportions is seen in many of the syndromes in which mental retardation is a dominating feature, described in Chapter 4. It is thus seen in almost all chromosomal aberrations, except those characterized by two or more X chromosomes and one or more Y chromosomes (*see* page 143). Retarded growth is found in many of the known metabolic disorders, e.g. mucopolysaccharidosis and phenylketonuria, and dietary treatment may make this feature even more marked. Children with sequelae after a fetal infection, e.g. rubella, or after intoxication, e.g. alcohol, are usually small and grow slowly. In most of the syndromes of unknown aetiology described in Chapter 4 and with mental retardation as a common feature, short stature is a typical finding. Many children with cerebral palsy and mental retardation due to a severe perinatal or early postnatal brain injury are of short stature with essentially normal proportions. Many short children with mental retardation also have delayed pubertal maturation.

Impaired growth with normal proportions and normal mental development may be seen in children with an affection of the hypophyseal–hypothalamic area. The cause may be purely a lack of growth hormone with no neurological symptoms, or a tumour in the area, e.g. a craniopharyngioma or an optic glioma. These conditions as a rule also produce neurological signs, particularly impaired vision and visual field defects, and the spinal fluid protein is often increased (*see also* page 368).

Chondrodystrophia myotonica, which causes several symptoms including short stature and myotonia, is described in Chapter 7 (page 216).

Short stature is a typical feature of many endocrine disorders, some of which are described in Chapter 20.

Abnormally rapid growth with normal body proportions or acromegalic features

Abnormally rapid growth is seen in various endocrine disorders, particularly those in which the production of sex hormones starts abnormally early; these patients thus have an early puberty with an abnormally early prepubertal growth spurt, but they stop growing soon after and are abnormally short in adulthood. This clinical picture, without neurological symptoms and signs, at least during the first few years of the disease, may be due to a slow-growing tumour of the posterior part of the hypothalamus – a possibility which must be kept in mind. A pinealoma may produce the same clinical picture (*see* pages 368–369), although in this type of tumour abnormal eye movements are more dominating findings than endocrine disturbances.

Children with acid mucopolysaccharidosis may grow abnormally fast during their first few years of life. During this period facial features and body proportions may be normal. Their rate of growth then slows down and during later childhood they are as a rule abnormally small for age.

The syndrome of *cerebral gigantism* consists of abnormally rapid growth during childhood, as a rule with acromegalic features (*Figures 19.1* and *19.2*), and mild to moderate mental retardation as evidence of a nonprogressive brain lesion. The

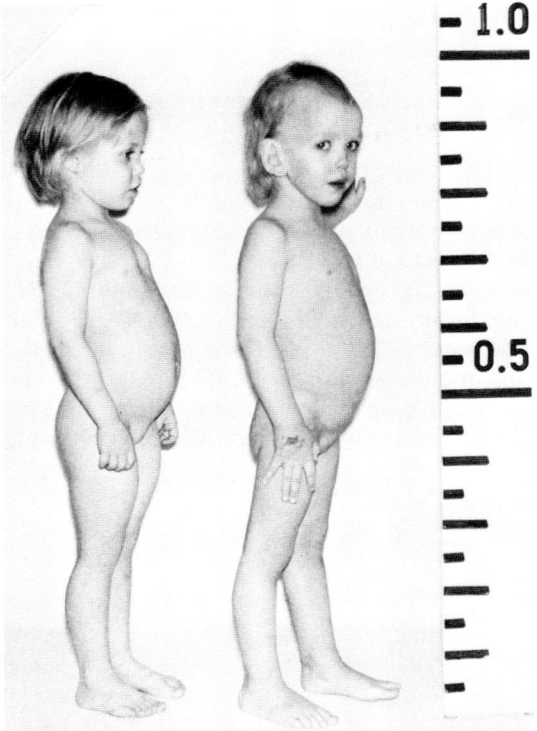

Figure 19.1. A 2½-year-old girl with cerebral gigantism (right) together with a 3½-year-old healthy girl (left)

hairline is often characteristic and unusual for a child, showing a receding angle at the temple (*see Figure 19.1*). Skeletal maturation is usually accelerated. The rate of growth slows down during later childhood. Computerized tomography of the skull reveals abnormally wide lateral ventricles. The aetiology of this syndrome is not known. Its course and its clinical symptoms and signs are similar to those caused by

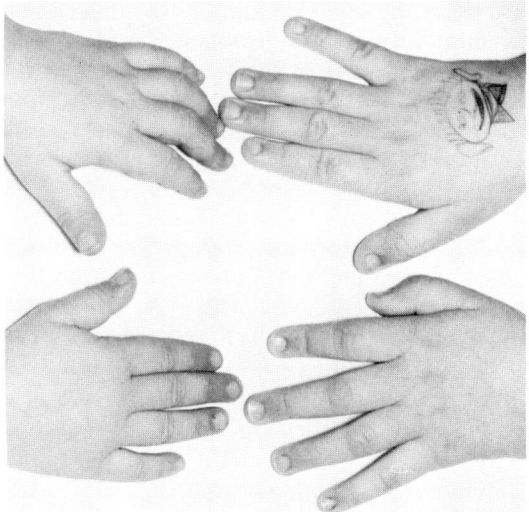

Figure 19.2. The hands of a 2½-year-old girl with cerebral gigantism (right) together with the hands of a 3½-year-old girl (left) of roughly the same height as the patient

a tumour in the posterior hypothalamic region; the likely localization is the same area (*see* page 391). Whether cerebral gigantism has a specific aetiology or is merely an expression of nonspecific brain damage is not clear.

The syndrome of *exomphalos*, *macroglossia* and *gigantism*, called the EMG syndrome or Beckwith–Wiedemann syndrome, is usually apparent at birth, with the infant showing these three cardinal signs. Also typical are peculiar parallel marks in the ear-lobes, resembling clips in a ticket (*Figure 19.3*). Infants with the EMG syndrome have a great tendency to develop hypoglycaemia which must be prevented or rapidly treated to prevent secondary brain injury. The omphalocele

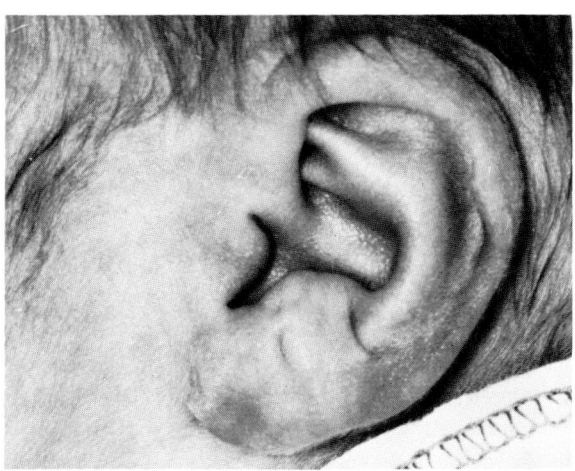

Figure 19.3. The ear-lobe of a boy with the EMG syndrome. Note the parallel marks in the ear-lobe, resembling clips in a ticket

must be surgically repaired. In all other respects the children appear healthy and develop normally, provided hypoglycaemic brain injury has not occurred. They remain big and the macroglossia (*Figure 19.4*) may require surgical correction. Hearing loss is common among children with the EMG syndrome; neurological findings are otherwise normal.

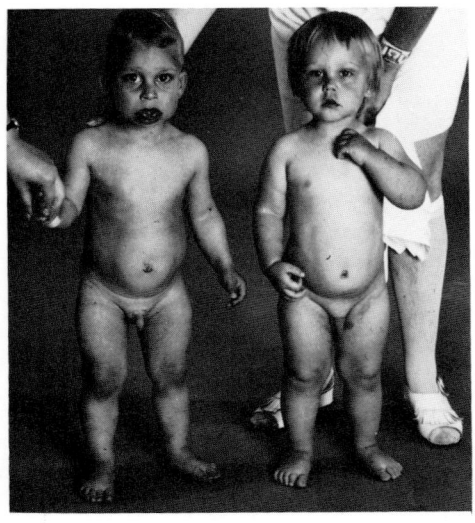

Figure 19.4. A 1½-year-old boy with the EMG syndrome (left) together with a healthy boy of the same age (right). Note the size of the boy, of his hands and feet, and of his tongue, compared with those of his peer

Individuals with two X chromosomes and one or more Y chromosomes are often tall with a normal male exterior. Most of them are neurologically and mentally normal, but as a group they have an increased incidence of mental problems, including retardation.

Patients with homocystinuria (*see* page 131) are usually tall with long limbs and spindle-like fingers and toes.

Obesity

Obesity complicates many neurological disorders because such disorders impair the patient's ability to work with his muscles but do not reduce his appetite to the same degree. When obesity is caused by a neurological disease, as may exceptionally be the case, its localization is almost always the hypophyseal–hypothalamic area; its nature may be a nonprogressive disorder or a tumour (*see* pages 158 and 368). A tumour usually produces other symptoms such as impaired vision and visual field defects but, for some time at least, obesity may be the main symptom.

Emaciation with normal body proportions or acromegalic features

A lesion in the diencephalic area may cause emaciation with normal body proportions or with disproportionately large hands and feet. Some children in this group have a severe loss of fat and muscles in spite of a reasonable food intake and little or no vomiting. In contrast to their poor physical condition they may appear happy and active. Other children in this group have virtually no subcutaneous fat, a strongly built skeleton, heavy muscles, and acromegalic features, particularly large hands and feet with thick coarse skin (*Figure 19.5*), and rarely a large tongue; hepatosplenomegaly is occasionally found. These children may be happy, almost euphoric, and show locomotor overactivity; they may also be irritable. Both types of disturbed growth are connected with an increased production of growth hormone, which may be demonstrated as an elevated blood level of the hormone.

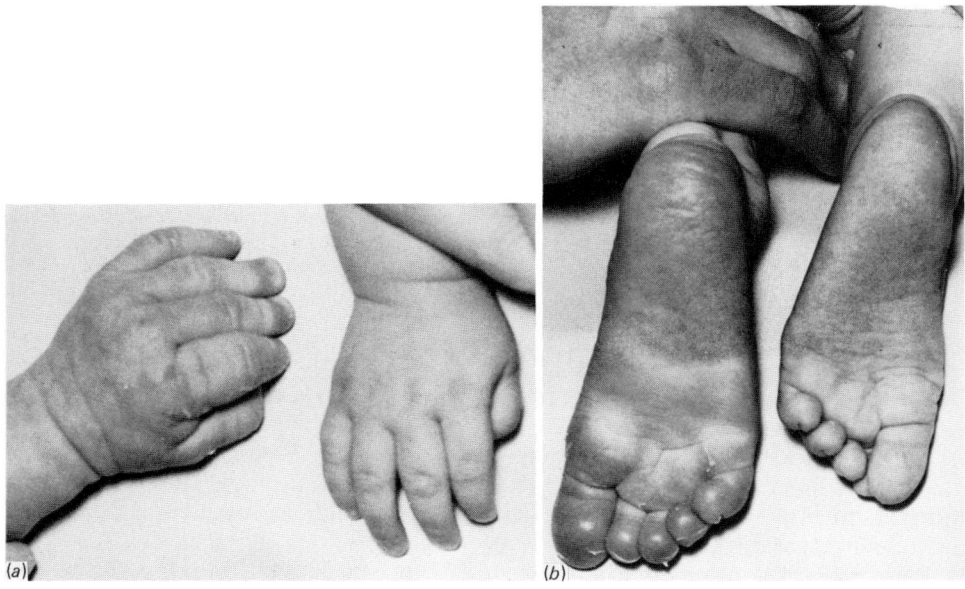

Figure 19.5. The hand (*a*) and foot (*b*) of a 5-month-old boy with a diencephalic syndrome (emaciation with acromegalic features), shown on the left in each picture, compared with the hand and foot of a healthy infant of the same age, shown on the right in each picture. Note also the coarse texture of the skin. (From Gamstorp, Kjellman and Palmgren, 1967, courtesy of The C. V. Mosby Co.)

This overproduction is caused by damage to the diencephalon, either a nonprogressive lesion or a tumour. The latter is usually an optic glioma (*Figure 19.6*), which will eventually produce neurological signs, particularly impaired vision and visual field defects, but these signs may be difficult to demonstrate in a young child and they may be absent for a long period. Thus, the clinical examination alone may not reveal the nature of the diencephalic lesion. The spinal fluid protein is usually normal when the lesion is nonprogressive but increased if it is due to a tumour (*see* page 368). With the growth of the tumour the clinical picture may change and the patient may become obese (*Figure 19.7*). Computerized tomography of the skull usually reveals the tumour; it must also be performed when the suspicion of a diencephalic tumour is slight, as optic gliomas grow slowly and even partial removal of the tumour may improve the patient's condition and give him some years of useful life. In rare selected cases a pneumoencephalogram may also be needed to prove or exclude the diagnosis.

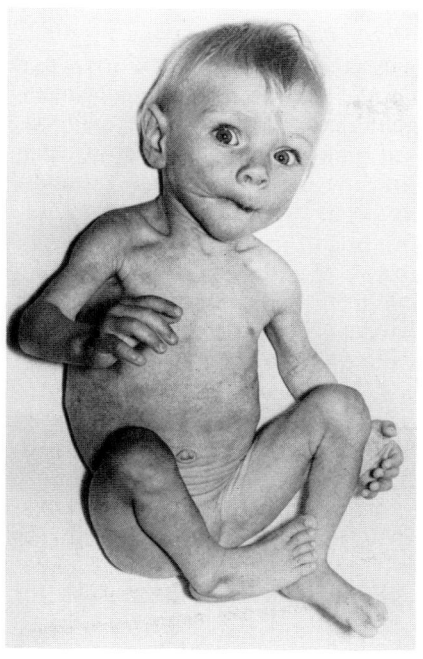

Figure 19.6. Diencephalic syndrome (emaciation with acromegalic features) due to an optic glioma in an 8-month-old girl. Note the depletion of subcutaneous fat, the disproportionately large hands and feet, and the expression of the face with its retraction of the eyelids (Collier's sign). (From Gamstorp, Kjellman and Palmgren, 1967, courtesy of The C. V. Mosby Co.)

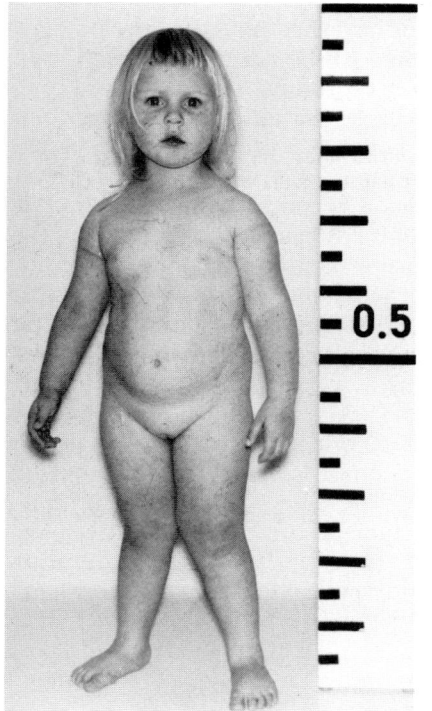

Figure 19.7. The same patient as shown in *Figure 19.6* aged 2 years and 10 months. The tumour was partially removed at 1 year of age. About a year later she started to become obese; severe progression of the tumour was noted on the pneumoencephalogram. (From Gamstorp, Kjellman, and Palmgren, 1967, courtesy of The C. V. Mosby Co.)

Other types of disproportionate growth

Patients with the Prader–Willi syndrome, which is characterized by proximal muscle weakness, muscular hypotonia, and mental retardation, are as a rule remarkably short and have disproportionately small hands and feet (*see* page 158). One of the syndromes in which mental retardation is an essential feature, i.e. that described by Rubinstein and Taybi, is characterized by remarkably broad thumbs and big toes with or without increased breadth of other digits (*see* page 149).

Impaired ability to move a limb leads to a retardation of its growth, regardless of the cause of the movement disorder. Retarded growth of a limb or of an arm and a leg on the same side is therefore a common finding in chronic neurological diseases with an onset in infancy and childhood; it is particularly noticeable in cases of infantile hemiparesis. Asymmetry of the size of the nails on the two hands is the smallest evidence of growth retardation (*see Figure 12.9*, page 283). Hemihypertrophy (or possibly hemihypotrophy of the other side, i.e. it may be impossible to tell which is the abnormal side) may rarely be found as a primary malformation with no neurological explanation and no neurological findings. Hypertrophy of one limb may be due to an arteriovenous malformation with increased circulation. Local gigantism, occasionally presenting as grotesque overgrowth of one or a few fingers or toes, may be a feature of neurofibromatosis von Recklinghausen (*see* pages 373–374); patients with local gigantism must therefore be examined carefully for other evidence of this disease.

Summary

Mentally retarded children may show all kinds of disturbed physical development with normal or abnormal body proportions. In some syndromes the abnormal body proportions constitute an essential feature of the syndrome.

Lesions of the diencephalic region may also cause various types of disturbed physical development with normal or abnormal body proportions. In nonprogressive lesions the spinal fluid protein is usually normal, whereas it is usually high when symptoms are caused by a tumour. From a practical point of view it is essential to stress that abnormalities of growth and physical development may for months or years be the only symptoms of a diencephalic tumour, which may for a long period be at least partially removable. Various types of abnormal physical development may be caused by lesions with slightly different localizations in the diencephalic region and may even follow each other in the same patient (*see Figures 19.6* and *19.7*) with further growth of the tumour.

References

FILIPPI, G. and MCKUSICK, V. A. (1970) The Beckwith–Wiedemann syndrome (the examphalos-macroglossia-gigantism syndrome). Report of two cases and review of the literature. *Medicine* (Baltimore), **49**, 279–298

FRASIER, S. D. (1979) Growth disorders in children. *Pediatric Clinics of North America*, **26**, 1–14

GAMSTORP, I. (1972) Neurological disorders and growth disturbances in infancy and childhood. *European Neurology*, **7**, 1–25

GAMSTORP, I., KJELLMAN, B. and PALMGREN, B. (1967) Diencephalic syndromes of infancy. *Journal of Pediatrics*, **70**, 383–390

KJELLMAN, B. (1965) Cerebral gigantism. *Acta Paediatrica Scandinavica*, **54**, 603–609

KJELLMAN, B., GAMSTORP, I., BRUN, A., ÖCKERMAN, P.-A. and PALMGREN, B. (1969) Mannosidosis. A clinical and histopathological study. *Journal of Pediatrics,* **75,** 366–373

RUSSELL, A. A. (1951) A diencephalic syndrome of emaciation in infancy and childhood. *Archives of Diseases of Childhood,* **26,** 274

SOTOS, J. F., DODGE, P. R., MUIRHEAD, D., CRAWFORD, J. D. and TALBOT, N. B. (1964) Cerebral gigantism in childhood. *The New England Journal of Medicine,* **271,** 109–116

WIEDEMANN, H.-R. (1973) Exomphalos-Makroglossie-Gigantismus-Syndrom, Berardinelli-Seip-Syndrom und Sotos-Syndrom – eine vergleichende Betrachtung unter ausgewählten Aspekten. *Zeitschrift für Kinderheilkunde,* **115,** 193–207

WU, N. F. T., KUSHNICK, T. (1974) The Beckwith–Wiedemann syndrome. *Pediatric Clinics of North America,* **13,** 452–457

20

Endocrine disorders causing neurological symptoms and signs

Only an outline of the neurological aspects of endocrine disorders will be given.

Thyroid disorders

Hypothyroidism

In hypothyroidism the rate of growth and of physical and mental development are decreased, as are pulse rate and body temperature. The clinical picture depends on the child's age at the onset of impaired hormone production.

ONSET IN THE NEONATAL PERIOD

When there is a lack of thyroid hormone from fetal life or the early postnatal period, the infant is short with a coolish, dry, pasty, wrinkled skin, dry hair, a protruding tongue (*Figure 20.1*), and an umbilical hernia. Constipation is a

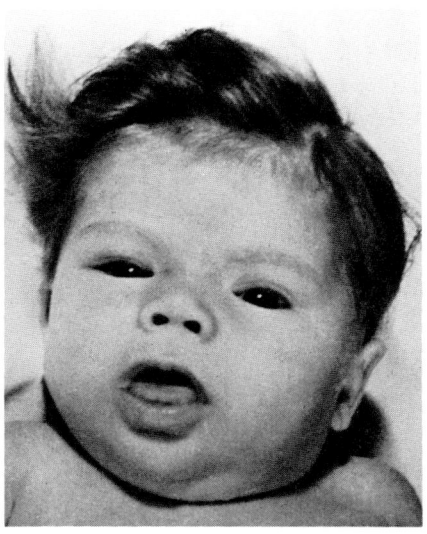

Figure 20.1. The face of an untreated hypothyroid infant at a few months of age

common symptom; pulse rate and body temperature are usually low. The infant is inactive with few spontaneous movements. Muscle tone may be decreased, but it is more common for the muscles to be stiff. Muscle reflexes have a normal strength, but the relaxation time after a reflex contraction is prolonged. Psychomotor development is delayed, often severely. Hearing may be impaired.

Delayed skeletal maturation is often found; it can best be demonstrated on X-ray of the knee. Anaemia is the rule. The measurement of thyroid-stimulating hormone (TSH), which is abnormally high in hypothyroidism, is the best laboratory test for establishing the diagnosis. It is also available as a screening method, applicable to all newborn infants; it is used in this way in several countries, and offers the best opportunity for early diagnosis and treatment.

Treatment must be started as early as possible; it consists of the administration of thyroxine in the highest dose that the patient is able to tolerate without developing side effects. Treatment is lifelong; the dose must be adjusted with increasing growth of the child. Physical signs of hypothyroidism usually diminish or disappear within weeks or months after the start of treatment. Mental development improves, but may remain permanently retarded in children with fetal or neonatal onset of hypothyroidism, particularly if treatment is delayed or inadequate. Cerebellar ataxia is another possible neurological complication of hypothyroidism.

ONSET IN LATER CHILDHOOD

When hypothyroidism has its onset in later childhood, the patient becomes tired and apathetic or irritable, loses his appetite, and becomes constipated, and his growth slows down. The muscles may become stiff and/or weak; true myopathy has been reported in hypothyroid adults. The confirmatory diagnostic procedures are the same as outlined for the neonatal group; after the neonatal period skeletal maturation is better evaluated from an X-ray of the hand than of the knee. The symptoms and signs usually disappear on substitution therapy.

Hyperthyroidism

ONSET IN THE NEONATAL PERIOD

Hyperthyroidism may occur in newborn infants of mothers with hyperthyroidism. These infants usually have exophthalmus; they are irritable and restless, have tachycardia, and may develop congestive heart failure. If the mother has been treated with antithyroid drugs during pregnancy, the first symptoms in the child may not appear until a few weeks after birth. A proven diagnosis of hyperthyroidism in the mother supports the child's diagnosis which can be confirmed by demonstrating a high level of thyroxine in the serum. The cardiac insufficiency must be treated and the child given sedatives; occasionally antithyroid drugs must also be administered. The symptoms and signs disappear, also without treatment, within a few months.

ONSET IN LATER CHILDHOOD

The dominating symptoms of hyperthyroidism in later childhood are mental symptoms with insomnia, hyperactivity, excitation occasionally intensified to psychotic behaviour, and cardiac symptoms such as severe tachycardia and congestive heart failure. Proximal muscular weakness and atrophy, which is frequently seen in adults with hyperthyroidism, has occasionally been reported in childhood (*see* page 203). Myasthenia gravis (*see* page 179) and periodic paralysis (*see* page 183) are conditions known to occur too often in hyperthyroidism, at least in adulthood, to be pure coincidence.

The diagnosis is confirmed by the demonstration of an abnormally high serum thyroxine level. An acute thyrotoxic crisis is treated with cortisone, sedatives, digitalis, and large doses of iodine. Prolonged administration of antithyroid drugs is the method of treatment after the crisis has been brought under control or in a less acute situation; partial thyroidectomy may be considered. Mortality is high in an acute thyrotoxic crisis, and prompt treatment may be life-saving.

Disorders of the hypophysis and adrenal cortex

Cushing's syndrome

Cushing's syndrome due to hyperactivity of the adrenal cortex, or, although rarely seen in children, of the hypophysis, causes as its main symptoms fatigue, abnormal body proportions, and increased blood pressure; proximal muscular weakness with atrophy has been reported in adults. Endocrine investigation is necessary to prove the diagnosis and to demonstrate its exact cause; therapy and prognosis depend on the cause.

Conn's syndrome

In hyperaldosteronism (Conn's syndrome) the main findings are elevated blood pressure and hypopotassaemia. The symptoms are usually general. Muscular weakness may be present, occasionally appearing intermittently; these attacks may be misdiagnosed as hypopotassaemic periodic paralysis (*see* page 183). This syndrome is rare in childhood. Treatment is surgical excision of the tumour.

Addison's disease

Hypoactivity of the adrenal cortex, Addison's disease, causes severe fatigue, loss of weight, increased pigmentation, low blood pressure, and electrolyte disturbances. One feature that often contributes to the fatigue is a moderate muscular weakness connected with mild atrophy. During an acute exacerbation of the disease, and particularly if the patient is given potassium-rich food or medication, the weakness may increase to a severe, occasionally life-threatening, paralysis. This possibility must be kept in mind when a patient has muscular weakness and hyperpotassaemia. Attacks of hypoglycaemia, possibly with convulsions (*see* pages 100–101), may, although rarely, occur in Addison's disease. An exact diagnosis usually requires extensive endocrine investigation. Treatment consists of substitution therapy, often combined with an increased intake of sodium chloride.

A syndrome known to occur only in boys consists of a combination of Addison's disease and leucodystrophy, termed adrenoleucodystrophy (*see* page 304). The first symptoms may be either neurological or endocrine. This syndrome must be kept in mind when a boy develops evidence of Addison's disease for no apparent reason. The endocrine abnormalities respond to substitution therapy but the neurological symptoms, for which no treatment is available, progress steadily.

Lack of somatotrophic hormone

Lack of somatotrophic hormone causes dwarfism with normal body proportions and may, although rarely, produce attacks of hypoglycaemia, occasionally with convulsions (*see* pages 100–101).

Tumour of the hypophyseal–hypothalamic area

A tumour of the hypophyseal–hypothalamic area, besides causing endocrine abnormalities, may also cause neurological symptoms and signs due to a direct effect on the surrounding brain structures. A tumour in this area may cause increased intracranial pressure, primary optic atrophy, visual field defects, abnormal growth and abnormal body proportions, diabetes insipidus, and various other endocrine abnormalities (*see* page 381).

Parathyroid disorders

Hypoparathyroidism

Hypoparathyroidism and pseudohypoparathyroidism both cause hypocalcaemia and tetany, occasionally with generalized convulsions which may be indistinguishable from epileptic fits (*see* page 100). Intracranial calcifications may be seen in conditions characterized by hypocalcaemia. Therapy and prognosis depend on the exact diagnosis. Fits due to hypocalcaemia have been reported in newborn infants born to mothers with hyperparathyroidism.

Hyperparathyroidism

Hyperparathyroidism causes symptoms mainly from the urinary and gastrointestinal tracts. Skeletal pains, muscular weakness, and mental symptoms, e.g. depression or bizarre behaviour, may, however, dominate the clinical picture and lead to neurological examination. The symptoms and clinical signs are usually vague, and there is often a long delay between the onset of symptoms of hyperparathyroidism and the correct diagnosis. Bone lesions are revealed on skeletal X-ray examination, and hypercalcaemia is demonstrated on chemical analysis of the blood serum. Treatment is surgical excision of the tumour.

Diabetes mellitus

In about 10 per cent of diabetic children, polyneuropathy can be demonstrated on neurophysiological examination although many of them lack clinical symptoms and signs. The incidence of polyneuropathy increases with increasing age of the patient and duration of the disease, and it is higher in diabetic children with poor control of their disease than in those with good control; the only available therapy is the best possible control of the diabetes.

There is also an increased incidence of EEG abnormalities in diabetic children. A connection between these abnormalities and an unstable diabetes mellitus with repeated attacks of hypoglycaemia is conceivable. The diabetes of some of these children becomes easier to control if they are given an antiepileptic drug, e.g. phenytoin, in the dose used in epileptic children (*see* page 112).

Occasional hypoglycaemic attacks almost inevitably complicate the treatment of juvenile diabetes; the diagnosis of them causes no difficulties. Rarely, spontaneous attacks of hypoglycaemia may be the first sign of juvenile diabetes mellitus and precede other symptoms by a couple of weeks or months.

Insulinoma

Insulinoma may cause attacks of hypoglycaemia, often with convulsions. It is a rare tumour in childhood and thus is only exceptionally the cause of the hypoglycaemic attacks, which may be mistaken for epileptic fits (*see* pages 100–101).

References

BERGSTRAND, C. G. and NILSSON, K. O. (1982) Treatment of Cushing's disease in children. *Acta Paediatrica Scandinavica*, **71**, 1–6

EEG-OLOFSSON, O. and PETERSÉN, I. (1966) Childhood diabetic neuropathy. *Acta Paediatrica Scandinavica*, **55**, 163–176

HAGBERG, B. and WESTPHAL, O. (1970) Ataxic syndromes in congenital hypothyroidism. *Acta Paediatrica*, **59**, 323–327

ROSENSTOCK, J., DOYLE, F. H., HALL, R., MASHITER, K. and JOPLIN, G. F. (1982) Childhood acromegaly successfully treated with interstitial irridiation using yttrium-90. *Acta Paediatrica Scandinavica*, **71**, 851–855

TSANG, R. C., NOGUCHI, A. and STEICHEN, J. J. (1979) Pediatric parathyroid disorders. *Pediatric Clinics of North America*, **26**, 223–249

ROSMAN, N. P. (1976) Neurological and muscular aspects of thyroid dysfunction in childhood. *Pediatric Clinics of North America*, **23**, 575–594

VIRTANEN, M., MÄENPÄÄ, J., SANTAVUORI, P., HIRVONEN, E. and PERHEENTUPA, J. (1983) Congenital hypothyroidism: age at start of treatment versus outcome. *Acta Paediatrica Scandinavica*, **72**, 197–201

21

Miscellaneous neurological diseases affecting infants and children

Syringomyelia

Syringomyelia is a chronic disease characterized by the presence of long cavities surrounded by glia in the grey matter of the spinal cord, most commonly in the cervical cord. They may also appear in the lumbar cord, and may extend upwards into the medulla oblongata (syringobulbia), and even into the pons. As a rule, the cavities seem to originate from the posterior horn. The expansion of the cavities, which contain a clear or yellow fluid, and the surrounding gliosis lead to compression of the anterior horns and the long tracts of the spinal cord with degenerative changes in these areas. The aetiology is unknown; a malformation, e.g. defective closure of the central canal of the spinal cord, is a possible explanation.

Symptoms usually start during childhood, but the onset is so insidious and the progression so slow that they are often present for years before the patients realize that something is wrong. Therefore, patients with syringomyelia seldom seek medical advice before their late teens or twenties, although they may then be able to date their complaints back to childhood.

Symptoms usually start in the hands. The first evidence of the disease is usually impaired pain and temperature sense in the fingers, leading to painless slow-healing wounds. The patient may, however, be unaware of these abnormalities until motor symptoms, i.e. weakness and atrophy of the small hand muscles, have also appeared. The same type of symptoms may eventually develop in the feet or, rarely, start there. Weakness, atrophy, and fasciculations of the tongue and weakness of the throat muscles are signs of syringobulbia. Painless dislocation and destruction of joints (Charcot's joints), particularly the shoulder joint, is another characteristic feature of the disease. Involvement of the corticospinal tract may eventually become apparent with spasticity and hyperactive muscle reflexes of the legs and the appearance of a positive Babinski sign.

The course of the disease is as a rule slowly progressive. Bouts of sudden deterioration, however, may occur due to a sudden increase in pressure within a cavity or bleeding into a cavity; such an event may be provoked by a trauma.

The full clinical picture of syringomyelia seldom develops before early adulthood. In establishing a diagnosis it is particularly important to look for the typical sensory disturbances, i.e. impaired pain and temperature sense with preserved touch sense. The motor symptoms and signs are the same as in amyotrophic lateral sclerosis (*see* page 173), in which disease sensation is normal. The conduction velocity of peripheral nerves is normal in syringomyelia, which helps to differentiate it from chronic polyneuropathy (*see* page 177). Syringomyelia and a slow-growing intramedullary tumour may produce the same clinical symptoms and signs and identical abnormalities on X-ray of the spine and on a myelogram; it may be impossible to differentiate between these two conditions. Amipaque myelogram and/or computerized tomography of the skull and the cervical cord are the best methods to establish the diagnosis of syringomyelia and/or syringobulbia.

Radiotherapy of the affected area gives some relief of symptoms and arrests further progress, at least temporarily. Occasionally surgical exploration is of value to relieve pressure on the cord.

Syringomyelia has little influence on the patient's ability to live a normal life during childhood. Adult patients may eventually become severely handicapped.

Vascular abnormalities of the spinal cord

These conditions are rare in childhood. Bleeding into the cord, haematomyelia, may be due to a trauma or to an arteriovenous malformation; it may be a haemorrhage into a cavity in syringomyelia (*see* page 393) or occur for no apparent reason. It causes the acute onset of neurological symptoms and signs, usually flaccid weakness at the level of the lesion and spasticity below the lesion (the weakness is flaccid at all levels during the first few days or weeks after the onset), impaired sensation below the level of the lesion, and sphincter disturbances. The spinal fluid is usually bloody. The peracute onset is followed by slow improvement. The severity of the permanent handicap depends on the extent and localization of the damage to the cord. An arteriovenous malformation may bleed several times. It is sometimes possible to diagnose such a malformation on angiography of the spinal arteries at the suspected level; rarely it may be neurosurgically accessible.

Occlusion of the anterior spinal artery at the lower cervical and upper thoracic level produces a typical clinical picture, characterized by the acute onset of weakness of the arms and legs, loss of pain and temperature sense and preserved vibratory and position sense, paralysis of the bladder and bowel, and often radiating pains at the upper level of the lesion. The anterior spinal artery supplies blood to the anterior two-thirds of the spinal cord; thus, occlusion of this artery does not affect the function of the posterior columns. The weakness is originally flaccid in both the arms and legs. After a few days tone and reflexes start to return in the legs, where the weakness eventually becomes spastic. It remains flaccid in the arms and hands, and muscular atrophy develops. The course after the acute phase is similar to that described for haematomyelia, as is the prognosis. Occlusion of the anterior spinal artery at other levels is rare; the ensuing clinical picture depends on the level of the occlusion. Occlusion of the anterior spinal artery appears to be a rare syndrome in childhood. Infection and trauma have been suggested as its cause, but often the cause remains unknown.

Hereditary sensory radicular neuropathy

This condition is inherited as an autosomal dominant trait. The first symptom often appears during the second or third decade and consists of a blackened crust over the head of the first metatarsal bone; this breaks down to form an ulcer which may be painless but is not always so. The ulcer heals if the patient stays in bed, but recurs when he again becomes ambulatory. The ulcer may then grow and new ulcers appear, causing destruction of subcutaneous tissue, osteomyelitis, and extrusion of bony fragments, until the foot is greatly shortened or even destroyed, with only a small stump remaining. Joints may also become deformed. The hands are rarely involved and, if so, always later than the feet. All sensory qualities are severely impaired. The conduction velocity of peripheral nerves, particularly on the sensory side, is low. Hearing may be impaired.

The clinical picture is similar in affected members of the same family but shows great variation between different families. In some reported families the sensory neuropathy has been combined with severe dysfunction of the motor nerves causing muscular atrophy and weakness (*see* page 177). In these families, foot deformities (high-arched feet and clawing of the toes) have preceded the development of ulcers and in some affected members have even been observed in infancy.

The ulcers and their complications are treated symptomatically. There is no treatment for the disease *per se*. In spite of the severe disability caused by the foot ulcers these patients may live until old age.

Congenital analgia

Congenital indifference to pain, analgia, is a rare condition, possibly inherited as an autosomal recessive trait. The symptoms are usually apparent from early childhood; they are most pronounced from the skin and mucous membranes. Patients are able to differentiate between sharp and dull objects and different temperatures, but they are unable to experience any traumata as painful and therefore do not trouble to avoid painful stimulation. They bite and chew on their tongue, lips, and fingers, and they always have wounds and scars in these areas. The hands are particularly traumatized with ensuing infected wounds which, in some cases, eventually lead to mutilations and spontaneous amputations of the fingers. Corneal sensation may be absent, and the patients may not try to avoid eye injuries, occasionally with serious consequences. Osteomyelitis, fractures and aseptic necrosis may occur without pain. The ability to record visceral pain has varied in reported patients; abdominal pains may be absent even in a case of appendicitis with perforation.

In a few patients weak or absent muscle reflexes have been reported. Epilepsy and/or EEG abnormalities have been described in some patients. They have otherwise been remarkably free of neurological defects.

In a few patients the ability to appreciate pain has been reported to develop with advancing age. All patients improve with age, as they learn about their defect and how to avoid its serious consequences. If severe injuries can be avoided during childhood, most patients survive and are able to live a fairly normal life as adults.

The only available therapy is protection against injuries and symptomatic treatment of them. The most important factor is the continuous education of the child about how to avoid traumata in spite of the lack of pain as a warning signal.

Porphyria

The porphyrias are metabolic disorders, two of which show neurological symptoms – the acute intermittent porphyria (Swedish type) and porphyria variegata (South African type). Both are inherited as autosomal dominant traits. The onset of clinical symptoms before puberty is rare in both types. The clinical picture in acute intermittent porphyria is dominated by attacks of polyneuropathy with severe paralysis, mental symptoms, occasionally psychotic behaviour, and abdominal pains; skin symptoms are absent. The urinary excretion of porphobilinogen is increased, particularly during acute attacks, when the urine may be red. Porphyria variegata is characterized by skin fragility and light sensitivity; attacks of polyneuropathy, bizarre behaviour, and abdominal pains also occur, but are milder and less frequent than in the Swedish type. Faecal porphyrin excretion is raised. Barbiturates may provoke attacks in both types and should be avoided.

Lead encephalopathy

Lead encephalopathy is a reaction to lead intoxication seen only in children. The most common cause is ingestion of absorbable lead salts present in paint on walls or toys; lead-containing paint has disappeared in most countries but still remains in some areas. Metallic lead can also, under unfortunate circumstances, cause lead intoxication by remaining in the stomach where it is dissolved by the hydrochloric acid and then absorbed. The acute episode is often preceded by vague symptoms such as irritability, fatigue, anaemia, poor appetite, and abdominal cramps. The main symptoms of lead encephalopathy are caused by oedema and increased intracranial pressure. They consist of headache, vomiting, a decreasing level of consciousness, and convulsions. A cracked-pot sound, stretched sutures, and papilloedema are often present, but their absence does not exclude the possibility of lead encephalopathy. The spinal fluid is under increased pressure, and its protein content is abnormally high. The presence of basophilic stippling of erythrocytes and anaemia supports the diagnosis. Heavy bands of increased density (lead lines) may be seen on X-ray examination of the growing long bones in cases of protracted intoxication; they are absent in the acute stage of the condition and are seldom seen in children below 2 or above 5 years of age. Plain X-ray of the abdomen may reveal the presence of leaden objects in the intestinal tract. The diagnosis can be proved by determination of the concentration of lead in the blood or the excretion of lead in the urine, but in an acute case treatment may have to be started before the results of these examinations are known.

The purpose of treatment is twofold: to lower the intracranial pressure and to remove lead from the body. If the child's general condition is good, efforts can be concentrated on the latter purpose and treatment started with the intravenous administration of the chelating agent calcium-EDTA (sodium calciumedetate) in a dose of 25 mg/kg for the first 24 hours, followed by 50–75 mg/kg per day during the following 2–4 days. Treatment is then stopped for a few days and resumed at the same dose if needed. During the first few days, however, there is a definite risk that this treatment may further increase the intracranial pressure and thus the neurological symptoms and signs. As a rule, therefore, the patient must be given corticosteroids, e.g. dexamethasone 1–4 mg orally four times a day. Subtemporal decompression may occasionally be necessary to reduce the increased intracranial pressure. The convulsions are treated symptomatically (*see* pages 109–111); the response, however, is often poor.

Lead encephalopathy carries a poor prognosis. Mortality is high, and cerebral symptoms and signs (impaired mental development, convulsions, and optic atrophy) are common in surviving children.

Malignant hyperthermia

Malignant hyperthermia is a syndrome connected with primary muscle diseases (*see* pages 197–203). The muscle disorder may be severe, as in Duchenne muscular dystrophy, or mild, as in central core disease, or it may be so mild that the patient is unaware of its presence. Malignant hyperthermia is provoked by general anaesthesia, particularly the combination of an inhalational anaesthetic such as halothane and a depolarizing muscle relaxant such as suxamethonium. During anaesthesia the patient develops rapidly increasing fever to 41–42°C, muscle rigidity, tachycardia, cardiac arrhythmia, tachypnoea, cyanosis, and respiratory and metabolic acidosis. Untreated, the patient will rapidly succumb. Treatment consists of the immediate and complete interruption of anaesthesia, ventilation with pure oxygen, cooling the patient, the prevention and correction of acidosis and electrolyte disturbances, and the administration of dantrolene sodium intravenously (1 mg/kg at intervals of 5–10 minutes until 10 mg/kg has been given or the symptoms are abating). It is advisable to continue with 1–2 mg/kg every 6 hours for the following 48 hours. Good urinary output must also be maintained.

As malignant hyperthermia is often inherited as an autosomal dominant trait, it is important to try to identify those relatives at risk. Most individuals at risk of developing malignant hyperthermia will show an increased serum level of creatine kinase, but approximately 30 per cent have a normal level. The safest way to identify a person at risk of malignant hyperthermia is to examine the *in-vitro* sensitivity of the muscle fibres (from a specimen taken at biopsy) to caffeine; this test is available in some specialized laboratories. Any individual at risk of malignant hyperthermia must have special attention at a surgical procedure. If possible, local or regional anaesthesia should be used. Thiopentone, opiates, and non-depolarizing muscle relaxants (such as tubocurarine and its derivates) are less risky than halothane and depolarizing muscle relaxants. It is also necessary to ensure that the level of anaesthesia is deep enough to avoid causing the patient distress; pains during a too-light anaesthesia may, albeit rarely, provoke the syndrome. Whether or not the prophylactic use of dantrolene sodium can prevent malignant hyperthermia is debated. It is, however, *necessary* that the drug is available and used immediately at the first sign of this severe condition.

References

DEAN, G. (1963) *The Porphyrias. A Story of Inheritance and Environment.* London: Pitman Medical Publication

FLETCHER, R., BLENNOW, G., OLSSON, A.-K., RANKLEV, E. and TÖRNEBRANDT, K. (1982) Malignant hyperthermia in a myopathic child. Prolonged postoperative course requiring dantrolene. *Acta Anaesthesiologica Scandinavica,* **26,** 435–438

FORSBY, N., FRISTEDT, B. and KJELLMAN, B. (1967) Acute lethal poisoning after ingestion of metallic lead. *Acta Paediatrica Scandinavica,* suppl. 177, pp. 107

GÖRKE, W. (1981) The differential diagnosis of congenital analgesia and other diseases with diminished pain perception in childhood. *Neuropediatrics,* **12,** 33–44

LINDQUIST, B. (1957) Syndrome of the anterior spinal artery. *Acta Paediatrica* (Uppsala), **46,** 380–386

RADWAN, H., BRAUN, H., BAR-SELA, S. and KOTT, E. (1982) Lead encephalopathy treated by Versenate (Ca-EDTA). *European Neurology,* **21,** 157–160

SCHULTE-SASSE, U. and EBERLEIN, H. J. (1983) Die maligne hyperthermie. *Anaesthesist,* **32,** 157–160

SMITH, M., DELVES, T., LANDSOWN, R., CLAYTON, B. and GRAHAM, P. (1983) The effect of lead exposure on urban children. *Developmental Medicine and Child Neurology,* suppl. 47

Index